THE NEW RULES OF LIFTING FOR Life

THE NEW RULES OF LIFTING FOR LIFE

An All-New Muscle-Building, Fat-Blasting Plan for Men and Women Who Want to Ace Their Midlife Exams

Lou Schuler and **Alwyn Cosgrove**

AVERY

A MEMBER OF PENGUIN GROUP (USA) INC.

NEW YORK

Published by the Penguin Group
Penguin Group (USA) Inc., 375 Hudson Street, New York, New York 10014, USA ·
Penguin Group (Canada), 90 Eglinton Avenue East, Suite 700, Toronto, Ontario M4P 2Y3, Canada
(a division of Pearson Penguin Canada Inc.) · Penguin Books Ltd, 80 Strand, London WC2R 0RL,
England · Penguin Ireland, 25 St Stephen's Green, Dublin 2, Ireland (a division of Penguin Books Ltd) ·
Penguin Group (Australia), 707 Collins Street, Melbourne, Victoria 3008, Australia (a division of
Pearson Australia Group Pty Ltd) · Penguin Books India Pvt Ltd, 11 Community Centre, Panchsheel Park,
New Delhi–110 017, India · Penguin Group (NZ), 67 Apollo Drive, Rosedale, North Shore 0632, New Zealand
(a division of Pearson New Zealand Ltd) · Penguin Books, Rosebank Office Park, 181 Jan Smuts Avenue,
Parktown North 2193, South Africa · Penguin China, B7 Jiaming Center, 27 East Third Ring Road North,
Chaoyang District, Beijing 100020, China

Penguin Books Ltd, Registered Offices: 80 Strand, London WC2R 0RL, England

First paperback edition 2012
Copyright © 2012 by Lou Schuler and Alwyn Cosgrove
Photographs © 2012 by Michael Tedesco

Most Avery books are available at special quantity discounts for bulk purchase for sales promotions, premiums,
fund-raising, and educational needs. Special books or book excerpts also can be created to fit specific needs. For
details, write Penguin Group (USA) Inc. Special Markets, 375 Hudson Street, New York, NY 10014.

The Library of Congress catalogued the hardcover edition as follows:

Schuler, Lou.
The new rules of lifting for life : an all-new muscle-building, fat-blasting plan for men and
women who want to ace their midlife exams / Lou Schuler and Alwyn Cosgrove.
p.   cm.
ISBN 978-1-58333-461-4
1. Weight lifting.   2. Muscle strength.   3. Physical fitness.   I. Cosgrove, Alwyn.   II. Title.
GV546.3.S39   2012   2012001268
613.7'13—dc23

ISBN 978-1-58333-513-0 (paperback edition)

Printed in the United States of America
1   3   5   7   9   10   8   6   4   2

BOOK DESIGN BY TANYA MAIBORODA

Neither the publisher nor the author is engaged in rendering professional advice or services to the individual reader.
The ideas, procedures, and suggestions contained in this book are not intended as a substitute for consulting with your
physician. All matters regarding your health require medical supervision. Neither the author nor the publisher shall be
liable or responsible for any loss or damage allegedly arising from any information or suggestion in this book.

The recipes contained in this book are to be followed as written. The publisher is not responsible for your specific
health or allergy needs that may require medical supervision. The publisher is not responsible for any adverse reactions
to the recipes contained in this book.

While the author has made every effort to provide accurate telephone numbers and Internet addresses at the time of
publication, neither the publisher nor the author assumes any responsibility for errors, or for changes that occur after
publication. Further, the publisher does not have any control over and does not assume any responsibility for author
or third-party websites or their content.

Acknowledgments

THE LONGER I spend in the publishing business, the more I appreciate the team effort required to make a book come together and ensure it gets the attention it deserves. The star of the team is Alwyn Cosgrove, my coauthor, whose work is literally at the center of each book in the New Rules of Lifting series. Alwyn puts a lifetime's worth of knowledge and creativity into all his workout programs, and his relentless search for better ways to train his clients at Results Fitness allows the project to continue.

It's a joy to work with my editor, Megan Newman, along with Miriam Rich, Andrea Ho, Anne Kosmoski, and the rest of the team at Avery; my agent, David Black, along with Gary Morris and Allie Hemphill; and publicist Gregg Stebben.

Photographer Michael Tedesco has become an invaluable partner in the NROL series. We push ourselves further with each book, and Michael always rises to the challenge, no matter the time or location constraints. Thanks also to Danelle Manthey, Michael's assistant, and our models, Dan Ownes and Rosemarie Hulbert. Dan is a veteran of hundreds of photo shoots, and his expertise made my job a lot easier. I'm profoundly grateful to Mike Cerimele, Chris Leavy, Brian Zarbatany, and the staff and members of Velocity Sports Performance and the Human Performance Center in

Allentown, Pennsylvania, where we shoot our exercise photos. I also want to thank Mira Kwon at Nike for her generous contribution of apparel for the shoot.

A long list of friends and colleagues helped me with research and shared their expertise, including Jon Fass, Martica Heaner, Mike Roussell, Lonnie Lowery, Alan Aragon, Mike Nelson, John Berardi, Billy Beck III, Jim Annesi, and Jacob Wilson. Every time I went back through my notes to figure out which studies I needed to review, or what the nuances of those studies revealed to people who know what to look for, I was surprised and humbled to see how much these experts helped me over the years.

Thanks to my friends Roland Denzel and Chris Bathke, who reviewed early chapter drafts and offered useful and much-appreciated suggestions; to Galya Ivanova Denzel, for the recipes she provided; to Adam Campbell and Nick Bromberg; and to my wife, Kimberly Heinrichs, for her love, patience, and catering services during the photo shoot (but mostly for her love and patience).

I'm also grateful to Jean-Paul Francoeur and my fellow members at the JP Fitness forum community, whose questions, suggestions, and comments make each book better than it otherwise would be. And of course I appreciate Otto and Aoife Hammersmith at werkit.com, whose custom-designed training logs give NROL readers a way to take the workouts with them to the gym.

I want to dedicate *The New Rules of Lifting for Life* to Hal Johnson, Jim Ross, and all the readers over the years who prodded, pleaded, and exhorted me to write a book for middle-aged, overweight, injured, or otherwise atypical enthusiasts. The series wouldn't continue if not for the dedicated lifters who've come to rely on Alwyn's programs to keep them motivated and excited about training, and this particular book wouldn't exist if readers like you hadn't demanded it. You make me want to be a better fitness writer.

—L.S.

As ALWAYS, my first thanks go to Lou Schuler. Thank you once again for believing in me and my ideas about programming and training. I don't think either of us expected this journey to reach book number four!

Thanks as usual to Adam Campbell. Your ability to convert my ramblings into gold has led to more opportunities than I could ever have imagined. We'll be on the same team forever, my friend.

It goes without saying that I'm profoundly grateful to the lecturers, coaches, authors, colleagues, and seminar hosts I've learned from over the years. Your willingness to teach has allowed me to grow. I'll forever be a student, and I'll continue to pay it forward.

To Chris Poirier and the Perform Better team, who gave me an opportunity to share what we do at Results Fitness with a wider audience. To Lee Burton, Michael Boyle, Gray Cook, Robert Dos Remedios, Todd Durkin, Jason Ferruggia, Jim Wendler, and Craig Ballantyne. You inspire me to get better each and every day. Thank you all.

To Derek Campbell, my tae kwon do instructor and original mentor. You are still the greatest coaching mind I've ever been fortunate enough to learn under. As I've said many times, you changed the direction of my life, and I have no idea where I'd be today if not for your influence. I have no doubt that I survived cancer because you taught me how to fight in that wee hall in Deans many years ago. I *still* want to be just like you when I grow up!

To my family at Results Fitness: None of this is possible without you guys. From our newest member to our longest-serving staff member, all of you are part of my journey.

To Mike Wunsch and Craig Rasmussen: You have taken my ideas and methods and run with them. As a result, they're now "*our* ideas and methods," and the programming at Results Fitness is at another level from the rest of the industry. PRO-grams, from PRO-grammers.

To Terry McCormack, my very first weight-training partner. Thanks for the encouragement and support and the traditional Sunday-morning sore head, and for not leaving me stuck under the bench press all those years ago. I don't think either one of us in those days thought that I'd be writing books on weight training. Thanks for the cunning plan.

To Darren Vella: Good friends will bail you out of jail. Great friends will be sitting next to you and will help you avoid getting shot in the leg.

To my mum: This time I *know* you're watching. I hope I've made you proud.

To Dad and Derek: Thanks for being the constant team in my corner this entire time. Dad, you were the one who inspired and encouraged me to move to the United States. I think it worked out okay. Dezi, as always, chin down, hands up, and no surrender.

To the loyal NROL readers and followers: Can they still be "new rules" when we're on book four? Thanks for supporting what Lou and I publish. Without you guys there would've been no book two, never mind book four!

To God, and in no small part to Dr. Sven De Vos and the elite team of doctors and nurses at UCLA who saved my life and gave me these extra days here. I don't know why I deserve these days, but I will never take them for granted and will always treat them as a gift. We know for sure that if it weren't for you, this book wouldn't exist.

To my life partner, Rachel: We're just a boy and a girl trying to take on the world one kiss at a time. Thanks for everything. "And they lived happily ever after."

—A.C.

Contents

PART 1

WHILE YOU WERE WORKING . . .

PART 2

THE PROGRAM

PART 3

THE WIDE ALBUM

PART 4

THOSE THINGS YOU DO

THE NEW RULES OF LIFTING FOR Life

Introduction
I'm Not a Geezer. I'm You

ALMOST EVERY DAY I GET an e-mail that starts like this:

"I'm ____ years old, ___ feet, ___ inches tall, and I weigh ____ pounds. I've been working out ___ years, with a combination of ___ and ___, but recently, I haven't been able to do ___ because of ____. Here's why I'm writing . . ."

Unless Microsoft has a new template for letters to fitness-book authors, virtually everyone who writes to me for the first time feels compelled to begin with these details. The order changes, but the uniformity is uncanny. The simplest questions about how to interpret workout charts, or whether it's okay to do one exercise instead of another, begin by telling me how old my correspondent is, along with his or her height, weight, and workout history.

I used to skim past the age/size/circumstances boilerplate so I could get right to the questions the reader wanted me to answer. Eventually, though, I realized I was misunderstanding my correspondents. Sure, they wanted answers to their specific questions, but there was a reason for the windup before the pitch. All of them, in one way or another, were asking me a different question entirely:

"I don't look like everyone else in the gym. I'm older/heavier/gimpier. But I still want to work out. What should I do?"

In my early years as a workout-book author, when I was more invested in the binary thinking of the troglodyte wing of the fitness industry, I took offense at questions like this. What does age have to do with anything? After all, I was in my forties, and I did all the workouts in my books with great success. If you were overweight, it was your own damned fault for eating too much and not exercising enough. And individual circumstances? Come on! You either want it, or you don't.

Then I turned fifty, and . . . well, I used the introduction to the previous book to describe in bloody detail the calamities that befell my suddenly middle-aged body. It's the reason I wanted to write *The New Rules of Lifting for Abs*: I needed to do something different, so I experimented with a new workout template and experienced remarkable improvements. Then I discovered that my coauthor, Alwyn Cosgrove, was using a similar template with his clients. They were coming to him in worse physical condition than demographically indistinguishable clients had just a few years before, so he changed his system to spend more time on mobility, core training, and metabolic conditioning, with less time in the weight room.

We wrote a book for a new type of exerciser: a man or woman whose body is starting to break down, or who has developed one type of fitness (strength, for example) at the expense of everything else.

That said, we also wrote *NROL for Abs* with the idea that we were producing a book for a broad swath of fitness-conscious readers. If you're serious about exercise in general and strength training in particular—and if you're especially interested in developing a lean, strong, athletic physique, highlighted by a flat and muscular midsection—that's the book for you.

Age? Size? Circumstances? Hey, none of us is getting younger, and we're *all* actors in a unique movie of life. Rough economy, complicated relationships, weird times all around.

And yet, as I wrote the manuscript in late 2009 and early 2010, the e-mails kept coming in. The details were always different, but a common theme emerged: "After doing X for years, I finally realized I'm too old / too fat / too *different* for X. I need to do X minus something, or X plus something. But what?" Sometimes the circumstances described by the reader came on suddenly, like an injury or illness. But most often, it was a gradual and grudging acceptance of the reality of age or weight or singularity. As someone in his fifties, I realized I had more in common with these special-circumstances readers than I did with the undamaged ones I've traditionally addressed in my books.

I asked myself some tough questions. Where's the book for someone who's middle-aged? Where's the book for someone who has a lot of weight to lose? Where's the book for someone who's not like all the other readers? Where's the book for someone like me—or, perhaps more important, for someone like my coauthor?

The Fight of His Life

Las Vegas, summer 2005. I met up with Alwyn at a strength and conditioning conference, where he was a presenter. We had mostly finished work on *The New Rules of Lifting*, our first book together; it would come out in six months. A lot had happened to both of us since we started the book two years earlier. For one thing, Alwyn had been diagnosed with Stage 4 lymphoma, undergone chemotherapy, and come out with a clean bill of health. For another . . . well, next to cancer, the rest doesn't really matter, does it?

Alwyn and I were having lunch with our friend Chris Shugart, an editor at T-nation.com, a popular bodybuilding site. It was the first time I'd seen Alwyn since his diagnosis, treatment, and recovery. He looked great, and felt so good that he told us he was thinking of fighting competitively again.

In his youth, Alwyn, a native of Scotland, had won seven national titles in tae kwon do, and was a two-time bronze medalist at the European championships, where he represented the UK. Despite the fact that he was a few years and one major illness removed from his peak as a martial artist, he was restless. He wanted a new challenge. "You have to remember," he told Chris and me, "I was still winning when I retired." At that moment, in his early thirties, Alwyn was 90 percent athlete and maybe 10 percent cancer survivor.

He never got a chance to resume his fighting career. Stage 4 cancer returned with a vengeance, and as Alwyn points out, there is no Stage 5. He checked into UCLA Medical Center on June 6, 2006, for a stem-cell transplant, an operation that completely dismantled his immune system and built a new one from scratch.

When he came out of the hospital, he was 100 percent cancer survivor. It took years to recover his strength and athleticism. He's never fully regained his ability to perform long, difficult workouts, and now it takes more time to recover from one workout to the next. Combat-sport athletes are notorious for their ability to manipulate their own body weight, but cancer had taken that away. He could maintain a stable weight, but his body fiercely resisted any attempt to lower it. Every aspect of his athleticism, even his flexibility, was suddenly, dramatically different.

The athlete who was thinking about a return to competitive tae kwon do at thirty-three was a middle-aged man at thirty-four.

Sizable Concerns

So that's where we start *The New Rules of Lifting for Life*: two longtime lifters who know what it's like to be forced by age or circumstances to change their approach to training. I had the luxury of reaching midlife the old-fashioned way—by pretending my age didn't matter until well past the point when it clearly did—while Alwyn got there overnight, courtesy of a deadly illness and a miracle of modern medicine. But we're both there now, and our first goal with this book was to provide a training system for people like us.

But what about item #2? What do we have to offer those who want to lose weight? I'll admit this right up front: I started *NROL for Life* with the idea that it would provide a useful guide to weight loss, in conjunction with the training program. After all, lots of readers of the first three *NROL* books told me they shed pounds while doing Alwyn's workouts and following the nutrition and lifestyle advice. Alwyn and I, it seems, had found a solid middle ground: We could help people lose weight without making it the sole focus of our books. I wondered what would happen if we made it a bigger part of the package.

Alas, almost from the first day of research, I realized we couldn't say anything with the prescriptive certainty you're supposed to have when you write about weight loss. The math and physiology appear simple only if you refuse to acknowledge complexity. There are too many individual metabolic variations, and they're too poorly understood. Then, when you look at weight loss from the behavioral side, you see an equally complex set of variables. Finally, good luck to anyone who tries to separate where physiology ends and behavior begins.

This would be really depressing except for one fact: People do manage to lose weight and keep it off. I know some of them, and I've probably corresponded with hundreds. Their secret? They figured out how they gained the weight, and did the opposite until they lost it. They can describe the process in simple terms, but it doesn't take much digging to get below the surface and see an infinitely complex set of personal, familial, and circumstantial variables that they learned to master over time. Exercise is always part of it, of course—too little before, the right amount now. But the desire to work out, the knowledge to do it productively, and the self-discipline to do it consistently were part of a long, often frustrating struggle to change physiology and behavior.

I don't think a diet or training program produces weight loss, any more than a hammer produces a house. It's the person. The best workout or nutrition plan in the world won't work unless it's used by someone who's ready to reorganize his or her life around the goal of losing weight. Even then, it's almost never simple or straightforward.

Intelligent Design

So if *NROL for Life* isn't a weight-loss book, what is it? More than anything, what you have in your hands is a workout book for people who like to work out, who enjoy challenging themselves with new exercises, new routines, new ways to get results. It's also a training program for men and women who want something they don't yet have—less fat, bigger muscles, more strength, more energy, more confidence—and are willing to work hard to achieve it. Finally, it's an exercise system for those who want to work out but for various reasons don't. Maybe you're recovering from an injury or illness and don't know how to modify a workout to fit your circumstances. Maybe you haven't found the right program, or don't feel confident that you understand the mechanics of training. Alwyn and I can't give you the motivation to show up and work hard, but we've done everything we can to pack *NROL for Life* with as much useful information and instruction as we could include without turning this into a multivolume encyclopedia.

About that information:

If you're looking for something so easy to understand that the entire thing can fit on a single page, this isn't the program for you. Not only does it require hard work once you get to the gym, it demands some effort on the front end. We ask you to choose your own exercises, based on detailed instructions, and fit them into the template Alwyn provides. Nothing here is beyond the comprehension of an adult who wants to train and whose mind is open to new information. But there is a bit of a learning curve.

You may wonder why we bother. Why not just tell you what to do? That's what we did in the first three *NROL* books. What's so special about this one?

The book may or may not be special; we'll have to wait for the reviews. But you are. From our earliest conversations about *NROL for Life*, Alwyn and I set out to create a product for readers who're challenged, in some way, by their age, weight, or circumstances. We had two choices: either we could imagine a composite of a challenged person, and have Alwyn design a program for that fictional reader, or we could assume that only individual readers truly understand what they can and can't do.

Obviously, we chose the latter. Our choice requires you to read carefully and follow the steps to assemble your own workouts, based on Alwyn's template. In return, you get a program that's fully customized to your individual strengths, limitations, needs, and goals.

But what if you don't have any limitations that require customized workouts? What if you simply need workouts that work? Even better. You now have the tools to create a program that moves as fast as you do. Get all you can out of an exercise, then move on to one that's more challenging. You don't have to wait for the next stage of the program.

This is how Alwyn designs programs for his clients at Results Fitness, the gym he owns with his wife, Rachel, in Santa Clarita, California. It's the first time he's opened up the playbook to show readers his methodology. You get more than a bunch of workouts. You learn how to customize *any* workout, or create your own from scratch. You learn, in short, how to be the trainer you've never had.

The Standard Disclaimers

Every workout book has some version of this boilerplate on a page demarcated with a Roman numeral:

> *"Not intended as a substitute for a physician's advice."*
>
> *"See a doctor before starting a program of strenuous exercise."*
>
> *"If you experience rapid weight loss or extreme muscle hypertrophy, be sure to give the authors credit."*

This time around, the standard disclaimers are more than legal indemnification. Alwyn and I beg you to exercise genuine caution before launching into this program. If you haven't worked out in a while, *please* get a checkup. If you're seriously overweight, *please* talk to your doctor about the program before you begin. If you're recovering from an injury or illness, *please* make sure you're cleared for training.

We ask you this because we have no intention of treating you like a weakling or invalid. No matter your age, your weight, or your circumstances, we want you to train hard, and to enjoy the benefits of hard training. We want you to do everything you can without fear or limitation. You'll customize the program to match your current abilities. But that's just the starting point. We want you to put your current abilities so far in the rearview mirror that you'll forget you were ever in the shape you're in now. We want you to be stronger, leaner, faster, and more athletic than you thought possible at this stage of your life. We just want to make sure you get there safely, with as few setbacks as possible.

With that out of the way, let's talk about how we're going to help you do this.

In Part One, I lay out the challenges as we currently understand them. Chapter 1 explains the goals of training while debunking some of the misconceptions common to men and women of a certain age. Chapters 2, 3, and 4 look at what our bodies can and can't do as we get older, how and where we're most likely to get injured, and why it's so ridiculously hard to manage our weight in middle age and beyond.

Part Two is the reason you bought this book. It has more exercise choices, information, and advice than any of the previous books in the *NROL* series. It explains every part of the program in full detail.

Part Three tackles the challenges of weight loss, explaining how we got here, the mathematical and physiological impossibility of traditional weight-loss advice, and the importance and challenges of weight maintenance following a successful downsizing. We'll wrap up with an easy-to-remember meal-planning system that can help you reduce calories without sacrificing nutritional necessities, along with some sample meals to put it into practice.

That's what we offer in *The New Rules of Lifting for Life*. What we don't offer, in this or any other *NROL* book, is a guarantee of specific results. We don't know where you're starting or how far you can go. All we know for certain is that we've given you the tools to get there, at your own speed, on your own terms.

It's your movie of life. Are you ready to create a masterpiece?

PART 1

WHILE YOU WERE WORKING . . .

It's Too Late to Say You're Sorry

I USED TO WORK with a guy who had a thing about baby boomers. My first few weeks on the job, he made comment after comment about how my generation had ruined everything for everybody. His biggest gripe was that we hoarded all the good jobs to prevent his generation from advancing into higher management. It didn't matter that he was closer to management than I was at the time. He was convinced the boom babies were conspiring to make his life undeservedly mediocre.

Funny thing is, up to that point in my life I'd always considered the year of my birth, 1957, to be a nontrivial handicap. From my earliest memories, it always seemed as if too damned many people wanted to do exactly what I was trying at the exact moment I was trying to do it. Too many kids wanted to play baseball, so I ended up on the bench. Too many kids wanted a limited number of seats in the Catholic school my older siblings attended, so I had to go somewhere else. (I went to four different elementary schools altogether.) Too many young men and women attended journalism programs in the late seventies, so when we graduated there weren't going to be enough jobs even if the economy had been booming, which it so totally wasn't.

The early eighties were one of the worst times ever to enter the workforce. "Stag-flation" was a word used in everyday conversations. Just when we started feeling better about things, the economy crapped out again in the late eighties. It dropped again in the early two thousands. Then, just for good measure, it nearly went down for the count in 2008.

Everyone who wasn't a boomer hated boomers. My parents and their friends are still bitter over the fact that some of us had long hair or walked around barefoot. My younger siblings and their friends saw us as caricatures, a privileged and useless generation who'd gotten our fashion cues from *The Brady Bunch* and our values from Gordon Gekko in *Wall Street*.

And what exactly did we boomers get out of the deal, aside from those four recessions, skyrocketing tuition costs for our children, falling home values, and the daily shock of realizing our parents still hate us despite the fact we're bankrupting the health-care system to keep them alive?

We're getting old and fat and broken down, three things we swore would never happen to us.

How did it come to this? How did the most fitness-conscious generation the world has ever seen turn out to be incapable of keeping ourselves lean and strong? I think it's because we've either forgotten or never learned these rules.

NEW RULE #1 • The older you are, the more important it is to train.

An untrained human body will reach its physiological peak in its early twenties. Sometime around age forty, bad things begin to happen. Muscles shrink. Fat accumulates. Starting at fifty, that untrained body will lose 1 to 2 percent of its muscle mass per year, and 10 percent or more per decade. Strength declines twice as fast as muscle tissue. And power declines even faster than strength.

So when I say it's more important to train as you get older, I'm not talking about establishing a best-ever bench press or winning a push-up contest or developing six-pack abs. If those things happen, great. But they aren't as important as regaining what you've already lost, or building what you never had.

You'll see in the next few chapters just how adaptable the human body is in midlife and beyond. Research shows that muscles can be built, strength can be improved, power can be restored, and fat can be lost at any age that's been studied. Alwyn's daily experience at Results Fitness confirms that hardworking men and women can make extraordinary improvements to their appearance and performance.

There's just one catch: Time is no longer on your side. If you already feel the encroachment of age, weight, or misfortune, you need to do something. You can't do anything about yesterday, but with each passing year "tomorrow" becomes a less attractive option.

NEW RULE #2 • The goal of training is to change something.

The hierarchy of physical training goes something like this:

1. *Physical activity* is everything you do when you aren't at rest. It's basic movement, with no goal beyond getting from one place to another.
2. *Exercise* is movement you do on purpose. It includes sports practice, jogging, yoga, backpacking, swimming, cycling, or anything else you think is important enough to take precedence over all the other things you could be doing at that moment. (New Rule #2a: If you can operate your cell phone while exercising, you aren't actually exercising. You're just proving you can walk and chew gum at the same time.)
3. *A workout* is an exercise session that's deliberately strenuous. You start with the goal of working up a sweat, pushing your muscles and your circulatory system toward their limit, and giving your body a challenge from which it will have to recover.
4. *Training* is a system of workouts designed to achieve specific biological adaptations.

The more physical activity you get, and the less time you spend sitting, the better. Some of that activity should be purposeful enough to qualify as exercise. More exercise is generally better than less. A workout is even better, but there are only so many true workouts you can do in a week, a month, or a year. A workout that's also a training session is usually best of all, because you aren't just testing yourself to see what you can do now. You're forcing your body to make adaptations that will produce better performances in the future.

NEW RULE #3 • Your body won't change without consistent hard work.

When was the last time you picked up a barbell or dumbbell with the goal of *training*, of changing the way your body looks, feels, and performs?

Maybe it's an unfair question. Maybe everybody in the gym, from the middle-aged guy who wears weightlifting gloves to do lat pulldowns with a padded bar to the clinically obese woman doing triceps kickbacks with a dumbbell that's smaller than her forearm, thinks they're training. They certainly see themselves as working out. But I have to tell you, most of what I see in the gym on a daily basis barely qualifies as exercise.

If you aren't out of breath at least some of the time, you aren't really working out. You certainly aren't working hard enough to build strength, power, endurance, or any other fitness quality beyond what you already have. And if you aren't getting better at *something*, you sure as hell aren't training.

I don't say this to scare you off. If you're new to training, or following a structured program for the first time, you're almost guaranteed to make rapid progress. You just have to show up and follow the directions. It will *feel* like hard work, and it will certainly take you out of your comfort zone. But in a month or two you'll be able to do so much more that the entry-level workouts will seem like child's play.

Conversely, if you have a solid base of strength and conditioning—you like to work out, and you're pretty good at it—then you have to push yourself to improve on that, starting with the first training session. Alwyn's workouts allow that kind of effort and reward you for it. I've been using his programs off and on since 2000, and each one includes exercises and techniques that catch me by surprise, showing me where I'm weak, unbalanced, immobile, or deconditioned, and giving me the tools I need to improve.

But no matter your level, you'll make only as much progress as your effort allows. Muscles don't get stronger without progressively more challenging weights. Fat won't come off until you force your body to use more energy than it currently does.

Remember, the shape you're in now is the result of everything you've done to this point. If you want to achieve something new, you have to do something different.

NEW RULE #4 • Hard work doesn't mean beating the crap out of yourself every time you train.

We all have two goals in common:

- Fix the problems we have
- Avoid new ones

The perfect training session gives your body a stimulus, a type of stress that forces an adaptation. You follow that stimulus with a recovery period that allows your body to adjust to the stress. My default setting as a fitness writer is to say, "This is when your muscles get bigger and stronger." But it's not just your muscles. The stress is trans-systemic. It affects your muscles, connective tissues, bones, nerves, hormones. It even changes your mood.

Like any good remedy, it works best when taken in limited, prescribed doses. Just as you wouldn't go to one of Wolfgang Puck's restaurants and try to improve your entrée by emptying the salt shaker on top of it, so you shouldn't try to improve Alwyn's workouts by adding extra exercises, sets, or reps, or doing too many of them in a week.

Too much work with too little recovery will bring down anyone, at any level. It'll put a pro athlete on the disabled list, and it'll leave you or me with worse aches and pains than we had when we started.

NEW RULE #5   •   You're not a kid anymore. Don't train like one.

When I was young, I thought middle age was the worst possible condition inflicted on our species. My parents and their peers represented everything I never wanted to be. Something puzzled me, though: If in my preteen estimation they should've been miserable, why did they seem so satisfied?

I had to reach middle age to realize it's not at all what I once feared. The world makes sense because you've seen more of it. Your own life is no longer a mystery because you've had enough time to figure it out. (Having children of your own accelerates the process.) You don't have to brood about what you're going to be when you grow up because you know. Middle age is the sweet spot. You still have room to grow in your life and career, and you now have the wisdom to help you get there.

Unfortunately, that wisdom vanishes the minute you come into contact with a weighted object and attempt to lift it. Strength training brings out the teenager in all of us.

A young guy cares about three sets of muscles: abs, biceps, and chest, probably in that order. So his workout begins with sit-ups, moves on to bench presses, and finishes with biceps curls. A more advanced or enlightened young lifter will know that other people can see his double-mirror muscles—the ones he can't see unless he stands with his back to one mirror while holding a second mirror to see his reflection—so he'll also do some exercises for his back. If he considers himself a bodybuilder, he'll probably have an entire day devoted to back exercises. Which means, alas, that he'll also have an "arm day"—a workout in which he does nothing but curls and extensions for his biceps and triceps.

A young woman cares about her butt, her belly, and perhaps her triceps. So her workout begins with dozens if not hundreds of crunches, followed by a series of high-rep, low-weight exercises for her lower-body muscles, and ending with a few sets of triceps extensions.

It doesn't really work for either gender.

The guy may rock a six-pack, but it's not much of an accomplishment. He just needs to be skinny and fit and human anatomy takes care of the rest. My teenage son has had visible abs for most of his life. The sit-ups he does in karate training probably have something to do with it now that he's sixteen and eats like a hyperactive wildebeest, but it doesn't change the fact that he had a six-pack the first day he stepped into the dojo. A teenage lifter's biceps will get slightly bigger, with the much-coveted cephalic veins running proudly up the middle, while his pectoral muscles will grow just enough to help hide his ribs. But all that repetitive pressing, curling, and crunching with his front-body muscles will eventually distort his posture, flattening his lumbar curve and rolling his shoulders forward. He'll look good when his shirt is off and he's consciously flexing. With the shirt on, he'll just look like every other kid who plays a lot of video games.

The girl, meanwhile, is terrified of getting "bulky." But she also wants a butt that looks like twin tortoiseshells. She's willing to do hundreds of sets and thousands of reps, but she'll do them with machines that limit the involvement of her glute muscles, while using weights that are too light to have any effect on the size or strength of the muscles she's trying to enlarge. Of course, she'd never acknowledge she's trying to *build* those muscles. Instead, she'll use words like "tone," "sculpt," and "shape," all of which are to be magically achieved without changing the muscles' strength, size, or performance capacity.

We don't expect teenagers to understand how anything works unless it involves a keyboard. If they did, the United States wouldn't have the highest rate of teen pregnancy in the developed world. But adults should know better. And almost every middle-aged adult I see in my gym trains like a teenager, even if he or she never picked up a weight before Y2K.

The men do their crunches, presses, and arm curls. The women do their crunches, leg exercises, and elbow extensions. And we wonder why we don't look any better than our parents did, back when we swore to ourselves we'd never be anything like those strange people we grew up with.

You can do better, and you will with Alwyn's workouts and an honest effort. But before we get to the tools of our future transformation, let's look at the changes we've already experienced, the ones that made us older, fatter, and more beaten up than we ever expected to be.

A Beginner's Guide to Gym Culture

My gym is owned by an orthopedic practice. A lot of the members are older and, judging by their wide-eyed bewilderment, exercising in a health club for the first time. The absolute beginners create some problems for the rest of us, including one near-disaster when an elderly woman stepped over a barbell that I was about to lift off the floor. If I hadn't seen her in my peripheral vision at the last second, I can't imagine the consequences of that weight slamming into her leg. But the real problems, in my view, are caused by people who think they know what they're doing, but don't.

The following aren't my pet peeves, although I have plenty of those I could share. (In fact, I do share them in the Notes on page 273.) They're behaviors and practices that create potentially dangerous or volatile situations.

Don't use an iPod your first year in the gym
In a crowded weight room, with people lifting heavy things in unpredictable ways, your ears are almost as important as your eyes. At best, your eyes cover 180 degrees in a 360-degree world. If you can't hear what's going on behind you, you might step right into a rising weight. Some of the most dangerous mistakes I've seen were made by people listening to music and oblivious to their surroundings.

Don't sit on the equipment between sets
This is a basic, timeless, no-excuses rule of gym etiquette: If you're resting and someone else needs to use your equipment, you let him or her use it. You don't have to let two or three people jump in, unless that's standard practice in your gym. But you do have to share. The worst that can happen is you rest a little longer between sets than you planned, which means you're stronger and can lift more. The best that can happen is you score points for courtesy. I see this as a pervasive issue with older lifters who have no exposure to traditional gym culture.

Don't block two pieces of equipment to do one exercise
At my gym it's not uncommon to see someone standing between two benches doing an exercise that effectively blocks both, even though the person doesn't need either and could

do that exercise anywhere else in the room. The one time I said something, the offender was so offended she stormed off and complained to the manager about how she was being bullied and harassed.

Don't tie up equipment you don't need

This one is the hardest to explain to novices. The classic complaint among gym rats like me is the guy who does biceps curls in the squat rack, which is typically the only place in a commercial gym where serious lifters can do barbell squats and deadlifts. Another example is the newbie who puts her training log and water bottle on a bench while she does an exercise that doesn't require a bench. Which leads to my final point . . .

You don't need a water bottle

The early nineties were the golden age of hydration. Carrying a water bottle meant you were hip to the fear-of-thirst Zeitgeist created and nurtured by Gatorade to sell its sports drinks. Today's gyms have plenty of drinking fountains. You don't need to lug your own supply around. It's just one more thing to burden you and inconvenience others. And you especially don't need to make everyone else wait while you fill your bottle at the fountain when you're never going to be more than ten feet away from it.

Middle Rage

GROWING OLD HAS NEVER BEEN POPULAR. Almost every religious tradition involves an element of immortality or eternal reward. And if you want to see how the anti-senescence sentiment plays out among today's youth, check out the young-adult section of your local bookstore (if you still have a local store). You can't keep track of all the popular series whose main characters have found ways to preserve their youth forever.

Personally, I'm in favor of aging. I compare more favorably with my age-matched peers each birthday. Since I turned fifty I catch myself mentioning my age whenever I find an opening, even if it's a complete non sequitur. "Speaking as someone who's fifty-five, I wonder if this rain is ever going to end." I don't expect people to respond, "You're over fifty? Really? I never would've guessed." But I appreciate it when they do.

One reason aging doesn't bother me is that I've never been particularly good at anything that diminishes with age. When I was really lean, guys made fun of me for being skinny. (If I'd been paying better attention I would've noticed that no girl ever suggested I bulk up.) As an athlete, a charitable assessment would put me in the bottom quartile for my age. I got pretty strong at one point, but now that I'm not as strong, I don't miss it all that much. Aches and pains? I guess I could complain, but I can't really remember a time post-puberty when I wasn't jacked up somewhere. I was vulnerable to ankle sprains and partial shoulder separations in high school, and I struggle with knee and shoulder issues now.

I say all this with tongue partially in cheek. I'm not a fan of the aesthetics of middle age; given the choice, I sure wouldn't check the box marked "thicker waist and wrinkled neck." But some aspects of aging, if not exactly optional, are at least modifiable. The goal of this chapter is to discuss what aging is and what we can do about it, starting with these rules.

NEW RULE #6 • Decline is inevitable.

Show me a world-class athlete in a strength-and-power sport who's better in his late thirties than he was in his late twenties, and I'll show you Barry Bonds. If nothing else, Bonds proved to the few remaining doubters that steroids work. The subsequent crackdown in baseball showed that the laws of human physiology didn't change in the late twentieth century.

Two types of people are guaranteed to reach their physiological peak in their twenties: those who do no exercise, and those who do little else outside of training and competition. From there, it's downhill for both groups. Elite competitive weight-lifters decline by about 1 percent per year after age thirty. After fifty, the decline is a little faster—16 to 21 percent per decade—and it goes all to hell after seventy. Different sports show different rates of decline at the elite levels, but the basic plot doesn't change. You see that the most talented and best-trained athletes in anything decline about 10 percent per decade. Doesn't really matter if we're talking about strength or endurance sports. The rate of decline is similar to that of adults who don't exercise at all. The athletes, of course, are still stronger and faster than the slugs at every stage. They're only getting weaker and slower in comparison with their younger selves.

I don't say any of this to limit your ambitions. You and I aren't elite athletes. Some of you reading this still haven't reached your physiological peak for strength, power, and muscle mass, even if you're middle-aged. I hit my peak in my forties. Friends and readers have told me they're still getting stronger in their fifties or sixties. There's only one way to go once you reach your peak, but that's no reason not to go for it in the first place. In a moment, I'm going to show you why that peak is so important.

NEW RULE #7 • How fast you decline is up to you.

Genes are totally overrated in the aging process. Let's start with how old you look—and by "you," I mean me. Balding is associated with looking older, but there's not much I could've done about it, back when I actually cared. It's about 80 percent genetic. (I'm also going gray, which is 90 percent genetic.) I've gone bald in the exact way my father went bald. If I had an identical twin, he would be stuck with the same monk's stripe. However, that hypothetical twin might look older or younger than me, depending on a long list of environmental factors and lifestyle choices.

He might have less sun damage than me (I was a lifeguard during my college summers), making him look younger. But if he smoked, his skin would look older. If he was a little chubbier than me, his face might look younger than mine, since the fat would minimize his wrinkles. However, if he lost that extra weight, his face might look older, with flaccid skin and more pronounced cracks and crevices.

All told, our genetic heritage accounts for 40 to 60 percent of the factors associated with perceived aging.

That's just the *appearance* of age, assessed from the outside. These differences, at best, make you look a couple years older or younger, and aren't always indicative of your health status. A fit, athletic man or woman could look older than a sedentary peer, thanks to sun damage and, in my case, an abdicating hairline. As your mother used to say, it's what inside that counts. Your workout routine and lifestyle choices can make you as much as two decades younger at the cellular level.

Those choices, and their consequences, are the main subject of this chapter. But first, let me get one thing off my chest.

NEW RULE #8 • You are not a rural Okinawan.

I'm highly suspicious of any longevity advice based on the lifestyles of isolated, agrarian populations. Here's what long-lived people tend to have in common:

- They live in temperate regions with year-round sunlight.
- They grow up in poor farming communities with very little social or economic mobility.
- They live in multigenerational households, including grandparents.
- Their daily lives include long hours of repetitive labor. Nobody truly retires.
- If they need to get somewhere, they usually walk.

- Their diets are mostly vegetarian, with a predominance of cereal grains. They don't overeat, but I don't know if that's by choice or necessity. You can't eat too much of what you don't have.
- They tend to have low-stress lives with a strong sense of community.

Some of that sounds appealing. But how does it apply to your life, or mine? Can you tell your boss, "You know, I think we should shift our best practices to the rural Okinawan model"? Would you want to live with your parents or grandparents? Would they want to live with you?

Like it or not, most of us live and work in a stress-filled world, with small families and long hours spent in technology-driven isolation. I think it makes more sense to look for the best ways to manage our health within the parameters of our own world than to try to replicate select features of another. How do we really know that any life-extending element of rural Okinawans or Sardinians or Costa Ricans would work without all the others? If it's a package deal—the low-calorie, low-protein diet doesn't work unless you live with your grandparents—then what's the point?

THE ROARING HUNDRED AND TWENTIES

The late, great Jack LaLanne is a perfect example of the inevitability of aging. He was there at the creation of modern fitness culture, hanging out at Muscle Beach in the 1940s with Vic Tanny (a guy who more or less invented the health-club chain as we know it), Joe Gold (founder of Gold's Gym), Steve Reeves (iconic bodybuilding champion who played Hercules in the movies), Harold Zinkin (a bodybuilding and weight-lifting champion best known for inventing the Universal Gym Machine), and Abbye "Pudgy" Stockton, the first woman to become famous for a body built with strength exercises. ("Pudgy" was a childhood nickname; as a fitness icon, she weighed a solid 115 pounds, with a tiny waist and beautiful curves.)

LaLanne was the first and longest-running fitness guru on TV; he invented exercise machines and owned gyms. In 1956, the year before I was born, he did 1,033 push-ups in 23 minutes on a TV show. Three years later, at age forty-five, he did a thousand jumping jacks and a thousand chin-ups in 83 minutes. By all accounts he had a close, loving family, and was the best advertisement for his own advice to live the healthiest, cleanest, most physically dynamic life that was humanly possible. He even refused to eat cake at his ninetieth birthday party.

He died in 2010 at the age of ninety-six, much loved and now much missed.

But here's something interesting: His brother Norman, who was an avid golfer and a former college athlete but nowhere close to Jack when it came to fitness fanaticism, died at ninety-seven. The guy who *didn't* exercise two hours a day or turn down birthday cake or tow barges through San Francisco Bay lived longer than his younger brother, who did all those things.

Make no mistake: Living a vigorous life into your nineties is a great accomplishment. And perhaps if LaLanne had gotten medical treatment for his ultimately fatal pneumonia, instead of trying to exercise his way through it, he might still be alive today.

The maximum human lifespan is thought to be about 120 years. Jeanne Louise Calment—born in 1875, died in 1997—is the only human whose claim to have lived 120-plus years is beyond dispute. What we know about her isn't any more helpful than what we know about LaLanne. She was independently wealthy and never had to work. She outlived her only grandchild and spent her final decade in a nursing home, including eight years in a wheelchair following a leg fracture. By her own account, she started smoking when she was twenty-one and didn't quit until she was one hundred seventeen. She says she drank port wine and ate two pounds of chocolate a week.

It's tempting to say that longevity is all in the genes, combined with the good luck to avoid catastrophic diseases and accidents. The latter explains how average human life span is increasing. We have less childhood disease, cleaner water, safer jobs, better medicine, and all kinds of expensive machines to keep us alive long past whatever our original expiration date may have been. Consistent exercise is estimated to add six to seven years to an individual's life expectancy.

But maximum life span, as far as anyone knows, isn't in play. A vigorous life might get you past a hundred, but it won't get you to 125. The best we can hope for is to get the most out of whatever years we have. Exercise, I'm happy to report, is the best tool we have for that project. And strength training may be the best type of exercise.

YOUR CELL-BY DATE

Parents and teachers know how hard it is to keep kids from running. It's their natural instinct when they want to get from one place to another. Then puberty comes around, and it's suddenly hard to get them to move at all, unless you count their thumbs as they text. As adults, few of us can remember the last time we ran all-out. We have to force ourselves to run because our bodies are telling us to walk.

It's all part of nature's plan: We have a high metabolism and high activity level in early childhood, and we gradually slow down until we're just barely shuffling along. Eventually that slow metabolism kills us. When we get less active, we lose fitness, both cardiorespiratory and muscular, and with lower fitness we move even less. At first our muscle tissue shrinks. Then the type IIb muscle fibers, the ones most responsible for strength and power, start to disappear. As we lose muscle cells we also lose motor units. A motor unit is a nerve cell and all the muscle fibers it's in charge of activating. Lose enough of these—especially the high-powered ones controlling type IIb fibers—and your body loses entire functions. It can't do things it used to be able to do.

Concurrent with these issues is a loss of appetite, as you know if you've cared for an aging parent. Many seniors, left on their own, will eat a low-calorie, low-protein diet that falls far short of what they need to maintain muscle tissue. That may be the biggest reason why the aging process speeds up so much around age seventy. Not only are untrained muscles getting smaller and weaker and losing motor units from disuse, they're being starved out of existence.

Of course this matches our memories and perhaps our experience, if we're pushing past middle age. The most energetic septuagenarian still looks old. Jack LaLanne, despite a lifetime of lifting, and despite a lifetime of eating to support his muscle tissue and activity level, was visibly much smaller in his later years. He may have lost more muscle than some people ever build.

The key to senescence is in parts of our cells called mitochondria. Mitochondria produce ATP (adenosine triphosphate, for those who've forgotten your high school biology), and ATP is where the action is. Or, rather, it's the juice that allows action. ATP fuels everything we do. We think of human energy as a product of carbohydrates and fat (protein is a minor energy source), but carbs and fat have to be converted to ATP before they can do squat.

The proteins that make up mitochondria have DNA, and within those DNA are structures called telomeres. I should point out that when we start talking about telomeres, we're getting down toward the most microscopic levels of human anatomy. But to understand aging, we have to go even smaller, to the tips of the telomeres. These get progressively smaller each time our cells reproduce. It's sort of like an eraser on the end of a pencil. You can erase only so much of your scribbling before the eraser gets down to the nub. When your telomeres get down to their own nub, the DNA stops reproducing, and bad things happen.

If I went through the list of bad things, I'd have to pretend I understand it in more depth than I do. So let's skip the fine print in our biological license agreement and return to the big picture: When parts of cells can no longer reproduce, those cells can no longer function as they once did. Cells mutate or die or otherwise malfunction. The cellular scrubbing system, which does such a great job of cleaning out the metabolic junk when you're young, doesn't work as well when you're forty or fifty as it did when you were twenty or thirty.

The work of mitochondria in muscle tissue is especially important. Muscle is where carbohydrates go to be used or stored following a meal. The carbs you eat are converted to a simple sugar called glucose, and 65 percent of that glucose is either used by skeletal muscles or stored there as glycogen. If the mitochondria in your muscle cells become smaller, weaker, or less active, you have a problem. Your body becomes less capable of handling all that glucose flowing through your bloodstream following meals. Excess blood sugar is typically accompanied by higher levels of the hormone insulin, which is in charge of pushing nutrients like glucose, fat, and protein into the appropriate storage centers. As insulin gets higher, your body becomes less sensitive to it. This is the path that eventually leads to type 2 diabetes.

But it won't be your path. Not if you train.

MUSCLE CHANGES EVERYTHING

"Sarcopenia" is one of those dry, nonjudgmental scientific terms that make the preventable and often self-inflicted loss of muscle in old age sound inevitable. It's inevitable that you'll decline from your peak—whatever it may be, and whenever you might achieve it—but it's not inevitable that you grow feeble. The more muscle mass you have at your peak, the more you'll have left as age takes its toll. The same goes for strength and power.

That's why it's so important to work harder and train more ambitiously than people our age are typically willing to do. If you've never pushed yourself in the weight room, you don't know what your muscles can handle. You can add size and strength at any age; the research is very clear on that point. It's also clear that the less you've pushed yourself to get to where you are now, the more room you have to grow.

Women reading this may be tempted to stop right here and ask for a refund. Who wants to get bigger, especially in middle age? Trust me on this: Bigger, stronger muscles don't mean a thicker, less attractive physique. (If you don't believe me, go online and find pictures of Pudgy Stockton from the 1940s. She was a knockout.) Muscle and fat are separate tissues. You can build muscle without increasing fat, or burn fat without losing muscle. Beginners can often do both at the same time. No matter your age or gender, you're better off with well-trained and well-developed muscles. You'll look better, feel better, and move better.

But if you've never done a serious training program before—including those of Alwyn's in the NROL series—you probably haven't developed your muscles to anything close to their full potential. I rarely see a middle-aged man or woman in a gym who appears to be working hard, and the research backs up my observation. Studies have shown that men and women, beginners and experienced lifters alike, typically choose weights well below those that would actually increase strength or size. Lifters rarely work with more than 50 percent of their one-rep maximum—the most weight they could lift once with good form—and when they aren't told how many reps to do with the weight they've selected, they inevitably stop well short of exhaustion.

When scientists conduct strength-training studies with older adults (or, really, with lifters at any age), they typically make them work with much heavier weights than they would choose on their own. Just to pick one example, let's look at a study titled "Resistance Exercise Reverses Aging in Human Skeletal Muscle." It was published in 2007 in a journal called *PLoS One* (the acronym stands for Public Library of Science). Among the authors is Mark Tarnopolsky, M.D., of McMaster University, one of the most innovative, prolific, and respected researchers in the field of exercise science. Dude's a rock star; his studies have changed the way we think about a long list of topics, including nutritional supplements, neuromuscular diseases, the aging process, and of course strength training.

In this study, he and his colleagues identified 596 genes found in skeletal muscle that change with age, hundreds of which are involved in metabolism and mitochondrial function. They took a group of healthy, older men and put them on a six-month strength-training program. Not only did the men increase their strength by 50 percent, but 179 of those genes shifted into reverse and started behaving like the genes of younger men.

Like magic, the biological clock is turned back by as much as twenty years at the cellular level.

There is, however, a catch: The older men in the study were doing a routine in which they used 80 percent of their one-rep max for three sets of eight repetitions of each exercise. They were working *hard*.

Getting to Know Max

Most of you reading this know exactly what I mean when I talk about sets, reps, and percentages of one-rep max. But for those who don't:

- A *repetition*, or rep, is a single performance of an exercise. So one push-up is a single repetition.
- A *set* is a series of repetitions. If you do three sets of eight reps (you might see it shortened to 3x8), you're doing eight reps three times, with rest in between each set.
- Your *one-rep max* (often abbreviated as 1RM) is the most weight you can lift once with good form. But it's not a weight you would ever use for training. Even competitive lifters rarely train with 100 percent of their 1RM.

For a practical example, let's say your one-rep max on an exercise is 50 pounds. Eighty percent of that max would be 40 pounds. If you try one all-out set with 40 pounds, you can probably do ten repetitions before your muscles become too fatigued to complete another one with good form. (We don't want you working with not-good form. Nobody is perfect on every rep, but deliberately changing your form to eke out one or two more is unnecessary and potentially dangerous.)

So if you see that subjects in a study did three sets of eight with 80 percent of their max, that means they were working very close to complete exhaustion on each set. Put another way, they were working their butts off to get stronger.

You see something similar in all the studies showing improvements in muscular strength and size in older men and women. Left on their own, these people wouldn't have lifted heavy enough, or pushed themselves hard enough, to get results. The researchers had to set parameters and then supervise them closely to make sure they lifted as much as they were supposed to. They also made sure they increased the weights as they got stronger.

When you do Alwyn's workouts, it's up to you to start with weights that challenge you, and to increase them as often as you can. Nobody's looking over your shoulder. You'll get some benefit from half-assed workouts—especially if you aren't currently lifting—but all the good stuff comes from full-assed training. That is, from forcing your body to do more today than it could last week.

HIGHER POWER

At this point, you might be wondering what's the best result you can hope to achieve. Research on this is consistent over the years. If you start lifting now, in middle age, and you push yourself hard, in six months you can be as strong as someone decades younger . . . as long as that person doesn't lift.

Here's a recent example: Researchers at the University of Regina, in Saskatchewan, took a group of healthy older men and compared them with a group of healthy younger men. The older men were between sixty and seventy-one years old. Neither group included men who were currently lifting. After twenty-two weeks, the older men matched the younger ones for strength and muscle mass, more or less. In some areas, like muscle thickness in their upper arms, the trained older men surpassed the untrained younger ones.

There are lots of studies out there with similar findings. Not every lifter in every study makes the kind of gains we're talking about; some don't make much progress at all, while others do considerably better than the averages show. The good news is that your chances of getting stronger—*much* stronger—and adding high-quality muscle tissue are pretty good. You can't stop the clock, but the evidence shows you can roll it back, if you're willing to work hard enough.

Hurt's No Good

WHEN YOU'RE A JOURNALIST, you quickly figure out whom to call when you need a certain kind of quote. Just as important, you learn which type of source to avoid. Some people see the worst of everything. It's not that they're dishonest or unfair. They'll honestly tell you about things that are so grim you want to start drinking before noon. These people come in handy when the goal is to paint a stark picture for your readers. Other sources are predictably sunny. If you need a hearts-and-rainbows, "everything is beautiful" kind of angle, you go to them, even if you know their optimism comes from assiduous refusal to consider any facts that would temper it. In politics they call it "spin," but in most other contexts we just call it B.S.

I decided early on that I didn't want to spend my career being depressed or lied to, which is why writing about health and fitness suits me so well. Almost everything I write is prescriptive. Experts are happy to talk to me, and readers are happy to find and use the information I get from my sources. Real controversies are so rare that you sometimes have to work hard to find them.

But there are some.

Take the barbell back squat. Although I was an enthusiastic back squatter at the time Alwyn and I wrote the original *NROL*, eventually I stopped doing them. They were hard on my knees and shoulders. I always felt worse for days afterward. Conversely, I could do front squats and not feel any joint pain at all. Whatever soreness I felt a day or two later was in the bellies of my thigh muscles—exactly where it's supposed to be.

There are two ways to look at my retreat from back squats:

I could try to extrapolate my problems with the exercise out to the entire population, and suggest nobody should do them. I can always find doctors and physical therapists who would be happy to portray dozens of exercises as injurious. They deal with injuries every hour of every working day, and their point of view, while honest, is tainted by the fact that they typically see people who are already in pain. The problem with this kind of reporting is that the same doctors and therapists might have similarly grim opinions about exercises that I think are safe and include in books and articles.

Or I could acknowledge that lots of people can do lots of things I can't. I've sucked at so many things in my life that it's easy to suppose an exercise I struggle with is just another brick in the wall. I can always find someone out there who'll agree with me on that as well.

Those two sides squared off in what I call the Squat Wars of 2009 and 2010, which began when Mike Boyle, a friend of ours, explained why he no longer uses the barbell back squat with the athletes he trains. The backlash was swift and furious. Even the National Strength and Conditioning Association got into the act, revoking Boyle's invitation to speak at its 2010 national conference.

The controversy illustrates my dilemma as an honest journalist whose reporting includes a mix of prescription and description. Is something dangerous because it doesn't work for me? Should Alwyn and I go so far toward the cautionary side that we tell middle-aged people like you and me to walk more and eat vegetables (although not at the same time, because someone might get hurt)? Or should we go to the opposite extreme and say no exercise is dangerous if you do it right (and if you don't, it's a sign of a serious character flaw)?

The rules of injury prevention and recovery, as you'll see, are simple and straightforward. How you apply them is infinitely more complex. I'll do my best to tell you what we know from research, but as I do keep in mind that your experience is the only one that really matters.

NEW RULE #9 • Everyone is injured. But not every injury hurts.

I was caught by surprise a few years ago when I suffered a deep chest bruise playing basketball. When it didn't get any better, I went to a doctor for an X-ray to see if it was more than a bruise. It wasn't, but the X-ray revealed a bizarre anomaly in my rib cage. One of my ribs stopped short of my spine. Was it an old and unhealed injury? A sign of the apocalypse? The orthopedist was equally baffled, but his advice was reassuring: If it doesn't hurt, don't worry about it.

It's not just me. When researchers go looking for injuries in people who are symptom-free, they find them. Just to pick one example, a study published in the *New England Journal of Medicine* in 1994 started with doctors at one hospital taking MRI scans of ninety-eight people who had no history of back pain. They sent the scans to another hospital, where they were examined by doctors who weren't told that the scans came from asymptomatic people. For good measure, the researchers mixed in twenty-seven scans of people who had back pain and whose scans showed abnormalities.

Just 38 percent of the people without pain had completely normal spines. Almost two-thirds had an issue that a doctor would expect to find in someone with back pain. Gender and activity level didn't seem to matter, although age did, as you'd expect. The study showed a steady increase in abnormalities in middle age and beyond.

Lots of things can go wrong. Aside from wear and tear, athletes in high-risk sports like football, mixed martial arts, gymnastics, cheerleading, and Olympic weightlifting are known to have higher risk of fractures in the tiny bones on the edges of their vertebrae. Those fractures may or may not cause pain at the time, but could show up as an injury later in life, when the former athlete is more sedentary and less fit.

That's just the spine. Add in shoulder, hip, knee, ankle, and elbow injuries, and chances are that none of us reach middle age without something going wrong. As my doctor said when looking at my inexplicably detached rib, if it doesn't hurt, don't worry.

NEW RULE #10 • If an activity hurts, stop doing it.

I guarantee this is the least original advice in this book, if not the entire NROL series. I've seen it countless times. I'm sure Alwyn has said it more times than he can remember. But it also needs frequent repetition because it's so easy to forget. I know because I sometimes push through discomfort in order to finish all the work I planned to do that day. I regret it every time.

Pain in the weight room will almost never be short, sharp, and shocking, unless you drop a plate on your foot. I can probably count on one hand the number of times I've gotten that kind of pain while lifting. And even then, I can think of only one time when it was an actual injury. The other times, nothing.

The really insidious injuries are the ones that you know you have but convince yourself you can work through anyway. There's no alarm-bell sensation that tells you to stop. You notice that an exercise aggravates your shoulder or knee or hip or elbow or back. But because it's a tolerable, familiar pain, you think it's okay to keep going. Trust me, it isn't. You're only making it worse.

NEW RULE #11 • If it hurts after you do it, it may or may not be a problem.

New lifters tend to overreact to delayed-onset muscle soreness, which is saddled with an unnecessarily ominous-sounding acronym: DOMS. Veteran lifters, on the other hand, sometimes overreact when they *aren't* sore a day or two after starting a new program. Both sides understand that muscles get sore in response to a new stimulus. One group assumes the pain is proof they worked too hard, while the other worries the lack of pain shows they didn't work hard enough.

They could be right. Or wrong. If DOMS persists more than two or three days, then yes, you probably overdid it. But that's almost inevitable for a new lifter, who doesn't yet know how to avoid doing too much of something she's never before done. Absence of DOMS might mean a new stimulus wasn't novel enough. Or it might mean that you're starting out at exactly the right level of intensity, giving you time to learn new exercises or sequences before you start pushing the limits.

Either way, general muscle soreness—the kind that leaves muscles tender in a uniform way—is a poor indicator of success or failure. But if you're not used to it, you probably wonder if it's okay to work out when you have lingering soreness.

You don't have to stop exercising altogether. The tissues still need to be nourished, and movement will accelerate the process by allowing enhanced blood flow. Jonathan Fass, DPT, a board-certified physical therapist, recommends this simple test to see if you're ready to exercise again:

- If a light touch is enough to trigger muscle pain, hold back at least one more day.
- If you feel pain only with deep pressure—like when you push your thumb directly

into the belly of a muscle—you're ready to train, although you should consider doing a little less total work than normal.

- If there's no pain or soreness, warm up thoroughly and have at it.

Once you start the workout, you have two rules: Use the full pain-free range of motion, but stop doing anything that hurts.

NEW RULE #12 • Never try to fix an acute injury by stretching it.

"Pain-free range of motion" isn't just the key phrase in the previous sentence. It may represent the five most important words in this chapter, if not the entire book. Your range of motion will shorten in the area surrounding an injury as your body tries to prevent further damage.

Imagine that you have a small tear in your shirt. If you pull on it, the tear gets bigger. Your shirt won't generate an inflammatory response to protect and repair the damaged area, so the analogy isn't perfect. But if you sew the shirt up, the stitching will leave a reminder that the shirt was once torn, just as a healed injury will have some residual scar tissue. That scar tissue changes the integrity and function of the connective tissues surrounding it, which is why you need to work injured muscles and joints through that pain-free range of motion early and often. The goal is to get back to full mobility without pain or limitation sooner rather than later.

But you can't reach that point ahead of your body's schedule. Soft tissue takes about six weeks to recover completely, although each of us ultimately recovers on our own schedule. Stretching an area while it's still sore and inflamed—depending on the severity, this could include the first week or two—will only create more pain and inflammation, extending the recovery rather than speeding it up.

With most common injuries, Fass says, you want to begin stretching within three weeks. That gives you a three-week window to work with the new tissue in its formative stage, before scar tissue has a chance to permanently alter its structure and function.

NEW RULE #13 • When in doubt, refer out.

Everything I've said about injuries so far is general information. Most of the time, for most mild injuries in most people, these guidelines are good enough. But you aren't a hypothetical person, and there's a chance your injury isn't a textbook example. Don't be stoic. If it's obviously a serious injury—severe inflammation, sharp pain, unabated soreness lasting five or more days—see a doctor. Even simpler: If you think you need a professional opinion, you probably do.

BACK OF THE LINE

You've read that 80 to 85 percent of adults will suffer back pain at some point in their lives. It may not be true, but it's close. According to the textbook *Rehabilitation of the Spine*, an American adult has a 56 percent chance of having lower-back pain in any single year, and a 70 percent lifetime chance. Almost half of us will experience some kind of back-related episode before we turn thirty, and at any given moment between 15 and 30 percent of us will be in pain.

But here's the stat of stats: More than 85 percent of back pain is caused by "non-specific" factors. Serious diseases and injuries (tumors, infections, fractures) cause less than 2 percent of back pain. Less than 10 percent is caused by nerve compression. The rest is classified as "nonspecific."

If it's nonspecific, you'd assume it's unlikely to be caused by a single event, which seems to be the case. We grind ourselves down over time. It could be too much of one kind of activity or too little overall activity. It could be genetic (there's a high correlation for combined back and neck-shoulder pain among identical twins), it could be occupational, or it could be linked to any number of personal characteristics or issues. Or it might be something else. The simple act of sitting in a chair for a long time is one of the riskiest activities we engage in on a regular basis.

Most acute back pain will subside on its own schedule, without intervention. But that doesn't mean you're off the hook. The number-one predictor of back injury is a previous back injury. More worrisome is this: Back injuries cause your body to use muscles differently. All your major joints protect themselves through muscular co-contraction. Muscles on one side of the joint contract in tandem with those on the other side to keep the joint in a stable position. When the normal firing patterns change or get disrupted, the previously protected joint is suddenly vulnerable. This is why bad posture—shoulders rolled forward, lower back flattened instead of naturally curved—is one of the best predictors of pain and injury, Fass says.

I don't think it matters which joints we're talking about. Those of you who read *NROL for Women* may remember the discussion on women and knee injuries. One cause is muscular imbalance; a woman's quadriceps are typically much stronger than her hamstrings, whereas men usually have a smaller discrepancy. Whether it's the lower back, shoulders, hips, or knees, if muscles on one side of a major joint are weaker or tighter than they're supposed to be, you have a greater chance of injury.

I'm not going to dwell too much here on specific problems, simply because Alwyn's entire program is designed to help you develop balanced strength and mobility. That balance is the key to everything.

What we don't know about injuries and persistent pain may still exceed what we do know. But we're pretty sure that the healthiest and most injury-resistant body is the one that can do the most things. It can lift heavy objects slowly but also complete explosive actions. It has steady-state endurance but also has well-trained reflexes for sudden and unpredictable movements. It can use your muscles as a coordinated movement system even when you aren't moving. When you run or jump or play, it protects itself by stabilizing key joints even when you're moving at full speed. At the same time, we know that the athletes and enthusiasts who push themselves the farthest in one or more directions are most likely to be hurt.

That leaves us with this directive: Do the entire program to the best of your ability, and you should end up with a body that's much stronger and more resilient from top to bottom. No body is ever 100 percent resilient, but if nothing else the more fit and functional body will be a lot more fun to have on a daily basis.

The Road
More Traveled

"I'M TRAINING FOR A MARATHON" is one of the more deflating sentences I hear in my life as a fitness professional. I have friends who run marathons and do it well. They're serious, gifted endurance athletes who've been training for years. The people who announce their long-distance ambitions to me are neither serious nor gifted. Most of the time, they're trying to lose weight. I don't even try to talk them out of it anymore because I know how it'll turn out:

1. They'll get angry and stop talking to me.
2. They'll do it anyway.
3. They'll get hurt.
4. They'll gain weight.

Once upon a time, the idea that you could gain weight on a serious endurance-training program was dismissed as physiologically impossible. Calories go in. Calories go out. If you're burning hundreds of calories a day that you weren't burning before, of course you'll lose weight. The only possible way you could gain weight is by eating substantially more food. And that's crazy. If people are overweight, they're already eating plenty of food to sustain an hour or two a day of running. Why in the world would they eat more?

At some point, the fact that many people were indeed training and gaining became too obvious to ignore. That's when a curious admonition started showing up in mainstream fitness articles. Often, the exhortation is right there in the headline: "Break the Work Out/Pig Out Cycle." The assumption is that men and women who're smart enough to exercise don't understand that too many post-workout calories will negate the effects of the workout.

This is, of course, part of a pattern among fitness and nutrition professionals. We always assume people lack the cognitive ability to understand they should move more and eat less. So we repeat it as often as we can, in as many different ways as our own cognitive skills allow. The goal is to convince any individual seeking advice that she's doing at least one of those things wrong. Two of my favorite scolds come from the bodybuilding world: "Great bodies are built in the kitchen" and "It's 90 percent diet."

The premise is absurd. You build a great body in the gym *and* the kitchen, and which is more important will vary from one person to the next. Imagine that you could take two identical twins, and have one eat perfectly without exercise while the other trains perfectly while eating her normal diet. Which would look better in a year? Of course it would be the one who spent hours in the gym lifting and sweating.

"Ah!" says the imaginary person I'm arguing with. "But what if the twin ate too much and her body got all flabby and shit?"

We now circle back to the original problem: Why would someone who's exercising to lose weight, or to get leaner and more muscular, eat so much food that he or she ends up gaining fat instead?

Let's take stupidity off the table. My career is based on the premise that if people are intelligent enough to seek out professional advice, they're intelligent enough to understand the basic math of calories-in, calories-out. That leaves us with this: There must be something about exercise that makes some people hungrier than they were before.

In fact, there is. That's the good news. The bad news: If you're remotely interested in the answer, you're probably one of them.

NEW RULE #14 • Exercise burns calories.
Sometimes that's a problem.

When researchers use the word "exercise," they don't use my definition. They mean steady-pace endurance exercise. "Strength training" or "resistance exercise" is something different, and "high-intensity interval training" is yet another thing.

And exercise, by their definition, is problematic. When researchers have used exercise as a short- or long-term intervention to help people lose weight, it doesn't work the way it's supposed to. Average weight loss in exercise-only studies is often minuscule. When the intervention includes a reduced-calorie diet, the people who diet and exercise don't lose any more weight than the people who diet without exercise.

What goes wrong? Why do people who are sometimes jogging for up to five hours a week not losing weight? A team of researchers based in Australia and the UK has been trying to crack the nut, and their findings are intriguing.

One study, published in 2009 in the *American Journal of Clinical Nutrition*, recruited several dozen overweight and obese adults between the ages of thirty and fifty. Their twelve-week exercise program was designed to burn 500 calories per session, and 2,500 calories a week. Most of the people in the study lost weight—seven pounds on average, virtually all of it from fat. But there was a huge gap between those who responded to the program and those who didn't. Responders lost an average of eleven pounds, which was close to 6 percent of their starting weight, versus two pounds and 1 percent for the nonresponders.

It gets worse. Fifteen percent of the participants gained weight. Daily hunger rose for the nonresponders, and their sense of fullness following a meal was lower. Some of the responders also ate more, which makes sense when their bodies are suddenly forced to burn off an extra 2,500 calories a week. But they didn't eat enough to negate the exercise. One responder ate an extra thousand calories a day and still lost nine pounds, while one *extreme* responder cut a thousand calories a day and lost more than thirty pounds. On average, the responders didn't report any change in their hunger levels.

So a hefty dose of exercise sure as hell works for *some* people.

At the other end, my heart goes out to the person who added 1,250 daily calories and gained seven pounds. And what are we to think of the nonresponder who added 2,000 daily calories—*four times* the amount of energy burned in each exercise session—but still managed to drop a pound?

The study left a very, very big question unanswered: Why were the nonresponders so . . . nonresponsive? The same team tackled that question in a review study, which led them to a fascinating possibility.

NEW RULE #15 • "Fat-burning" exercise doesn't always burn fat.

Human bodies burn a combination of fat and carbohydrate for energy. A healthy body will burn more fat than carbohydrate at rest and in low-intensity exercise. The harder you go, the higher the percentage of carbs you burn, until you're burning almost all carbs during those short bursts of all-out exertion. But when you recover from a sprint or a set of heavy lifts, you burn almost all fat, and you burn a lot of it because your heart is thumping and your metabolism is as high as it can go.

There's only so much of this activity you can do, as I noted in Chapter 1. But if you do three of Alwyn's workouts a week, and push yourself to work harder and get stronger, you'll spend enough time with an elevated metabolism to see a real difference. Your body will burn a lot of fat during and after the workout as it recovers. The term for this is *metabolic flexibility*. The easier your body can switch from burning fat to carbs and back again, the more metabolically flexible you are, and the easier it will be for you to train hard and to enjoy the results of training, all else being equal.

Alas, some people don't burn fat the way they should. They burn a higher percentage of carbs at rest, during exercise, and while they're recovering. Because the human body has limited ability to store carbs—as opposed to its unlimited ability to store fat—this metabolic inflexibility presents a serious problem.

Humans can store carbohydrate three different ways: There's the glucose in your blood (typically from recently digested food), glycogen in your muscle tissues, and a smaller amount of glycogen in your liver. Your body will never let the supply run out completely. Even if you're starving on the frozen tundra, your body will use fat and muscle tissue for energy before it wrings the final grams of carbohydrate from your system. You'll die of starvation first.

Logically, if your body places that much value on its carb reserves, it's extremely sensitive to carb depletion. The lower it goes, the hungrier we get. Somebody who burns too many carbs all the time, at rest and in motion, will feel that depletion sooner, and respond with greater hunger.

No one can say exactly how this process works, or even say with 100 percent certainty that it happens at all. When we do have a clearer picture, it won't be as simple as what I just described; nothing ever is. The most we can say now is that some evidence suggests that those who burn a higher percentage of fat calories during exercise will be less hungry afterward than those who burn less fat. This has been shown in studies in which all the participants, male or female, were lean.

We also know that obese adults typically burn a higher percentage of carbs all day, every day. If burning too many carbs during exercise indeed provokes more hunger afterward, then we have an explanation for why endurance exercise doesn't do much to help people lose weight. It works for healthy, lean people, or those predisposed to be lean, but they were that way before they started running or riding or swimming. Thus, when friends and relatives who're slim and fit tell you that a morning run is their secret to staying slim and fit, they're telling the truth. Endurance exercise works for them because their bodies burn more fat during exercise and are less hungry afterward.

If you're not one of them, if you're predisposed to gain weight easily and conventional exercise doesn't work for you, the carb-depletion theory might explain why.

NEW RULE #16 • Alwyn figured this out a long time ago.

Alwyn would be the first to tell you that he's not an inventor. He's an integrator. He figures out the best ways to do things based on what others have done successfully. But by the time he finishes integrating, the programs he creates don't typically look like anyone else's.

Take the idea that endurance exercise is the best weight-loss tool for the people who most need to lose weight. It was gospel when I started writing about fitness back in the early nineties. But by the time I worked with Alwyn in the early 2000s, several prominent trainers had already shared their skepticism about steady-state cardio. Alwyn's skepticism didn't seem unique.

Over time, though, the way he *applied* that skepticism started to look very different from what other trainers I knew were doing with their clients. For one thing, he rejected the idea that extremely overweight clients needed an easier training program. He worked them hard. He understood that fatigue gave him two potent fat-loss tools:

- Fatiguing exercise burns calories.
- Fatiguing exercise leaves you with an elevated metabolism and a need to recover.
- Endurance exercise is also fatiguing, and the more fatigued you are from any individual bout, the more recovery you need. But there are two problems with endurance training as a primary weight-loss tool:

○ Your body becomes more efficient at running or cycling or swimming, and burns fewer calories per unit of work.

○ Weight loss slows down your metabolic response to both food and exercise. Your body becomes biased toward regaining the lost weight.

Those two outcomes are the best-case scenario. That's your reward for *successful* weight loss when you use a combination of diet and endurance exercise. You need to exercise even more and eat even less just to break even and not regain the weight.

Alwyn went to the other extreme. He created fatigue through the widest possible variety of movements: forward, back, sideways, up, down, and every angle in between. But it wasn't just fatigue that he was after. He used every intervention he could think of to force a body to make adaptations, to do or be something it couldn't or wasn't before. The most important of those adaptations is tissue remodeling.

Your body breaks down and rebuilds its own tissues all day, every day. Without exercise, you have three stages of tissue remodeling throughout your life. When you're young, there's a net protein accretion. That is, your body builds more muscle and other tissue than it tears down. In your twenties and thirties, if you aren't training and you aren't eating in a way that adds to or reduces your weight, you achieve net protein balance. You break down and rebuild tissue at the same rate. Finally, starting in midlife, you break down more than you put back, unless you take specific actions to prevent it from happening.

Alwyn's goal is to maximize every part of the adaptive process while stopping short of the point at which fatigue does more harm than good:

1. First, you will do enough work to burn a lot of calories.
2. Some of the work will be difficult enough to jack up your heart rate and get you breathing hard. Your body will use the anaerobic energy systems, during which your muscle cells will be forced to create ATP without oxygen. It's a less efficient and thus more metabolically expensive way to create energy.
3. You'll almost always stop long enough to catch your breath between sets or intervals of anaerobic exercise. That enhances metabolic flexibility by forcing your body to switch back and forth between fuel sources—burning carbs during the set and then burning fat as you recover.
4. Most of the exercises employ your body's biggest muscles, which takes more energy and requires more recovery.

5. The strength exercises will break down muscle tissue. That would be a bad outcome if you didn't rebuild at least as much as you break down. (Chapter 18 covers post-workout nutrition.) The goal is a net gain in muscle protein. Stronger, thicker muscles allow you to train harder, which is the best kind of adaptation you can achieve. But even without bigger muscles, simply forcing your body to break even can be a win, as long as it takes a lot of energy to get there.

More than anything, Alwyn makes sure his clients—and by extension our NROL readers—don't become so efficient that they stop seeing results. That's why there are so many different movement patterns in every workout, why there are so many ways to make the movements more challenging, and why the programs change every few weeks. You want to get good at doing individual exercises, but you never want to repeat the same exercise in the same way so many times that your body goes from adaptation to efficiency.

And yet, all those interventions, by themselves, don't guarantee weight loss. Some of you will probably lose a few pounds of fat on Alwyn's program, and that can be substantial if you're already close to your fighting weight—whatever makes you feel like you're at the top of your game. Some of you will gain a few pounds, especially if your body responds well to strength training and you add solid muscle. Again, that can be a great outcome if you were relatively lean and a few pounds of muscle makes you look and feel better.

But if you aren't particularly lean right now, and your goal is to lose more than a few pounds of fat, even Alwyn's workouts won't get you there without a change in your diet. Alwyn will be the first to tell you that. I can't specify what you need to change—although I'll give it my best shot in Part Three—but if you're heavier and fatter than you want to be, you'll have to change *something*. There's no scientific evidence that exercise alone will create enough of a calorie deficit to produce substantial weight loss. Exercise can certainly create a calorie deficit in isolation, but our bodies will typically find a way to compensate for that, as I explained earlier.

There are outliers, of course. They show up in almost every study, including the one I described. Every trainer has worked with them. They exist at both extremes: Some gain more muscle or lose more weight than expected, while others lose muscle when trying to gain, or gain weight while trying to lose.

The first kind of outlier makes my life a whole lot easier. They get extraordinary results, attribute them to Alwyn's programs, and convince their friends to buy our books. The truth is that the program put into motion something that was waiting to happen. The reader's preexisting propensity to gain muscle or lose weight just needed the right stimulus. Don't get me wrong: We still deserve credit for providing what they needed. I just want to make it clear that there's nothing magical going on. It's the right program applied by the right person at the right time in the right way. (Then again, given how rare it is for all this to come together, maybe it *is* magic.)

As for the other type of outlier, it's easy to say that he or she just didn't work hard enough to get the expected results, or didn't follow directions. Either or both might be true. But there's also the possibility that it wasn't the right program for that person. We'll never know.

All we can do is present the program, starting on the next page, and hope it works exactly as expected for you. If not better.

PART 2

THE PROGRAM

Every Workout Tells a Story

Alwyn and I began this book with the premise that each lifter is slightly different from every other lifter. I can't remember the last time I went to the gym with a workout that I hadn't modified in some way to accommodate my tragic inability to do every exercise in the canon, including the workouts in my own books.

That's why Alwyn came up with what he describes as a "Chinese menu" system. Instead of giving you a series of workouts with all the exercises filled in, he's putting the power to create a customized program in your hands. It's the most important and unique feature of *NROL for Life*, and we've done everything we can to make it easy for you to choose.

But before we get to the exercises, it's important to understand the system itself.

ELEMENTS OF THE PROGRAM

I'll introduce them here in the order in which you'll perform them during each workout. Each is explained in full detail in its own chapter.

1. RAMP (Chapter 15)

Each book in this series has emphasized the importance of getting your body warmed up and ready to lift. In fact, Alwyn's concept of warming up has grown to the point that he doesn't even use that term anymore. "Warming up" implies that there's a moment when your body is fully prepared for training, and there's nothing else you need to do. You're there, and you can stay there as long as you want.

RAMP—an acronym for *Range of motion, Activation of muscles*, and *Movement Preparation*—suggests something slightly but meaningfully different: You've *begun* the process of training your body. Each challenge leads to the next. There's nothing static or finite about the process. It ramps up your metabolism and your mood to ensure you're ready for challenges that will ramp them up even more.

This part of the workout will usually take about 10 minutes.

2. Core Training (Chapter 6)

We define the core as including all the muscles that attach to and help stabilize the lower back and pelvis. Starting out, you'll do two core exercises each workout, drawn from two categories: *stabilization* and *dynamic stabilization*. Each category has five levels of exercises.

3. Power Training (Chapter 7)

I've already noted that power—the ability to rapidly exert force—declines faster in middle age than strength or muscle mass. We also know from research that it's possible to reverse declines in power. That process is relatively straightforward, and Alwyn has provided five levels of power exercises to get you there.

But there's more to power development than doing a single, power-specific exercise per workout. Alwyn has incorporated exercises throughout the program that lend themselves to fast, powerful movements. You can't and shouldn't do everything fast, certainly, but throughout the following chapters I'll note places where it's appropriate for readers who're ready to push themselves. Physiological benefits aside, I think you'll find that it's just more fun to work fast once you have the green light.

4. Strength Training

Readers of the original *NROL* will recall that we reduced all exercises to six basic categories: squat, deadlift, lunge, push, pull, twist. The concept is the same in *NROL for Life*, but Alwyn has changed some of the terms to better describe the way he designs programs. Each of these categories has five levels of exercises.

- **Squat (Chapter 8)**. These are exercises in which you bend at the knees and hips, usually with your feet shoulder-width apart and parallel to each other. They work all your lower-body muscles.
- **Hinge (Chapter 9)**. These are deadlift-type exercises in which you bend forward at the hips and then return to a standing position. The muscles on the back of your body, mainly your glutes and hamstrings, do most of the work.
- **Lunge (Chapter 10)**. You perform these exercises with your feet split apart and your torso upright. They activate most of your lower-body muscles.
- **Single-Leg Stance (Chapter 11)**. These exercises are variations on the previous three movement patterns—squat, hinge, and lunge. But because you're doing them with one foot off the floor, they're different enough to merit their own designation. They're crucial for improving balance, coordination, and joint stability.
- **Push (Chapter 12)**. The push-up is the most obvious and important exercise in this category, which also includes bench and shoulder presses. Your chest, shoulders, and triceps are the prime movers.
- **Pull (Chapter 13)**. These are the opposite of push exercises. They work the muscles on the back of your shoulders and torso, primarily the trapezius and lats, with assistance from your biceps. The category includes rows, chin-ups, and pulldowns.
- **Combination (Chapter 14)**. Some of the best exercises, and coincidentally the most challenging, involve two movement patterns: a squat with a press, for example.

Every workout includes a pull, a push, and either a lunge or single-leg-stance exercise. You'll do hinges and squats every other workout. Combination exercises first appear in Phase Two and then feature prominently in Phase Three. (I'll explain the three phases of the program in the next section of this chapter.)

5. Metabolic Training (Chapter 16)

The exercises in these drills are pretty simple; you might do gym-class staples like push-ups and squats in one workout, or a newer but easy-to-learn exercise like kettlebell swings. You want them to be simple because your body is too exhausted to do anything requiring a high attention to form. But don't confuse "easy to learn" with "easy." The goal is to work hard and make your body even more exhausted in these 5 to 10 minutes.

I should stop here and note that the categories I've just described, for all their distinctive qualities, have just as much in common. From RAMP to metabolic training, they all work to increase your overall conditioning level along with strength, power, stability, coordination, mobility, athleticism, and efficacy. Each thing makes you better at lots of things.

Metabolic training has all the aforementioned crossover qualities. You could even argue that it's redundant, since you might end up repeating exercises you've already done in that very workout.

The big difference: You're doing the exercises in a deeper state of fatigue. Ten push-ups or squats in the 45th minute of a workout are exponentially harder than 10 push-ups or squats in the 25th minute. Your heart is pounding, it's hard to catch your breath, and your metabolism is at its limit. It's going to be elevated for many hours after you leave the gym, which is exactly what you want from one of Alwyn's workouts. Of course you want to burn a lot of calories while you're training, but you also want that accelerated metabolism while your body recovers.

6. Recovery (Chapter 18)

No workout is complete until you've started preparing your muscles for the next workout. As you'll see, the recovery process includes stretches and foam rolling. This chapter also offers a look at post-workout nutrition, the most important aspect of recovery.

THE PHASES

Alwyn's program has three phases, each of which should last four weeks on average for most readers.

Phase One: Transform

Experienced lifters will look at the workout charts in Chapter 17 and ask themselves, "Is that *it*?" It looks easy on paper. But if it's easy to perform, you're doing it wrong. You're either using the wrong exercises for your level, or too little weight, or both. Conversely, many of you will choose exercises and weights that are too challenging for this phase, and end up with more soreness than you've had since the last time you underestimated one of Alwyn's workouts.

The goal of the phase is in the title: During the first four weeks of the program, you're going to train your body to do things it has forgotten how to do, never learned to do, or can only kinda-sorta do. You'll improve your fitness in almost every area. RAMP will boost your mobility. The core training will improve the strength, stability, and endurance of your mid-body muscles. The power exercises will teach your muscles to work fast, improving your rate of force development. The four resistance-training exercises in each workout will build strength and muscle size in those of you who're new to this, and improve muscle endurance and tissue quality in veteran lifters. Metabolic training will give everyone a fat-burning stimulus. Recovery will be whatever you make it. For those who've never used a foam roller to smooth out the knots and adhesions in muscles, it can be a workout all by itself. All of it combines to improve your total-body conditioning and athleticism.

Phase Two: Develop

By now you're familiar with the exercises and system, and it's time to push yourself. If you're relatively new to lifting, that'll happen with heavier weights and more challenging exercises. Weight-room vets will advance with heavier weights and higher volume: up to four sets of 10 reps of each resistance exercise. Everyone will strive to increase some aspect of performance each workout.

Phase Three: Maximize

The big change in this final phase is that you'll do five resistance exercises each workout, instead of four. The added move is a combination exercise, which requires a higher level of effort and will induce a deeper level of exhaustion. No matter how well you prepare for it, you'll still notice a difference.

THE WORKOUTS

Each phase has two total-body workouts, labeled Workout A and Workout B. You'll alternate between these workouts until you finish the phase. You will never, ever do both workouts on the same day, and if you're even slightly tempted to do A and B on consecutive days, it means you aren't working hard enough to get the results you want. You should need, and your body should *demand*, at least one day of recovery between workouts.

Three workouts each week is ideal for most readers, although it may be too much for you if you're especially challenged—coming back from an injury or a long layoff, for example. Two workouts a week is still a decent volume of exercise if you're starting from zero. One is too few to see results, no matter your present condition, and four of Alwyn's workouts are too much for anyone. If you have that much time and energy, there are better ways to use it (see Chapter 22).

Here's what a month of training will look like if you follow the classic Monday-Wednesday-Friday workout schedule:

	Monday	Tuesday	Wednesday	Thursday	Friday	Saturday	Sunday
Week 1	Workout A	off	Workout B	off	Workout A	off	off
Week 2	Workout B	off	Workout A	off	Workout B	off	off
Week 3	Workout A	off	Workout B	off	Workout A	off	off
Week 4	Workout B	off	Workout A	off	Workout B	off	off

Most readers should do workouts A and B six times each, which, as you can see in the chart, will take four weeks on a typical schedule. Some exceptions:

- If you train twice a week, you'll need six weeks for each phase.
- If you're an absolute beginner, coming off a long layoff, or returning from a serious injury, you may want to do A and B eight times each. This is tricky, though; I tend to get bored with any workout after three weeks, and I usually make my best gains in the first and second weeks. Then again, I started lifting before some of you were born. You know it's time to move on when you stop making gains. You should see an improvement in *something* from one workout to the next—each week, each phase—throughout the program. (At first you'll see improvements in everything, which is fun while it lasts.)
- If you're an NROL veteran, and you've done the entire program in at least one of our books, you may want to do each workout in Phase One four times, instead of six. You'll know you're ready to move on if the fourth time through workouts A and B feels exactly like the third time. At that point, there's nothing more to gain from Phase One, and it's time for Phase Two. The same guideline applies to Phase Two and Phase Three, but I doubt if many of us will adapt to those workouts so quickly.

Now that you understand the program's goals and parameters, it's time for what might be the most important step: selecting exercises.

HOW TO CHOOSE THE BEST EXERCISES FOR YOU

Here's how Alwyn explained the Chinese-menu system to me: "You pick something from every column—a soup, a meat, two vegetables, a sauce, and rice or noodles." The most important rule, Alwyn says, is to make sure you pick just one from each column. "You can't mix beef and shrimp, or two sauces. You'll come up with something nasty."

The key to a tasty workout—or at least one that gives you all the benefits of a good training program without any of the sour aftertaste of one that exacerbates your weaknesses and limitations—is to select the best exercises for you in each phase of the program.

1. Stay true to the category.

As you know, the strength workouts include six categories of exercises: squat, hinge, lunge, single-leg stance, push, pull. There's also a seventh category, "combination," which blends two distinct movements into one exercise.

You have two categories for core training—stability and dynamic stability—and two more for power exercises—upper-body and lower-body.

Alwyn gives you five levels of exercises in each category, arranged according to the difficulty of the technique and the amount of training experience it requires. You'll often have variations on those choices to modify the difficulty in either direction, or to accommodate different equipment preferences. The next few chapters will show all your options in each category.

You can also bypass the decision-making process altogether by following the done-for-you sample workouts in Chapter 17. If you choose to choose, make sure you select each exercise from the proper category.

But how do you know which exercise is best for you?

2. In Phase One, pick the easiest exercises you can do with full intensity but without discomfort.

Most categories give you simple self-tests to help you figure out the right level. But the tests aren't definitive. You still need to make choices. Let's use the squat category as an example. Here are the five levels:

Level 1: Body-weight squat

Level 2: Goblet squat (holding a weight against your chest with both hands)

Level 3: Front squat (supporting a barbell or dumbbells on your front shoulders)

Level 4: Back squat (supporting a barbell behind your shoulders)

Level 5: Overhead squat (holding a barbell at arm's length overhead)

Chapter 8 begins with a self-test to see if you can skip past Level 1. If you're a strong, experienced lifter with no injuries to hold you back, Level 2 might also be a nonstarter. You'd have to hold a pretty heavy weight in front of your chest to work your lower-body muscles to exhaustion; when you're doing 15 reps, your arms and shoulders would give out before the bigger, stronger muscles in your hips and thighs. Levels 3, 4, and 5 present no such problem. Any lifter can build a serious workout with the front, back, or overhead squat.

But what if you can do the workouts as written with *any* of the exercises, including the overhead squat, one of the most challenging in any category? You might want to start with the front squat in Phase One, move up to the back squat in Phase Two, and save the overhead squat for Phase Three. If you're that good a lifter, you can certainly trust your own judgment and instincts.

Conversely, if you've never done any of these exercises and feel like you've stumbled into a foreign movie without subtitles, don't worry. The next few chapters will explain and illustrate all of them.

3. In Phase Two, pick the exercises that allow you to work with the heaviest weight for multiple sets.

It may not be the most difficult exercise in the menu. You might even go back a level in some categories. The goal is to use an exercise that's easy to load without discomfort.

4. In Phase Three, pick the exercises that kick your ass.

I don't think this needs explanation.

5. Don't feel pressure to get through all the levels.

A pure beginner, or someone who's never used free weights, will do well to get to Level 3 on everything by the end of Phase Three. You might not even get to Level 3 across the board. No problem. Simply repeat the program, using higher-level exercises.

If you're more advanced, I'll explain in Chapters 17 and 22 how to repeat the program, using the same exercises with higher intensities for strength and size development.

Chapters 8 through 16 show you all the exercise choices. Chapter 17 explains Alwyn's system, with step-by-step guidance on how to create your own custom workouts. By the end you'll have two full programs, one each for beginners and advanced lifters. (The latter is my own program, which I put together with Alwyn's guidance.) If either looks like it fits your needs and abilities, you can simply take it to the weight room and get started.

Finally, Chapter 18 shows you a sample set of exercises for recovery. I put them last because they need so little explanation. You just do what's on the page.

STUFF YOU NEED, AND STUFF YOU'LL PROBABLY WANT

With each book, a few readers will drop down from the cyberclouds and ask if it's possible to do the workouts without any equipment. There's always an excuse that makes sense to them: They can't afford it, they don't have room, they can't find a barbell to match the drapes. So let this be our final word: You have two choices. Either buy equipment for your home, or join a gym that has everything you need. You can't do a resistance-training program without some form of external resistance.

Some of the exercises require nothing more than your body weight (a formidable challenge on chin-ups and many of the core exercises), but you won't find bodyweight exercises in every category. And even when you do, those exercises may be too easy or too advanced. *That's why you need equipment.*

And *please* don't e-mail requests to revise the program because the gym you belong to doesn't have standard gear like barbells or dumbbells heavier than a five-year-old. Alwyn has provided the most flexible strength-training program in the history of publishing, and I've done the best I can to explain how to modify it for your own needs, limitations, or equipment options. But if your gym doesn't have basic training tools, you have to find another gym, or buy your own equipment for home workouts.

Let's start with what you need:

1. Dumbbells

For home exercise you can buy a range of dumbbells, or a single set of adjustable weights. Either works just fine. If you're buying individual dumbbells for the first time, shop for price. We're just talking about hunks of inert iron; fancier stuff is nice but completely unnecessary. Keep in mind that as you get stronger you'll need bigger dumbbells. Make sure you set up your workout space with room to add more. If you're getting adjustable dumbbells, I've always liked the original PowerBlocks (powerblock.com). They're pricey—over $400 for a set that goes up to 50 pounds per block, when you add shipping—but easy to use and convenient.

2. Barbell and weight plates

Weight plates, by themselves, can be a handy form of resistance for some of the exercises. Weight plates secured to a barbell are your only option for some, particularly the deadlifts. We recommend an Olympic barbell set, with a 45-pound bar. It's certainly the best choice for male readers. You'll never outgrow it, and you'll never wear it out. You can pass it on to your grandchildren. A woman working out at home might want to consider a 35-pound Olympic bar, which is shorter as well as lighter. The only drawback is that you'll probably have to buy the bar and weights separately, instead of getting a discounted set.

You can also consider a 10-pound standard barbell. It's narrower, making it easier to grip for women with small hands. I don't recommend it for most lifters; it's less versatile than the Olympic bar. Then again, I started out with a standard barbell set when I was thirteen, so I can't really knock it.

As with dumbbells, you can shop for price. Iron is iron, whether it's new or used. Start with yard sales and Craigslist. If you buy online, check out performbetter.com or fitnessfactory.com. Get on their mailing lists and, if possible, wait for a sale that includes free shipping.

3. Squat rack with chin-up bar

The chin-up is a somewhat advanced exercise for middle-aged men and for women of any age, and not even an option for those who're overweight or recovering from shoulder or back injuries. But the bar is crucial. By design it's strong enough to support several times your weight, which makes it the perfect attachment point for elastic bands or a suspension system like the TRX, both of which are described below.

A good squat rack also has adjustable supports for the Olympic bar. They obviously allow you to perform barbell squats. Less obviously, you can set the supports closer to the floor for the deadlift variations shown in Chapter 9. And even less obviously, you can set the bar in an optimal position for push-up variations.

4. Cable machine, elastic bands, or resistance tubing

If you have access to a cable machine, you don't need bands or tubing. (Bands and tubing are the same thing, functionally, but tubing comes with handles, which make it easier to use and more comparable to cable exercises.) But you have to have one or the other. It's nearly impossible to do the program without this type of resistance.

5. Bench, box, and/or steps

You don't *need* a traditional weight-lifting bench, but it helps. Aside from the obvious bench presses, a good bench gives you a platform for elevating your hands or feet on a variety of exercises. (If you're going to get a bench, you may as well make it adjustable so you can do incline presses and chest-supported rows.) A perfect workout room gives you a variety of boxes and steps, from 6 to 24 inches high. Most of the boxes you see in our photos are industrial-quality, designed for big athletes to perform jumping and landing exercises. They're also expensive. (If you're curious, you can find them at performbetter.com.) A home lifter can get just about the same benefits from a set of adjustable aerobics steps. I've used the ones at my gym for years and never worried about my safety.

6. Mats or a padded floor

You don't want to try some of Alwyn's core and power exercises on a concrete or wood floor. If you don't have a carpeted or padded surface, find something that will protect your elbows on core exercises and your hands on explosive push-ups. You'll also want to find a forgiving landing spot for the jumping exercises in Chapter 7.

7. A clock or timer

The core-stabilization exercises in Chapter 6 call for timed sets, as do the metabolic-training drills in Chapter 17. That means you'll need either a timer or a workout space that allows you to see the second hand on a wall clock. I used to use a timer called the Gymboss (gymboss.com). When it gave out a couple years ago, I switched to the free Gymboss app for my iPhone. Another great app is the iWorkout Muse Pro (workoutmuse.com).

Here's some stuff you might want:

8. Swiss ball

You can find one at any sporting-goods store or big-box retailer, and it comes in handy for core exercises and push-up variations.

9. Suspension trainer

These are straps with handles that hang from a doorway, chin-up bar, or ceiling attachment and allow you to do body-weight exercises with your hands or feet suspended above the floor. You don't need one for this program, but it's good to have. Alwyn uses the TRX, the best-known system. It's also the one you see in our photos. The TRX is expensive, at $190 for a package that includes a DVD and instruction booklet. You can do all the same things with a Jungle Gym XT at half the price. There are other options with their own advantages and drawbacks, and by the time you read this there may be new choices that are even better.

10. Kettlebells

I was surprised to see kettlebells in Walmart in early 2011. I knew they were increasingly popular, but I didn't know they were ubiquitous. Maybe next they'll be in the checkout line of my grocery store, next to the Tic Tacs and gossip mags. Serious kettlebell enthusiasts will tell you that there are big differences from one type to another; some have smooth handles that make them tough to grip, while others are so rough they'll tear your skin off. I'll take their word for it, and advise you to do some research before you purchase one or more for your home gym.

More important, though, is that you get the weight right. My friends tell me that women should start with a 15-pound kettlebell for swings (a terrific exercise for power and metabolic training), and go up from there. For men, the minimum starting weight is 25 to 30 pounds. There are certainly great exercises you can do with lighter weights, but they aren't in this program, and dumbbells are just fine for some of them.

11. Sliding discs

I like the $30 Valslides, which have slick plastic on the bottom and a rubber grip on top. I use them for a variety of exercises, and find they work equally well with my hands or feet controlling them. Many readers have told me that cheap furniture sliders, available online or at Home Depot and Lowe's, work just as well at a fraction of the price. I can't confirm or refute. I'm a lot more comfortable using equipment that's designed for training. Alwyn says that some gyms don't allow you to use homemade or off-label gear. And here's something I didn't know until Alwyn told me: If you're a trainer, and you use something like furniture sliders with a client, and that client gets hurt, you could be looking at a lawsuit, one you have little chance of winning.

Core Training

IF YOU'RE LOOKING FOR CRUNCHES HERE, you won't find them. Alwyn and I believe the crunch is a useless exercise the way most people perform it, with high reps and low intensity. There are certainly other ways to do it, and you can argue their merits, but in our view they present their own problems. Our biggest concern: Many of us already have postural problems from sitting all day. Why use your valuable workout time on an exercise that, at best, does nothing to improve your posture, and at worst may exacerbate an existing problem?

The goal of core training is to increase the endurance, stability, and strength of the muscles that are responsible for keeping your lower back safe and coordinating upper- and lower-body movements. We don't like to make extravagant claims for what core training gives you in isolation. It does something—particularly for those recovering from back injuries—but it's hard to measure. We're a lot more comfortable saying that when you combine core training with all the other elements of Alwyn's training programs, you end up with a body that looks better, feels better, and does better. The synergistic effects are far more important than whatever you get out of the individual components.

There's almost certainly a point of diminishing returns with core training. I can't tell you where it is, but when I see someone in my gym doing core exercises for a half hour or more, I have to think he's well past that point. Five to ten minutes per workout should be plenty.

THE PROGRAM

Alwyn divides the core exercises into two categories: stabilization and dynamic stabilization. For stabilization, you'll get into a position and hold it for a timed set (up to 30 seconds, although you can go longer, as I'll explain). Dynamic stabilization involves getting into a position and holding it while doing repetitions of a movement with one or more limbs. The challenge is to keep the original, stable position while your center of gravity changes. For these exercises, you'll count reps the traditional way, rather than holding them for a predetermined amount of time.

Both categories have five levels, but the way you advance through the levels is slightly different. Advanced lifters (especially *NROL for Abs* veterans) may move quickly through the stabilization levels. If you can hold the position for maximum time, there's no reason to do it more than once. You'll spend more time at each level for dynamic stabilization. Alwyn chose exercises that allow you to increase weights and/or reps from one workout to the next.

Next, we'll look at how you'll advance through the exercise levels, then move on to the exercises themselves.

Stabilization

Start the program with the Level 1 stabilization exercises. That is, in Workout A do a basic plank, and in Workout B do a basic side plank. If you hit or exceed the time limit for both sets of both exercises, move up to Level 2 the next time you do workouts A and B. If you again hit or surpass the time limits for both exercises, then do the Level 3 stabilization exercises the third time you do A and B. Thus, if you do each workout six times, and you advance through a level each workout, you'll hit all five levels, and only in your final two workouts will you repeat a level.

I realize that what I just wrote is confusing. So let's look at this in chart form, assuming you do three workouts a week and follow a traditional Monday-Wednesday-Friday schedule:

	Monday	**Tuesday**	**Wednesday**	**Thursday**	**Friday**	**Saturday**	**Sunday**
Week 1	Workout A: Level 1 (basic plank)	off	Workout B: Level 1 (side plank)	off	Workout A: Level 2	off	off
Week 2	Workout B: Level 2	off	Workout A: Level 3	off	Workout B: Level 3	off	off
Week 3	Workout A: Level 4	off	Workout B: Level 4	off	Workout A: Level 5	off	off
Week 4	Workout B: Level 5	off	Workout A: Level 5	off	Workout B: Level 5	off	off

Realistically, I don't know if any readers need to move that fast through the levels. By the time you get to Level 4, you have enough options to keep you busy for multiple workouts. Even advanced lifters may want to save Level 5 for your second time through the program.

Final point: You may not advance through the plank and side-plank levels at the same speed. You may get to Level 5 on planks while you're still doing the Level 3 side planks.

Dynamic stabilization

With these exercises, which involve movement rather than getting into one position and holding it, you can advance within each level by increasing weights on some exercises, and increasing reps on others. The body-weight exercises make it easy to know when it's time to move up to the next level. When you hit the maximum reps, you move up. But when you're doing one of the cable exercises, and you can increase the weight from one workout to the next and still hit all the reps, it's harder to know when to move up. Here's your guideline: When you can't use a heavier weight with perfect form—that is, when you have to twist your shoulders or shift your weight to do the exercise—it's time for the next level.

This assumes that you've mastered the form and maxed out the reps on each set. If you haven't, keep working at the same level for the duration of that phase of the program. (When you advance from Phase One to Phase Two, or from Two to Three, you probably want to start with all-new exercises. If nothing else, you'll have more fun with something new to try.)

And keep in mind . . .

All training is core training. When you do the exercises in Alwyn's program with perfect form, you're working your core along with the specific muscles the exercise targets. The combination exercises, shown in Chapter 14, are the best illustration of this. You can't do them at all without stabilizing the muscles in your hips and abdomen.

STABILIZATION LEVEL 1

✳ Plank

- Get into plank position, which is also called a modified push-up position: You're facedown, with your weight resting on your forearms and toes, forearms aligned with your torso, elbows directly beneath your shoulders, and your body in a straight line from neck to ankles.
- Hold that position for at least 30 seconds, and as much as 60 seconds.

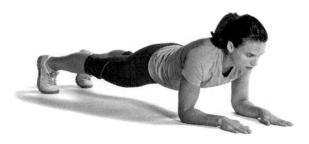

DIAL IT BACK

✳ Torso-elevated plank

If you can't hold the basic plank for 30 seconds, or at least get close, rest your forearms on a padded bench or step. The rest of the exercise is the same. Elevating your upper torso makes the exercise easier, allowing you to build strength and endurance until you're ready for the traditional version.

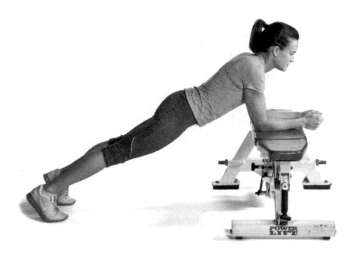

✳ Side plank

- Lie on your left side with your legs straight and your right leg on top of your left. Position yourself so your weight rests on your left forearm and the outside edge of your left foot. Your left elbow should be directly beneath your shoulder, with your upper arm perpendicular to the floor.
- Lift your hips until your body is in a straight line from neck to ankles. You want your shoulders square and on a plane that's perpendicular to the floor, as if your back was supported by a wall.
- You can place your right hand on your right hip or left shoulder.
- Hold that position for at least 30 seconds, and up to 45 seconds, then switch sides and repeat.

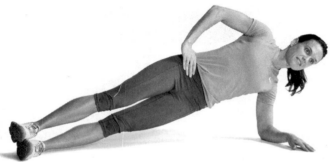

DIAL IT BACK

✳ Modified side plank

If you can't hold the side plank for at least 15 seconds, try this modification: Bend your knees so your weight rests on your left forearm and the inside edge of your left knee. Align your body so it forms a straight line from neck to knees. Other than that, it's the same exercise.

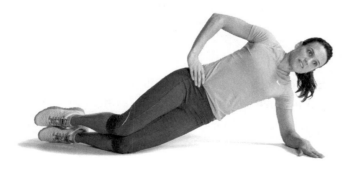

STABILIZATION LEVEL 2

✳ Plank with reduced base of support

You have three options here:

- Plank with one leg elevated
- Plank with one arm extended in front of you
- Plank with one leg elevated and the opposite-side arm extended in front of you

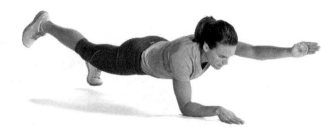

Or you can switch from a plank to the push-up position, and run through the same list of options: one leg elevated, one arm extended in front of you, or one leg elevated and the opposite arm extended.

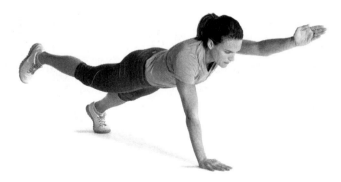

With any of these options, you want to hold one leg or arm (or both) off the ground for half the time, then switch to the opposite limb or limbs for the rest.

✳ Side plank with reduced base of support

You have two options. One is hard. The other is *really* hard.

- For the side plank with leg raise, get into side-plank position, and lift your top leg so your legs form a V shape.
- For the side plank with knee tuck, lift your bottom leg off the floor, bending your hip and knee so your bottom foot is near your top knee. Your weight will rest on your forearm and the inside edge of your top foot.

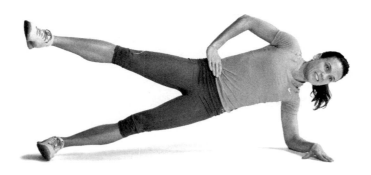

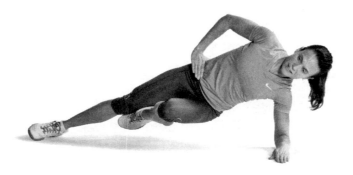

STABILIZATION LEVEL 3

✳ Feet-elevated plank

Same exercise, only with your toes resting on a bench or step. You can also do this from a push-up position.

✳ Feet-elevated side plank

Again, same exercise, only with your feet elevated on a bench or step. As with Level 2, this side-plank variation is much harder than the matching plank variation.

STABILIZATION LEVEL 4

✳ Feet-elevated plank with reduced base of support

Options include:

- Elevated plank with one leg raised
- Elevated plank with one arm extended in front
- Elevated plank with one leg elevated and the opposite arm extended
- The same three options in the push-up position: one leg elevated, one arm extended in front of you, or one leg elevated and the opposite arm extended

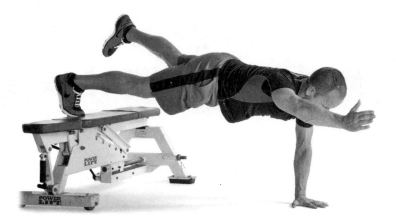

✳ Feet-elevated side plank with reduced base of support

You have the same two options for reducing your base of support: lift your top leg (which is hard) or lift and tuck your bottom leg (which is *extremely* hard).

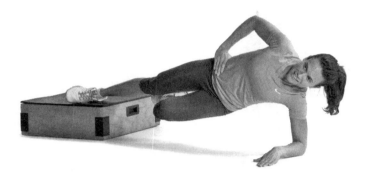

STABILIZATION LEVEL 5

✳ Feet-elevated plank with unstable point of contact

You can rest your toes on a Swiss ball, or put your feet into a TRX or comparable suspension system. With the Swiss ball, you probably want to use the push-up position instead of the plank, although either position works fine with your feet suspended. You can also get creative and elevate your feet on a stable surface, like a bench, and put your forearms or hands on something unstable, like a Swiss ball or medicine ball.

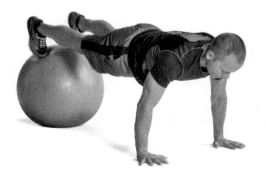
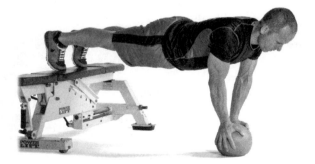

✳ Feet-elevated side plank with unstable point of contact

Same idea: Get into the side-plank position with your feet on a medicine ball, or suspended.

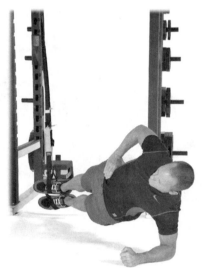

STABILIZATION BEYOND LEVEL 5

✳ Feet-elevated plank with reduced base of support and unstable point of contact

Clunky name, great exercise options. You can use any variation described so far, and reduce your base of support by lifting a leg, an arm, or an arm and a leg. You can put your hands or feet on the unstable object.

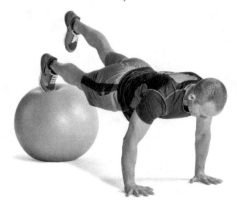

✳ Elevated side plank with reduced base of support and unstable point of contact

Same two options: Elevate your feet on a Swiss ball or with a suspension system, and either lift the top leg or lift and tuck the bottom leg.

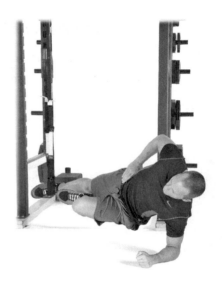

DYNAMIC STABILIZATION LEVEL 1

✳ Plank and pulldown

- Attach a D-shaped handle to the low cable pulley.
- Set up in the plank position facing the cable machine.
- Grab the handle with your nondominant hand, using a neutral grip (your palm facing in, neither underhand nor overhand). You want tension in the cable when your arm is fully extended in front of you, which will probably require some maneuvering to get the right distance from the machine.
- Pull the handle until it's just below your shoulder, keeping the rest of your body in the plank position, with everything from chest to ankles on a plane parallel to the floor.
- Do all your reps, then switch sides and repeat.

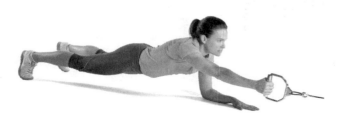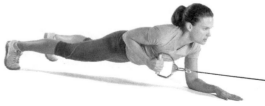

✳ Side plank and row

- Attach a D-shaped handle to the low cable pulley.
- Get into side-plank position facing the cable machine, supporting your weight on your dominant side.
- Grab the handle with your nondominant hand, palm facing down, and adjust your position so your arm is fully extended toward the machine with tension on the cable.
- Pull the handle to your rib cage, keeping your body aligned on a plane perpendicular to the floor.
- Do all your reps, switch sides, and repeat.

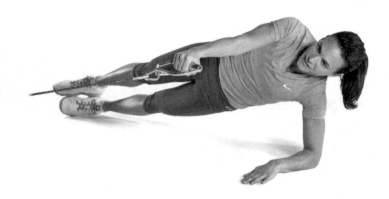

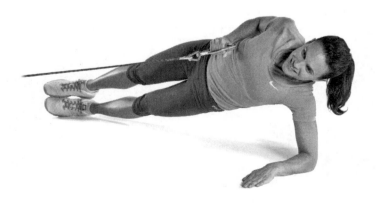

DYNAMIC STABILIZATION LEVEL 2

✳ Push-away

- Grab a pair of Valslides, furniture sliders, or anything else that will slip across your floor with minimal friction while supporting your weight. (Towels should work on a wood or tile floor, while plastic works best on a carpet.)
- Get into push-up position with one slide in each hand.
- Slide your nondominant arm as far forward as you can, keeping your arm straight and your core in a stable, neutral position. If you feel anything move in your lower back, shorten your range of motion.
- Pull it back, then slide the dominant arm forward.
- Alternate until you finish the set. If the workout calls for 10 reps, do that many with each arm.

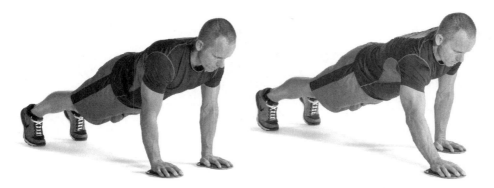

✳ Side plank and row with reduced base of support

- Get into position for the side plank and row, as described earlier, and lift your top leg.
- Do all your reps (following the previous instructions), switch sides, and repeat.

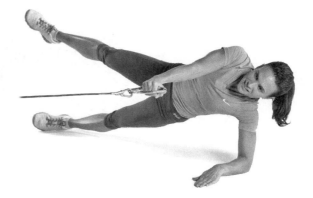

DYNAMIC STABILIZATION LEVEL 3

Starting with this level, Alwyn switches things up. Instead of exercise pairs, with one based on the plank and the second based on the side plank, you have multiple variations on the same basic movement, and multiple ways to use them. Let's say you're in Phase Two, and you're doing a dynamic stabilization exercise in Workout B. You can try the Level 3 variations one at a time, and then decide which, if any, you want to repeat. Or you can pick one and work on it each time you do Workout B until you max out. Then you can try another Level 3 variation (which we recommend) or move up to Level 4.

But let's say you're in Phase One or Phase Three, and you need to do a dynamic stabilization exercise in both workouts, A and B. You should do one of these from Level 3 in your A workout and a Level 4 exercise in your B workout. These Level 3 exercises challenge your core by moving your legs while your upper torso remains stationary. In Level 4, you stabilize your lower body while moving your arms and shoulders. Thus, the two levels work in a complementary way within the same phase.

✴ Spiderman plank

- Get into plank position.
- Lift your left knee toward your left elbow, keeping everything else in the same position.
- Return to the plank, then lift your right knee toward your right elbow.
- Alternate until you do all the reps to each side.

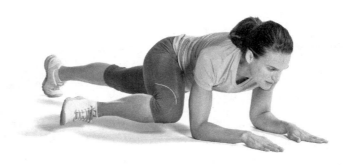

✳ Swiss-ball mountain climber

- Place your hands on a Swiss ball, roughly shoulder-width apart.
- Set up as you would for a push-up hold, with your body forming a straight line from neck to ankles.
- Raise your nondominant leg off the floor and bring your knee up toward your chest.
- Lower it, then repeat with your dominant leg.
- Continue alternating until you do all your reps with both legs.
- Once you can hit all your reps, work at increasing your speed. You'll be surprised at how challenging it is to maintain good form at a faster tempo.

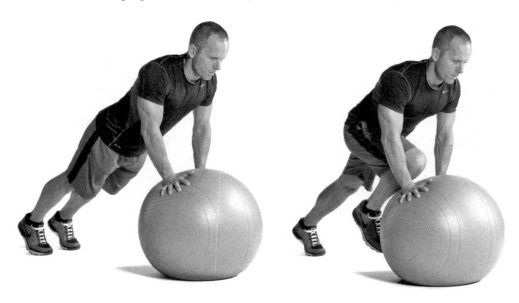

✳ Mountain climber with slides

- Get a pair of Valslides (or anything else that slides on your workout floor, as described on page 63 for the push-away), and set them on the floor next to your feet.
- Bend forward at the hips and place your palms on the floor.
- Place your feet on the slides, and push your legs back until you're close to the push-up position, with a slight hinge in your hips.
- Slide your nondominant leg toward your chest, bending your knee.

- Slide back, then slide your dominant leg forward.
- Continue alternating until you do all your reps with both legs.
- You can also elevate your hands on a bench or step.

This version of the exercise gets easy in a hurry, so you'll want to make a couple of modifications after the first or second workout:

- You can increase the reps, up to 20 per leg on each set.
- You can place your hands on an unstable surface, like a medicine ball or Swiss ball.
- You can do all that and also move your legs really fast, which is more fun than you might expect. (I enjoy it, anyway.)

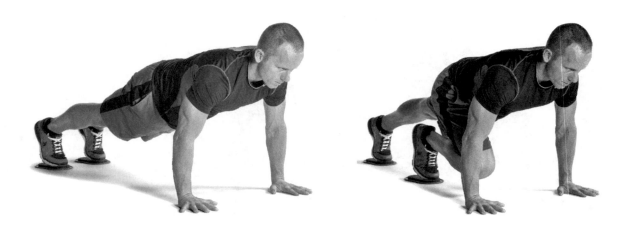

DYNAMIC STABILIZATION LEVEL 4

These two exercises are a progression, and you should work through them in order. When you master the half-kneeling chop, advance to the kneeling chop. Then you're ready for the standing exercises in Level 5.

✳ Cable half-kneeling chop

- Affix a rope handle to the high cable pulley. Pull the rope through its metal attachment ring as far as you can, giving you about 24 inches of rope to grasp.
- Grab the rope with an overhand grip, one hand at each end.
- Kneel sideways to the machine, with the knee closest to the machine up and the other one down. Your weight is resting on your inside foot and outside knee.
- Straighten your torso to make yourself as tall as possible, holding the rope between the machine and your shoulders.
- Square your shoulders and focus your eyes straight ahead.
- Pull the rope down and across your torso. The hand closest to the machine should end up in front of your outside hip. Keep your arms straight and your midsection and hips stationary, moving only your arms and shoulders.
- Do all your reps, switch sides, and repeat.

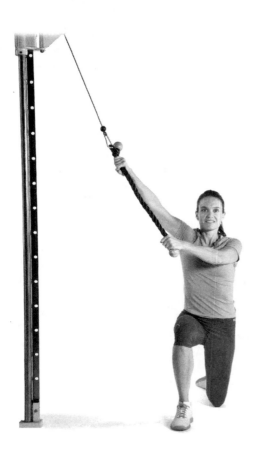
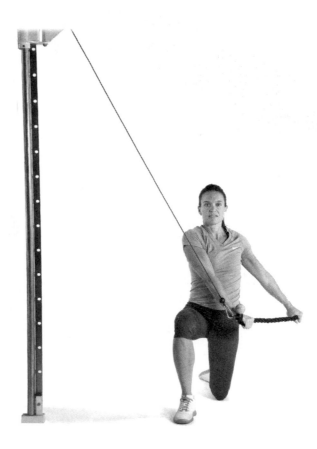

✳ Cable kneeling chop

This is the same exercise, only with both knees down and your body in a straight line from neck to knees. It's harder than you think to keep your hips and midsection in a stable position as you pull the rope down and across your torso.

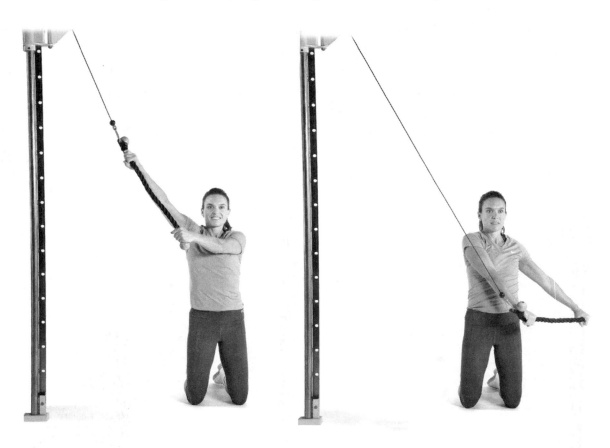

DYNAMIC STABILIZATION LEVEL 5

Again, the two exercises are a progression. Master and max out on the first before moving on to the second.

✳ Cable split-stance chop

- Affix the rope attachment to the high cable pulley, as described earlier.
- Stand sideways to the machine, holding the rope between your shoulders and the cable machine, and take a long step back with your outside leg. You want your torso upright, arms straight, and both knees bent slightly.
- Pull the rope down and across your torso until the hand closest to the machine is in front of your outside hip.
- Do all your reps, switch sides, and repeat.

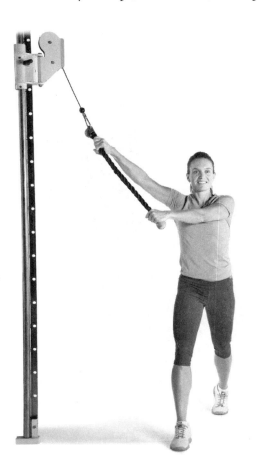
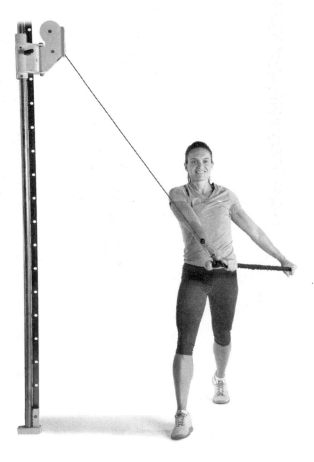

✳ Cable horizontal chop

- Attach the rope, as described earlier, and lower the pulley so it's at about waist height.
- Stand sideways to the machine with your feet parallel to each other and spread wide apart. Hold the rope between your shoulders and the machine with straight arms and your torso upright.
- Pull the rope straight across your torso until the hand closest to the machine is just past your chest and shoulders.
- Do all your reps, switch sides, and repeat.

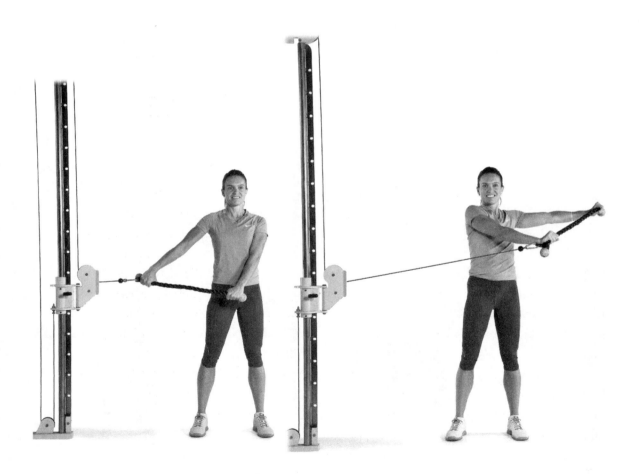

7

Power Training

At the highest levels of nerdery, power is defined as work divided by time, or the speed at which you can do some specific thing. Which, I'll admit, isn't particularly helpful in the context of a workout book. So let's start by defining something else: strength. Strength is the amount of force you can generate at a specific speed. Power, by contrast, is how fast you can generate that force. Two corollaries: The bigger the object you're trying to move, the slower you can move it; the smaller the object, the faster you can move it. Power peaks somewhere in the middle, when you're moving something that's neither tiny (like a baseball) nor huge (like your maximum weight on a deadlift).

We know this is important because, as I explained in the opening chapters, human bodies lose power with age, and lose it more precipitously than we lose strength or muscle mass. Bad things happen when we can no longer generate force quickly. We fall more, and fall harder.

True power, according to its technical definition, is something you can develop in a systematic way with the exercises in this chapter. But if we use the term loosely, a shorthand way to describe the rate of force development, that's something you can work on every day, in or out of the gym. Walk up the stairs faster. Jump over puddles instead of stepping over them. In the gym, once you're confident of your form, you can do just about any exercise faster. Not every exercise can or should be done truly *fast*, but moving faster than you do now is a good way to make any part of your workout harder, which is to say more exhausting, with a more profound conditioning effect.

Plus, all else being equal, fast lifting is just more fun than slow lifting. Work your way through the following exercises and you'll see what I mean.

THE PROGRAM

In Phase One and Phase Three, you'll do a power exercise in Workout A and B. That configuration gives you a lot of options. Ideally, if you do a lower-body power exercise in A, you should do an upper-body move in B. That's why they're paired up in levels 1 through 4: one each for lower and upper body.

In Phase Two, however, you'll do a combination exercise in A—which involves both upper- and lower-body work—and a power exercise in B, for which you want to choose a lower-body movement.

You probably won't advance through the lower- and upper-body exercises at the same pace. The exercises move on separate tracks until you get to Level 5, the dumbbell single-arm snatch, which is a total-body exercise. You're cleared to try it when you've mastered the first four levels of the lower-body power exercises. It doesn't matter if you haven't yet finished all four levels of upper-body training. You can always catch up your next time through the program.

One unique feature of power training is that it's done with low repetitions and a moderate weight, neither heavy nor light. You'll use your own body weight on some of the exercises (which, I know, may or may not be "moderate"). When using weights on the higher-level exercises, you want to start light until you learn the exercise. After that, a moderate weight is defined as about 40 to 60 percent of your one-rep max, or the most you could lift on that exercise at any speed. But that's not much help, considering that none of us has a clue what our maxes are on these exercises. So it's up to you to decide what "moderate" means, relative to what you think your max might be.

But that's part of the fun. Power performance is the undiscovered country for most lifters, young and old, beginner and advanced. Let's go there now.

LEVEL 1, LOWER BODY

✳ Box jump

- Stand in front of a box or step that you're sure won't move or collapse when you land on it.

- With your feet set shoulder-width apart, bend at the hips and knees as you swing your arms back, then swing your arms forward and jump up onto the box.

- Cushion your landing with "soft" knees—that is, land with the knees slightly bent, and let them bend a little more to absorb the impact of the landing.

- Stand up, step off the box, and repeat.

- When you can do all your reps with good form, advance to a higher box. When you run out of boxes to jump onto, move up to Level 2.

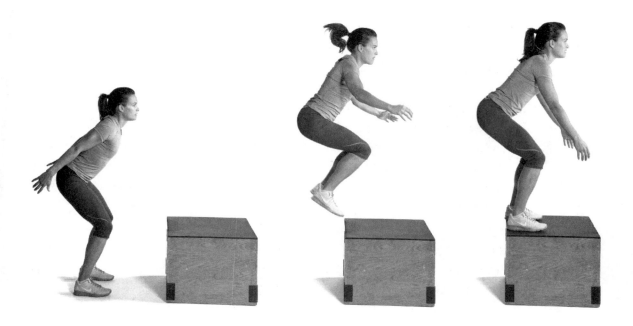

LEVEL 1, UPPER BODY

✳ Elevated explosive push-up

- Get into the elevated push-up position, with your hands higher than your feet and resting on a padded bench.
- Lower your chest toward the bench, then quickly and powerfully push yourself up so your hands come all the way off the bench.
- Catch yourself and immediately go into the next push-up.

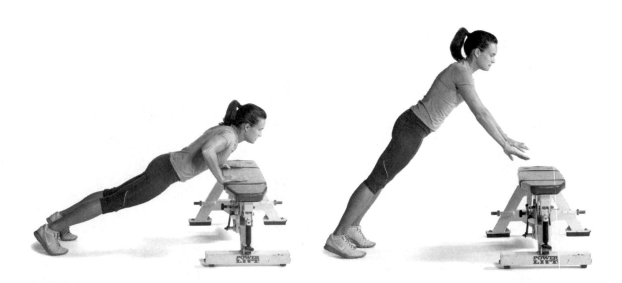

LEVEL 1, UPPER BODY OPTION

✳ Medicine-ball push pass from knees

- Hold a medicine ball with both hands against your chest and kneel a few feet in front of a solid wall, or in front of a training partner who'll catch the ball.
- Push the ball straight out from your chest with as much force as you can generate.
- Retrieve the ball and repeat.

LEVEL 2, LOWER BODY

✳ Body-weight jump squat

- Stand with your feet shoulder-width apart, hands behind your head in the prisoner grip.
- Push your hips back, allowing your knees to bend, and jump.
- Land with soft knees and immediately go into the next jump.

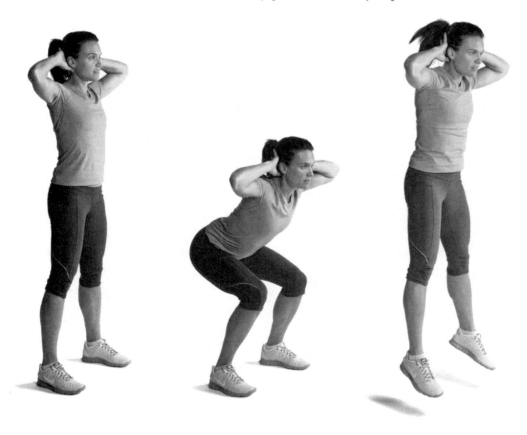

✳ Explosive push-up (first photo)

Same as the one described on page 74, only with your hands on the floor.

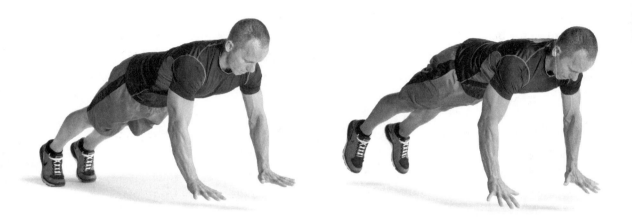

FUN ALTERNATIVE

✳ Levitating push-up (second photo)

When a friend told me about this exercise, I didn't think it was possible: you push off so hard that your hands *and feet* leave the floor. Then I tried it. It's really not much harder than a regular explosive push-up.

LEVEL 2, UPPER BODY OPTION

✳ Medicine-ball push pass

Same as the kneeling push pass, but this time you're standing, and you want to get a bit farther from your target, whether it's a wall or a training partner. Start with your feet about hip-width apart, and stride forward with one leg as you push the ball away from your chest. Alternate legs on each throw.

LEVEL 3, LOWER BODY

✳ Kettlebell swing

Here you'll take a temporary break from the jump-squat sequence and work on the swing. Take a workout or two to get used to the basic two-handed swing if you've never done it before. Once you're comfortable with the movement, you want to use a fairly heavy kettlebell, and move it explosively. For most guys, the minimum weight for a two-handed swing would be 16 kilograms/35 pounds. Women will probably need at least 12 kilograms/25 pounds. I know that sounds obscenely heavy to some readers, and I certainly don't want you to jump right into those weights if the movement still feels awkward or unnatural. But when you feel you've got it, heavier weights aren't much harder to move. You're using your body's biggest, strongest muscles. Your arms and upper-torso muscles are just along for the ride.

- Grab a kettlebell and hold it with both hands in front of your torso, with your arms straight.
- Set your feet wider than shoulder width, your toes pointed straight ahead or angled out slightly.
- Push your hips back, lowering your torso toward the floor as the kettlebell swings back. Your forearms should touch your inner thighs on the backswing, and your knees should bend slightly.

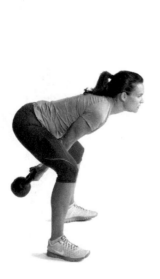
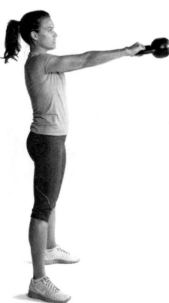

- Snap your hips forward as you come back up, propelling the kettlebell up and out in front of your torso. Don't raise it with your shoulders; the height of its trajectory should be determined by the power of your hip thrust.
- Let the kettlebell swing back between your legs as you push your hips back for the next repetition.
- If you don't have a heavy enough kettlebell for the two-arm swing, you can do one-arm swings. The technique is the same. Do the recommended reps with each arm.
- You can also swing two kettlebells at once, a variation called the power swing.

LEVEL 3, UPPER BODY

✳ Dumbbell push press

- Grab a pair of dumbbells and stand holding them at the sides of your shoulders. You can turn your palms in or out, whichever feels more natural.
- Stand with your feet shoulder-width apart, toes pointed forward, knees unlocked.
- Push your hips back slightly, as if you were about to jump.
- Snap your hips forward and use that momentum to push the weights up off your shoulders.
- Lower the weights and go right into the next repetition.

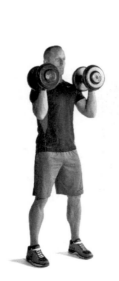 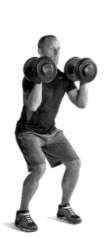 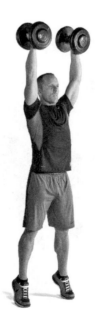

LEVEL 4, LOWER BODY

✳ Dumbbell jump squat

- Grab a pair of dumbbells and hold them outside your legs. Set your feet shoulder-width apart.
- Push your hips back and bend your knees.
- Jump as high as you can, using all three lower-body joints—hips, knees, ankles—to power the movement.
- Land softly on the balls of your feet (not flat-footed!), bending your knees and hips to start the next rep.
- You can also use a barbell, holding it across the back of your shoulders. It's probably a more effective power exercise, but I wouldn't do it that way; there's so much that can go wrong with a higher center of gravity, starting with the fact you're doing a ballistic movement with a weighted object near the top of your spine. However, for lighter, smaller lifters, this variation may be easier.
- Whether you use dumbbells or a barbell, the key is to jump as high as you can on each rep. You should be winded after 5 or 6 reps. If it's easy, you're not doing it right.

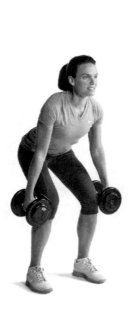
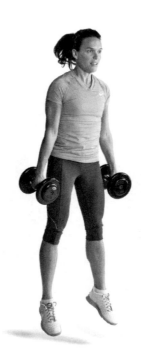

LEVEL 4, UPPER BODY

✴ Explosive push-up from boxes

- Set up two equal-size steps or boxes, each about 6 to 8 inches high, so they're just outside where your hands will be in the push-up position.
- Get into push-up position with your hands between the boxes.
- Do an explosive push-up, landing with your hands on the boxes.
- Do another explosive push-up, this time landing with your hands on the floor.

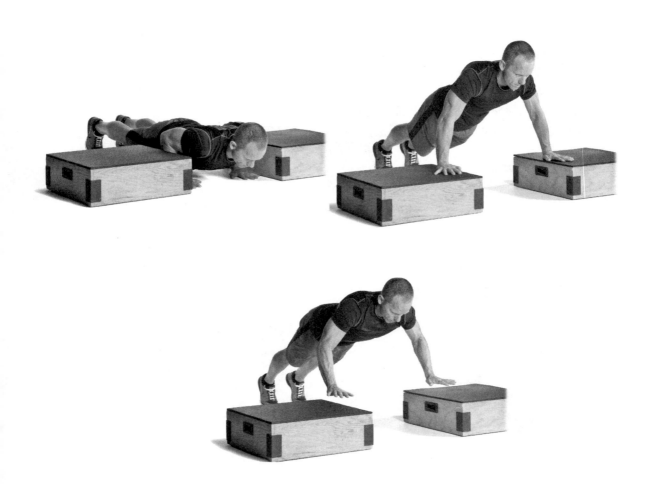

- Caution flags:
  - Make sure the floor is well padded. You don't need the impact shock of wood or concrete. (This of course applies to every ballistic push-up variation.)
  - Don't do this variation if you have current shoulder issues. It's too much risk for the minor benefit of doing a cool-looking exercise.
- For the heaviest readers, this one is a non-starter. The form will be difficult, and the damage caused by the impact could negate any potential benefit.
- You need a strong and stable core to pull this off. If you can't keep your lower back and pelvis in a neutral position on takeoff and landing, the exercise may be too risky for you.

LEVEL 5

✳ Dumbbell single-arm snatch

- Grab a dumbbell with your nondominant hand and stand with your feet shoulder-width apart, toes pointed forward.
- Push your hips back and bend your knees, with the dumbbell hanging straight down from your shoulder between your legs, palm facing behind you.
- Jump, powering the movement with your hips, knees, and ankles, and coming all the way up on your toes, or even off the floor slightly.
- Shrug your shoulder as you come up, which will pull the weight up the front of your torso. The weight will be near your chin at the top of the jump.
- As your body comes down from the jump, straighten your arm so the weight ends up overhead. Your knees and hips will be bent slightly, as they would when you land following a jump.
- Catch your balance and stand up straight to complete the repetition, then drop the weight back to the starting position and begin the next snatch.
- Do all the reps with your nondominant arm (your left if you're right-handed), then repeat the set with your other side.

Some style points:

- It should never feel like you're *lifting* the weight. I like to think of it as *throwing* the weight without letting go. If the movement is slow and you feel your arm and shoulder muscles working, focus on speeding up the movement until it feels like jumping and throwing.
- The great thing about a one-arm snatch is that you really can't do it with dangerous form unless you hit yourself (or someone else) with the weight. It takes some practice, but if you keep your focus on jumping and throwing, your body will eventually get the idea.
- When I was younger and braver, I used to do single-arm snatches using an EZ-curl bar. (It's the barbell with zigzag bends in the middle, allowing you to hold it with an angled grip, which is easier on your wrists and elbows than a straight bar.) More advanced lifters sometimes snatch an Olympic barbell with one arm. (You can go to YouTube and see guys do this with as much as 200 pounds.) I've never been that bold or ambitious, but I will tell you that this is a fun exercise to test your limits with relatively little risk.

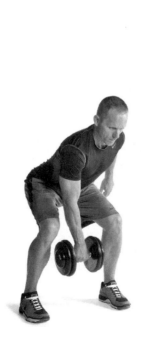
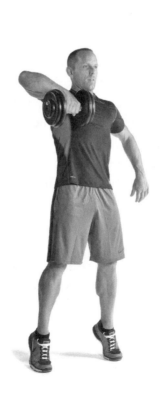
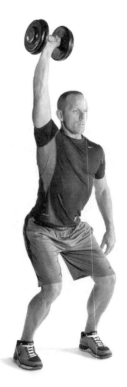

8

Squat

THERE MAY NOT BE AN EXERCISE that works more muscles in a more functional movement pattern. The squat hits all the major muscles in your hips and thighs, and the advanced variations also force your lower-back muscles to work hard. It's one of the first coordinated movements in human development—babies learn to squat before they learn to stand—and it's one that the elderly miss the most when they can no longer get up from a chair.

It's also a movement that most adults have to relearn when they begin a strength-training program. A full squat requires core stability as well as mobility in the hips and ankles. Moreover, it requires these qualities while the body is moving, which presents a coordination challenge as your body's biggest, strongest muscles shorten and lengthen. As Gray Cook notes in *Athletic Body in Balance*, if you can't squat well, you can't really do *anything* well. It's the key to fluid movement, to athleticism itself.

LEVEL 1

✳ Body-weight squat

Set down the book and get out of your chair. (Come on, you know you've been sitting too long.) Stand with your feet shoulder-width apart. Extend your arms out in front of you for balance. Push your hips back and sit back as far as you can while keeping your feet flat on your floor. Don't worry about your knees; just let them bend whenever they need to. The key is to start the movement with your hips, and descend until your upper thighs are parallel to the floor, if not lower.

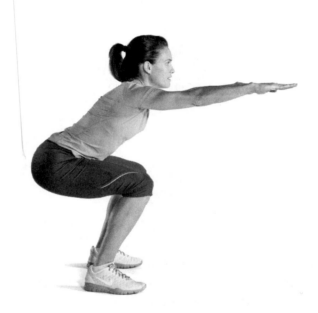

If you have a full-length mirror, look at yourself first from the side. This is what you should see:

- Your feet are flat on the floor.
- Your ankles and torso are bent forward at the same angle, more or less.
- If you weren't looking at yourself in the mirror, your eyes would be looking forward, not up or down.
- If you were to look down, you'd see that your knees are directly over your toes—not inside or outside of them.

From that position, you should be able to stand straight up. Now turn 90 degrees, squat down again, and look at yourself from the front. Check for symmetry. Are your toes either straight ahead or turned out slightly at the exact same angle? Are your knees and feet equidistant from the midline of your torso?

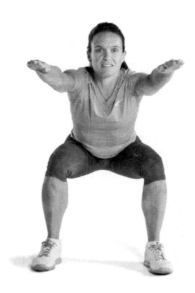

- If so, congratulations. You can squat.

Next question: Can you perform 15 of these body-weight squats with perfect form? If so, you're cleared to move ahead to Level 2.

If not, can you at least achieve good form on multiple body-weight squats? If the answer is yes, then this is the exercise you'll start with in Phase One of Alwyn's NROL for Life program. Your goal is to work your way up to two sets of 15 repetitions.

But what if you can't yet do multiple body-weight squats?

DIAL IT BACK

✳ Supported body-weight squat

Stand next to something sturdy—a pole or the edge of a solid piece of furniture work equally well. Rest one hand lightly on the support. Set the other hand on your chest or alongside your ear. Push your hips back and descend into a squat as described above, then return to the starting position, using the support as little as possible. Do as many as you can, up to 15. For your next set, switch sides and support yourself with your opposite hand.

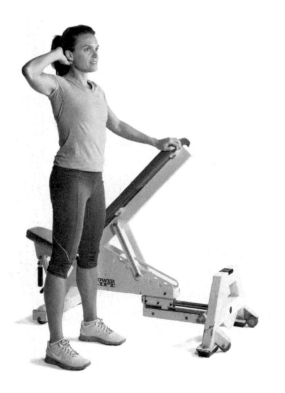
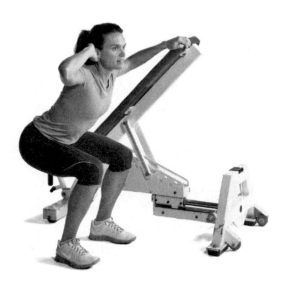

✳ Suspended body-weight squat

Attach the TRX (or any suspension-training system) to a chin-up bar or overhead support. Take a light grip on the handles and stand with your feet shoulder-width apart, leaving some slack in the straps. Push your hips back and descend into a squat, then return to the starting position. If you can do a few reps without using the straps to pull yourself up, you're ready for unsupported body-weight squats.

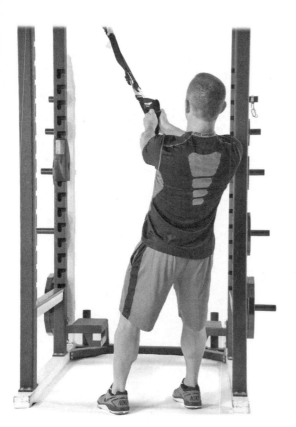
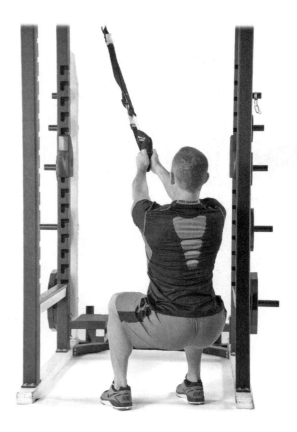

LEVEL 2

✳ Goblet squat

Traditionally, the first progression from a body-weight squat is a squat holding dumbbells at your sides. But there are two problems with the dumbbell squat: First, the weights start low to the ground, below your center of gravity, so they have to be pretty heavy to present any kind of challenge. Holding heavy weights outside your legs is awkward. Second, if you do try holding heavy dumbbells outside your legs, you might find that your grip gives out before your lower-body muscles do. Even if you can handle the weights for the required number of reps, the gripping muscles in your hands and forearms will be exhausted, leading to compromised performance in subsequent exercises.

The goblet squat is the perfect alternative. You'll get more from holding a lighter weight above your center of gravity than you will with heavier weights at arm's length.

Grab a dumbbell or weight plate and hold it with both hands against your chest, just below your chin. (It's called a goblet squat because if the weight were a cup, you could drink out of it.) Stand with your feet shoulder-width apart, push your hips back, and squat as described above. Keep your eyes focused forward and your torso as upright as possible.

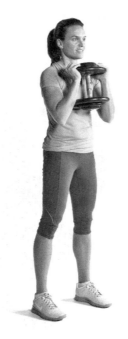
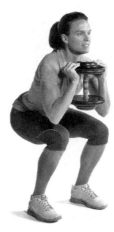

LEVEL 3

✳ Front squat

This is an easy and important progression from the goblet squat. You have to hold the weight higher, which means farther from your center of gravity. That increases the challenge to your core. (It's also an example of a *self-limiting exercise*, which I explain in the sidebar.)

- Set a barbell in the supports of a squat rack just below shoulder level. Grab the bar overhand, with your hands just outside shoulder width, and step up to the bar so it sits on your front shoulders. Lift your elbows until your upper arms are parallel to the floor and your palms are on the underside of the bar.
- Lift the bar off the supports and guide it back until it rests just above your collarbones. It will probably roll to the ends of your fingers, rather than staying on your palms. This is a safe and stable position as long as your upper arms stay parallel to the floor and your torso remains upright.
- Step back from the supports and set your feet shoulder-width apart. Your toes will probably point out slightly. (Just make sure they point out at the same angle.)
- Push your hips back and descend until your upper thighs are parallel to the floor, or even lower. Push back up to the starting position.

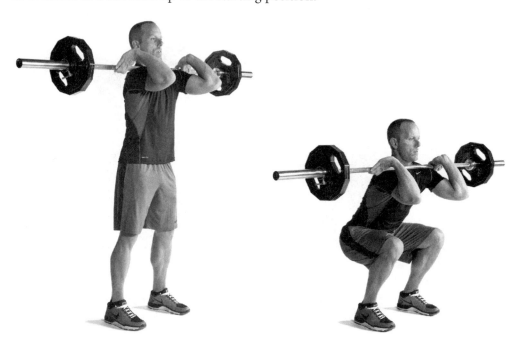

LIMITED-EQUIPMENT OPTION

✳ Dumbbell front squat

- Grab a pair of dumbbells and hold them so one end of each rests on your corresponding shoulder. Your palms should face each other, with your upper arms parallel to the floor.
- Push your hips back and squat as described.
- The only problem with this variation is the awkwardness of putting heavy dumbbells on your shoulders as you get stronger. But on the bright side, it puts the load well above your center of gravity, giving you both a core challenge and a workout for the stabilizing muscles in your hips and lower body.

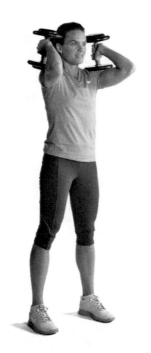 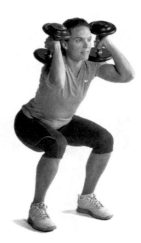

Self-Limiting Exercises

My high school weight room in the early seventies had two pieces of equipment. The first was a Universal multistation gym, the presence of which supported the crazy idea that machines were better than free weights. America was still an industrial power, and we put our faith in chrome. Plus, the Universal machine was efficient. Six or eight guys could work out in the space you'd need for a single squat rack and a bench.

The second was an ancient chin-up bar embedded in the doorway.

Strange as it sounds, I used to do pull-ups to prepare my body for lat pulldowns on the machine. At my peak I would do two sets of 15. If I'd known anything about lifting back then I would've found a way to add resistance and made those pull-ups the highlight of my workouts. It was by far the best strength- and muscle-building exercise I did, and probably accounted for most of the modest results I attributed to the Universal machine.

Pull-ups and chin-ups are perfect examples of a self-limiting exercise, a category I didn't know existed until Alwyn told me about it shortly before we started working on this book. You can't pull your chest up to the bar without using the right muscles in the right way. (Okay, you *can*, but you'd have to try pretty hard to mess it up.) Contrast them with lat pulldowns, the exercise that most people do instead. A beginner will often use a light weight and try to pull the bar down to her belly button, engaging small rotator-cuff muscles instead of the big latissimus dorsi muscles—which, after all, are the target of the exercise; it's right there in the name. A musclehead might do the old-school version of the lat pulldown, when you pull the bar down to the back of your neck. It puts your shoulder and neck joints into their most vulnerable position, and then forces them to strain against a heavy load.

The front squat is also a self-limiting exercise: not always easy to do right, but nearly impossible to do wrong. If you don't keep your torso upright and head up, you'll drop the bar. You need near-perfect form on every rep.

The hallmarks of a self-limiting exercise are the hallmarks of any good exercise. The basic movement is natural—squatting, pushing, pulling, or bending—and includes a challenge to your strength, stability, and balance. Your form and strength are co-equal partners. When you reach the limit of one or the other, you're forced to stop.

Most exercises are not self-limiting, including many in this book, or any other. Take, for example, the barbell back squat. As I said in Chapter 3, I had to concede sometime after my fiftieth birthday that I simply couldn't do it anymore. It hurt to hold the bar behind my shoulders, and my knees ached for days after doing heavy squats. But that's not to say it's a "bad" exercise, or one that none of you can or should do. It's an exercise that stopped working for me, probably because I did it long enough that I learned to lift heavy loads while injuring myself.

Common sense remains your best defense against injury in the weight room. If you're doing something that hurts while you're doing it, don't. If it leads to excessive aches and pains in the days after you do it, move on to another exercise variation, and see if the problem is the exercise or the movement pattern. If it's the latter, you need professional guidance. An experienced trainer may be able to identify flaws in your form. A physical therapist might be able to free up restricted muscles or connective tissues that affect your performance. Trainers and PTs can also tell you if you have a bigger problem that requires medical intervention.

LEVEL 4

✳ Back squat

Alwyn has changed his view of the back squat in the past few years. We used it as the default exercise for this movement pattern in earlier books, for good reason: No other squat variation allows you to use as much weight, making it ideal for both strength and size development. But as you get older, the fact that you have to support that weight on your back becomes increasingly problematic. There's a high risk to the structures of your cervical spine, which have direct pressure from the barbell. The stronger you get, the greater the load on the discs in your lower back.

All that said, if you can handle the back squat without pain—immediate or post-exercise—it's a terrific exercise for rapid strength gains and muscle growth. Here's how to do it:

- Set the barbell in the supports just below shoulder level.
- Grab the bar overhand, your hands just outside shoulder width, and duck under the bar so it rests on your upper trapezius. If you squeeze your shoulder blades together, your upper traps will form a nice little shelf for the bar.
- Lift the bar off the supports and take a step back, setting your feet shoulder-width apart (you can also go a bit wider; the best position is whatever gives you the strongest platform and feels most natural), with your toes pointing forward or angled out slightly.
- Push your hips back and descend as far as you can without your heels coming off the floor or your lower back shifting out of its neutral position.
- Return to the starting position.

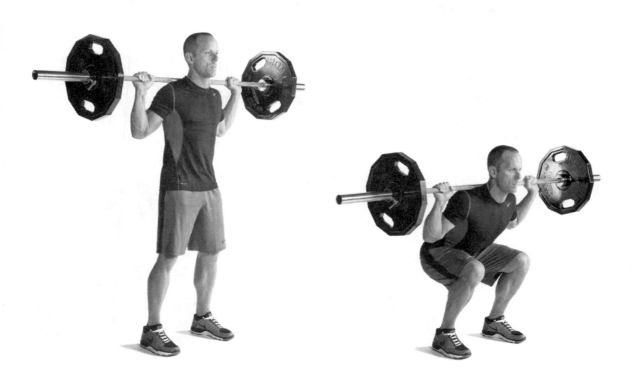

COOL OPTION FOR ADVANCED LIFTERS

✳ Hex-bar deadlift

Gyms set up for serious lifting often will have a barbell that's shaped like a hexagon in the middle. (It's also known as a trap bar, since the original design, patented by Al Gerard, used a trapezoid-shaped frame.) You stand in the center and lift the bar by grabbing the handles just outside your legs, with your palms facing each other. It's probably the safest position for heavy lifting. There's no barbell pressing down on your upper spine, and your lower back stays in a strong, stable position.

The open question is whether the exercise should be included with the squats, or if we should honor its name and put it with the other deadlifts in Chapter 9. Alwyn thinks it's more of a squat, as you have a lot of knee bend at the start of the movement and thus use your quadriceps more than you would on a traditional deadlift. It most resembles the dumbbell squat, only without the awkwardness of trying to hold heavy dumbbells outside your legs.

That said, you can use it as a heavy-duty alternative for either squats or deadlifts, and you won't miss out on any benefits of Alwyn's program. For accounting purposes, keep in mind that there's no standard weight for this piece of equipment. The original trap bar weighed 30 pounds, while newer versions, such as the hex bar sold at performbetter.com, are typically 45 pounds. But the one in your gym could weigh more or less.

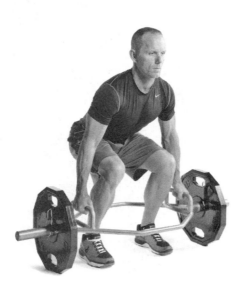

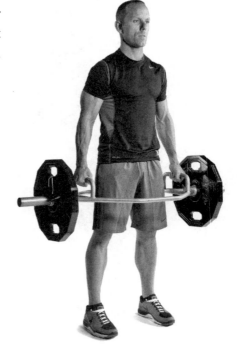

LEVEL 5

✳ **Overhead squat**

- Grab a barbell overhand with a very wide grip, probably double your shoulder width.
- Stand holding the barbell with straight arms over the back of your head. Set your feet as described earlier. Your goal is to keep your arms perpendicular to the floor throughout the movement.
- Push your hips back and descend as far as you can while keeping your feet flat on the floor, your knees steady and aligned with your toes, and the bar over the back of your head, or slightly behind it.
- Return to the starting position.
- As you get better at the movement, first aim to improve your depth—going lower while maintaining perfect form and completing all the repetitions. Then add more weight.

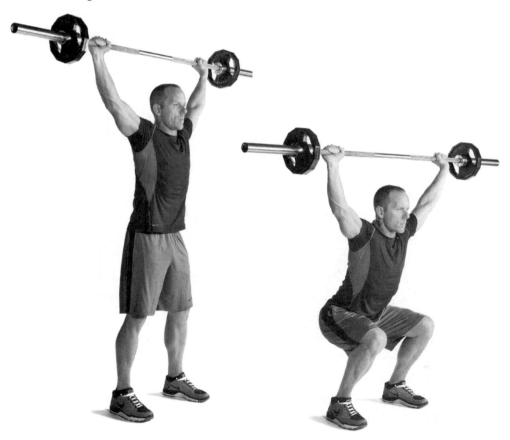

Hinge

To UNDERSTAND THE BENEFITS of this exercise category, we have to talk about the muscles we don't normally discuss in polite company. That's right: We're going to have a frank conversation about your hamstrings.

And your glutes. Mostly your glutes.

We're all adults here. If we think about our glutes at all, it's probably to chastise ourselves for their size, appearance, or consistency. Negative self-talk doesn't actually make them smaller, smoother, or less gelatinous, but that's not my concern right now. I want you to think about your glutes in the non-aesthetic sense—specifically, how your glutes come into play during your workouts. The stronger they are, and the more reliably they engage when you need them, the more productive your workouts will be, with a lower risk of back injury.

Let's try a test to see how well they work. Lie on your back, knees bent, feet flat on the floor, arms out to your sides. Squeeze your glutes and lift your hips until your body forms a straight line from knees to shoulders. Did you feel anything else tighten up along with your glutes and hamstrings? Some of you probably felt a contraction in your lower back. That's a problem.

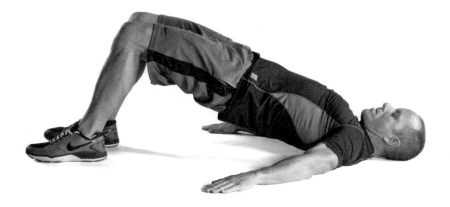

The basic movement we're after is called hip extension—straightening your hips when you're bent forward. Do it right and all the action takes place in your hip joints, driven mostly by your glutes with support from your hamstrings. Other muscles will engage to keep your lower back and pelvis in a neutral position, allowing them to move as a unit as your hips hinge and straighten. But if your glutes can't do their job, your body will compensate by using your lower-back muscles to pull your lumbar spine into a deeper arch (aka hyperextension). Someone who sits in a chair for most of the day is at high risk for gluteal dysfunction. Even advanced lifters can develop something the experts call "gluteal amnesia"—glutes that have forgotten how to do their primary task. Someone with a "bad" back often has a very strong back, the result of those muscles compensating for a butt that can't get into gear.

Let's try one more test, called the Cook hip lift (after physical therapist Gray Cook), to see if your glutes are doing their job. Find a tennis ball, or anything that's round and roughly that size. Get into the same position as the previous test. Put the tennis ball at the bottom of your left rib cage, and pull your left knee to your chest to hold it in place. Put your hands out to your sides, as before, so your left thigh is all that holds the ball against your abdomen. Now try a series of hip lifts, powered solely by your right glute. Repeat with the opposite leg. (If any part of this exercise causes pain, stop immediately.)

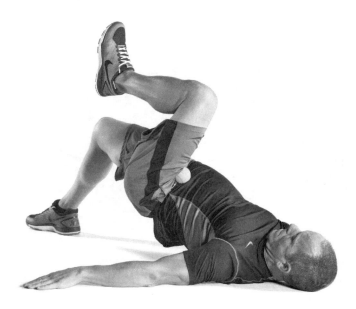

Congratulate yourself if you can do a few reps on each side without losing your hold on the ball. Even if your range of motion is tiny, the fact you can hold the ball means you used your glutes to lift your hips off the floor, rather than your lower-back muscles. Conversely, if you can't hold the ball, it's a sign that you're using your lower-back muscles to compensate for poor glute activation.

Feel free to repeat this drill as often as you like, or not to repeat it at all. I don't know if it has any kind of nondiagnostic benefit. But do keep in mind the goal of glute activation. The better your buttocks work during hip-extension exercises, the more productive your workouts will be. And if they end up smoother or less gelatinous in the process, thanks to a combination of fat loss and muscle development, so much the better.

LEVEL 1

✳ Swiss-ball supine hip extension

This is the same idea as the first hip-raise exercise you tried on the floor, only with your heels on a Swiss ball instead of having your feet flat on the floor. Everyone starting the NROL for Life program should try this exercise at least once, even if you're a relatively advanced lifter. If you can do 15 reps for at least one set, great. You're ready for a higher-level exercise. If not, work at this one until you can get two sets of 15, or until you finish Phase One.

- Lie on your back with your heels on a Swiss ball and your arms out to your sides.
- Lift your hips until your body forms a straight line from ankles to shoulders.
- Lower your hips until they're close to the floor but not touching, and repeat until you finish the set.
- If you feel any discomfort in your lower back, go back to the basic hip extension on the floor described at the beginning of this chapter.

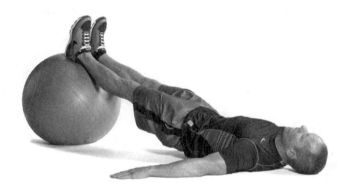

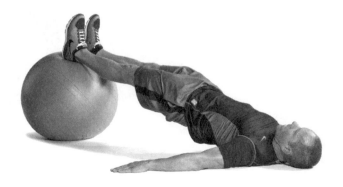

LEVEL 2, OPTION 1

✳ Cable pull-through

To be honest, this can be kind of an obscene-looking exercise. So if you take one look and say, "No way in hell am I doing that in a crowded gym," you'll get no argument from us. However, if you can try it just once in an uncrowded gym, or at home if you have a cable machine or elastic bands, you'll see that it's a really good exercise for two reasons:

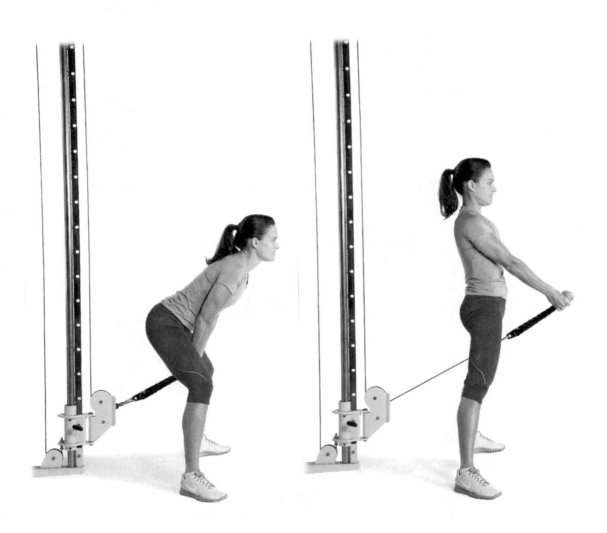

- It helps your body "get" the basic action of loading and then firing your hip muscles from a standing position. You can certainly learn this with free weights, but with the cable there's some drag as you push your hips back to start each repetition, so you get a sense of your hip muscles preparing themselves for a powerful movement in the opposite direction.
- If you train with this exercise, and get comfortable with it, you can move pretty fast without much risk to your lower back. Thus you get a trifecta of benefits: You learn to load and fire your hips, you learn to do this with speed and confidence, and you develop power that will translate to more advanced exercises in this movement category.

Here's how to do it:

- Attach a rope handle to a low cable pulley. (You can also do the pull-through with a band attached to a pillar a few inches above the floor.)
- Holding the ends of the rope attachment between your legs, stand with your back to the cable machine.
- Push your hips back, feeling them load, until your knees bend and your torso is near parallel to the floor.
- Fire your hips forward to straighten your body.
- Keep your back flat and arms straight throughout the movement.

LEVEL 2, OPTION 2

✳ Romanian deadlift

The Romanian deadlift—usually abbreviated to RDL—is the same movement described in the previous exercise, only this time you'll have to work a bit harder to control the descent of the weight as you load your hips. It's a skill we all need to learn anyway, so you may as well learn it here. Many of you will do this exercise in Phase One (after passing through Level 1 by doing 15 supine hip extensions), and let me tell you, when you're doing 15-repetition sets of deadlifts with a barbell, you'd better be very, very sure of your form.

- Grab a barbell with an overhand grip. Your hands should be about shoulder-width apart, or just a bit wider. Stand holding it with straight arms in front of your thighs.
- Push your hips back until the bar is just below your knees. Your knees will bend slightly, and your torso will probably be at a 45-degree angle to the floor. Keep your arms straight and back flat.
- Fire your hips forward to straighten your body.

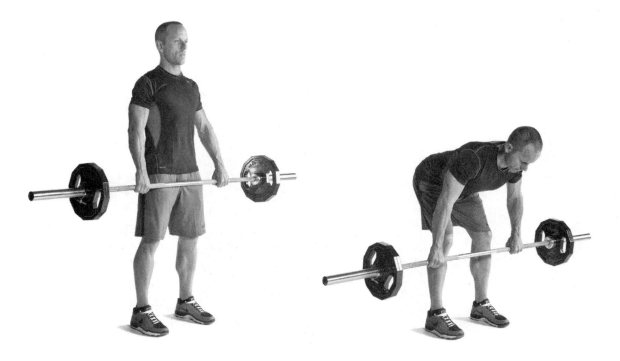

<u>LEVEL 3</u>

✳ Rack deadlift

The Level 2 exercises are both based on momentum. That is, you start upright, with your hips fully released, load your hips, and then release them again. When you do this with high repetitions, there's a rhythm to it. Load, fire, load, fire. Even if you do it fast—Load, fire! Load, fire!—you still end up following whatever rhythm you create. Now you're going to take the musicality out of it and start each repetition from a dead stop. You'll adjust your grip, load your hips, fire them, and slowly return the bar to a dead stop.

- Set the pins or rails of a squat rack just below knee height. If you don't have a rack, you can also set up the bar so it rests on a pair of equal-height boxes. Anything that allows you to start each lift with the bar just below your knees will work.
- Set the Olympic barbell on the pins or rails. Most of you will need to add weights to the bar, but for some the 45-pound Olympic bar may be enough to start with.
- Grab the bar overhand, with your hands just outside your knees.
- Push your hips back, grip the bar as hard as you can, and tighten up everything, from hands to feet. Lift your chest up and focus your eyes forward.
- Fire your hips as you pull the weight off the supports and straighten your body.
- Lower it slowly to the pins or rails, reset your body, and repeat.

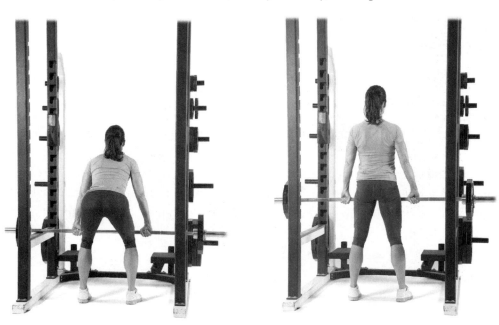

LEVEL 4

✳ Deadlift

This is the exact same exercise as the rack deadlift, only with the bar starting at about mid-shin height.

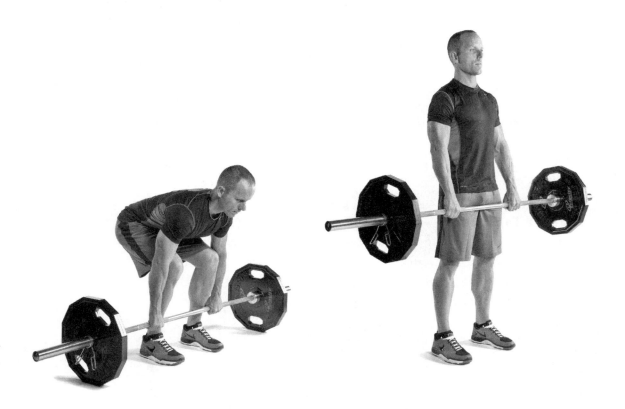

But there is an important nuance that I haven't discussed in previous books. Male readers who qualify for Level 4 should be able to deadlift at least 135 pounds— a 45-pound Olympic bar plus a 45-pound weight plate on each side. Since 45-pound plates are about 18 inches in diameter, and the bar runs through the middle, that puts the bar about 9 inches above the floor, which will hit an average-size guy at about mid-shin height.

But not every woman who's ready for Level 4 will be able to use 135 pounds. A lower weight means smaller plates; the bar will start out a couple inches closer to the floor, which means each repetition begins with your back in a more compromised position. Thus, female readers have a couple of options to start the bar out at mid-shin height.

The best option is a pair of bumper plates. These are lighter, rubber-coated plates with the same 18-inch diameter as 45-pound Olympic plates. But few commercial health clubs will have these, and they're expensive to buy for a home gym. The second-best option is to start each rep with the bar or plates resting on supports that lift it a few inches off the ground and put it at mid-shin height.

Final note: This advice also applies to guys who're significantly taller than average. A guy who's six-foot-three will start with the bar lower on his shins than someone like me, who stands five-foot-ten.

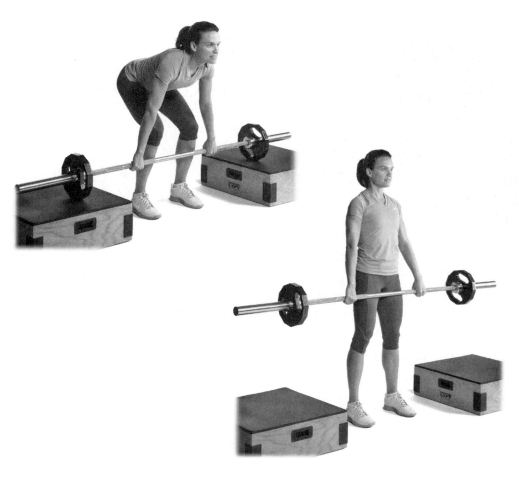

LEVEL 5

✳ **Wide-grip deadlift**

This is probably my favorite exercise in Alwyn's arsenal. Start with a grip that's about twice shoulder width. To do this, you'll have to bend over farther, which is a more challenging position for your lower back. But the benefits are outstanding. The wider grip creates more work for the stabilizer muscles in your shoulder girdle, especially the middle part of the trapezius muscle. The longer range of motion means more work for your glutes and hamstrings.

But the benefits come with risk. You have to build up to this. You really don't want to move to this level until you have at least a year's experience doing deadlifts. I'm tempted to say that men shouldn't train with wide-grip deadlifts until they can deadlift at least their body weight the conventional way, as shown in Level 4. But I don't think the rule needs to be that hard and fast. You don't need to be especially strong; you just need to be really good at deadlifts.

To execute the lift:

- Load the bar and grab it overhand with your hands about twice shoulder-width apart.
- Push your hips back as far as you can. You'll start with your hips hinged at a more severe angle and your knees bent more than in other deadlifts.
- As described for the rack deadlift, tighten your entire body, from your hands to your ankles. Lift your chest and focus your eyes straight ahead.
- Make sure your feet are flat on the floor. If you can't push down through the middle of your feet to start the lift—that is, if you come up on your toes—you aren't qualified for Level 5.
- Fire your hips as you stand and pull the weight off the floor. Finish with your hips and knees straight and your shoulders back.
- Lower the weight to the floor and repeat.

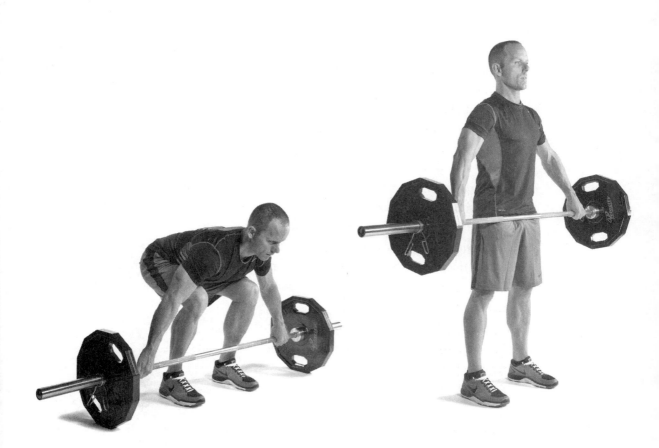

BEYOND LEVEL 5

✳ Wide-grip deadlift from deficit

Although it's a simple progression from the wide-grip deadlift—you're adding a couple inches to the range of motion by allowing the bar to start from a lower position on each repetition—don't mistake simplicity for ease. This is an aggressive, advanced exercise for those who qualify to do it.

I've used the wide-grip deadlift from a deficit successfully in fat-loss programs. It's hard to do, and harder is almost always better. But it also takes a lot of skill and experience to get to the point at which this exercise offers more benefit than risk. You need full mobility in your hip and ankle joints, coupled with advanced-level core strength and stability to keep your back safe. Upper-back and shoulder stability come into play as well.

- Set up a box or step that's sturdy enough to stand on and about 3 to 4 inches high.
- Grab the barbell with a wide grip and step up onto the box. Stand with your feet shoulder-width apart and toes pointed forward.
- Push your hips back and lower the bar until the edges of the weight plates are below the top of the box. The bar will be at or near the bottom of your ankles, and your hips might be lower than your knees. Your feet should remain flat on the box.
- Straighten your knees and fire your hips forward, finishing the movement with your shoulders back.
- Lower the bar and repeat.

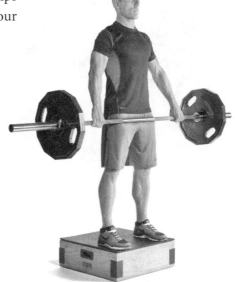

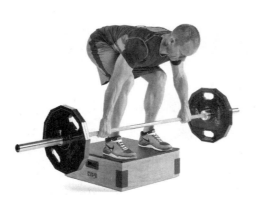

10

Lunge

THE SQUAT AND THE DEADLIFT—the subjects of the previous two chapters—offer you simple, efficient ways to increase the strength, size, and endurance of your lower-body muscles. Both movements start and end with your feet parallel to each other and about shoulder-width apart. But most of the things you do in life—from walking or jogging to tennis, basketball, or rock-climbing—involve putting one foot in front of the other. You would think the symmetry of the movement would even out over time; you'd take the same number of steps with each leg, with more or less the same level of difficulty, and the two legs would end up with more or less equal strength and range of motion.

Ha!

My guess is that everyone reading this has a series of imbalances. One leg is stronger than the other. One hip has more mobility. One knee bends and straightens more easily. One ankle is more likely to roll in or out.

These aren't character flaws. They're the cost of doing business as an ambulatory human. But they are a problem, and the problem doesn't fix itself. It goes one direction until the asymmetry leads to chronic pain or an injury that requires surgical intervention. Many of you are already there.

The good news is that these imbalances can be modified. Alwyn's workouts, by themselves, will go a long way toward rebalancing your strength and mobility, and improving your overall coordination and athleticism. But before we get to the exercises, let's try a test called the in-line lunge (yet another from Gray Cook) to see where you are now.

You'll need a light, straight object, like a broomstick or dowel rod, and some masking tape. Measure the distance from the bump just below your kneecap to the floor. (It's about 17 inches for me.) Tear off that much tape and stick it to the floor in a straight line.

Stand over the tape and place your left heel at one end and your right toes at the other. It's crucial that both feet are on the same line. Hold the broomstick vertically against your back with both hands so it touches the back of your head, the space

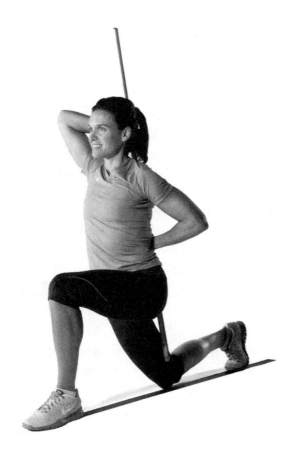

between your shoulder blades, and the midline of your glutes. Your right hand will hold the top of the stick behind your neck and your left hand will hold it in the small of your back.

Lower your right knee so it touches the tape on the same line as your left heel and right toes. Rise to the starting position. The goal is to descend and rise without wobbling or leaning to either side. The broomstick should remain in contact with all three spots and perpendicular to the floor. Do as many as you can, then switch legs, reverse your hands on the broomstick, and repeat.

Consider that your trial run. Rest for a minute, then try it again, this time shooting for 10 to 15 slow, controlled reps with each leg. If possible, have a partner watch for form. In the absence of an observer, use the focus test: Keep your eyes focused on a single spot directly in front of you; if your eyes slip off target, you can bet that you lost your alignment at some point.

How did you do? If you got more than 10 perfect reps with each leg, and your body feels fine (not stiff or cramped), you're qualified to do any exercise in this chapter. Your challenge is to use them in a way that allows for higher reps in Phase One, a heavier load in Phase Two, and combination of higher reps and faster tempo in Phase Three.

Those who didn't fare as well will need to start at Level 1 and work your way up.

LEVEL 1

✳ Split squat

The exercise itself is simple enough, as you can see. The trick is figuring out what to do with your arms. If you can do at least one set of 15 with your body weight, you'll need to do the exercise with dumbbells, which you hold at arm's length at your sides. But if you need to work up to that point, you can either start with your arms at your sides, your hands on your hips, or your hands behind your head in the prisoner grip, as shown here.

- Stand with your feet hip-width apart, and take a long step back with your right leg. This is your starting position.
- Lower yourself until the top of your left thigh is parallel to the floor and your right knee nearly touches the floor.
- Return to the starting position and repeat until you finish all your reps. Switch legs and repeat the same number of reps. That's one set.

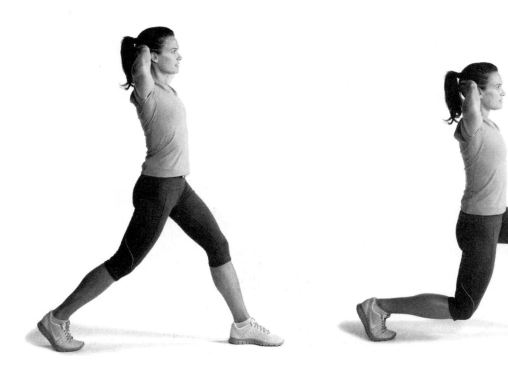

DIAL IT BACK

✳ Supported split squat

Can't yet do the basic split squat? Stand next to something sturdy—a pole or the edge of a solid piece of furniture. When your left leg is forward, as described earlier, rest your left hand lightly on the support. Lower yourself until the top of your left thigh is parallel to the floor, and then return to the starting position, using the support as little as possible. Do as many as you can, up to 15. For your next set, switch sides and support yourself with your right hand.

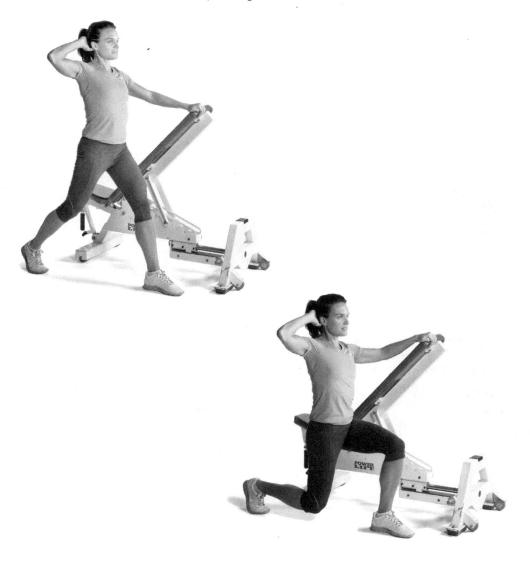

LEVEL 2

✳ Dumbbell reverse lunge

This is a terrific Phase Two exercise because it allows you to use fairly heavy weights without knee strain.

- Grab a pair of dumbbells and stand holding them at your sides, with your feet hip-width apart.
- Take a long step back with your right foot and lower yourself until the top of your left thigh is parallel to the floor and your right knee nearly touches the floor. Keep your torso upright.
- Step back to the starting position and repeat until you finish all your reps. Switch legs and repeat. That's one set.

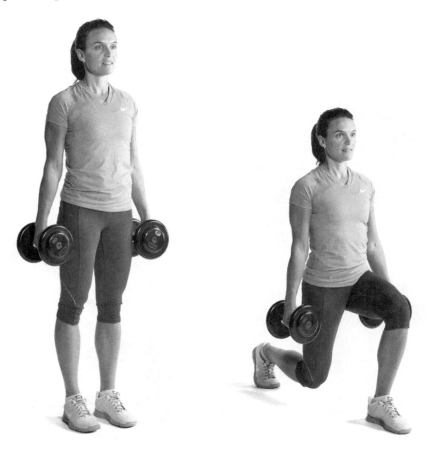

COOL VARIATION #1

✳ Goblet reverse lunge

Holding dumbbells at your sides for high-repetition sets can do a number on your gripping muscles. You can get around that by holding a dumbbell or weight plate against your chest with both hands.

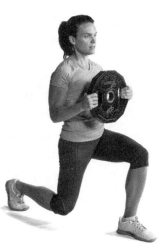

COOL VARIATION #2

✳ Reverse lunge from step

Start with both feet on a box or step that's about 6 inches high. Step back with your right foot and lower yourself into a deeper lunge. Your left thigh will end up below parallel to the floor. Finish the set as described above. The extra range of motion challenges your mobility and balance, and potentially leads to faster muscle development. You'll certainly use your lower-body muscles in a different way, with a bigger role for your supporting muscles. For some reason, I always seem to get better calf development when I include this variation in my workouts.

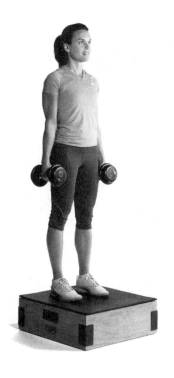

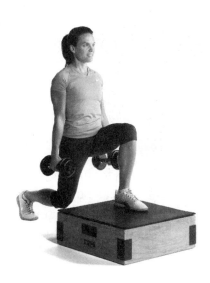

COOL VARIATION ON THE VARIATION

✳ Offset-loaded reverse lunge from step

This time, hold a single dumbbell in your left hand at shoulder height as you step back with your right foot. Switch the weight to your right shoulder when you step back with your left. The offset weight develops core stability along with the challenges to your balance and mobility.

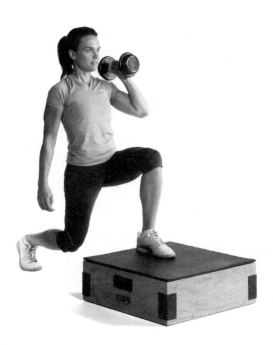

LEVEL 3

✳ Split squat, rear foot elevated

If you're doing this for high reps in Phase One, you might want to start with just your body weight. You can put your hands at your sides, on your hips, or in the prisoner grip behind your head. If you use weights, you can either hold dumbbells at your sides or hold a dumbbell or weight plate with both hands against your chest.

- Get into a split-squat position, with the toes of your back foot resting on a low step.
- Lower yourself until the top of your forward thigh is parallel to the floor, keeping your torso upright.
- Push back to the starting position, and do all your reps before switching legs and repeating.

Most lifters doing this for the first time will feel an uncomfortable stretch in the quadriceps of the trailing leg. You want to go easy at first with the range of motion, gradually expanding it to give your lower body a better workout.

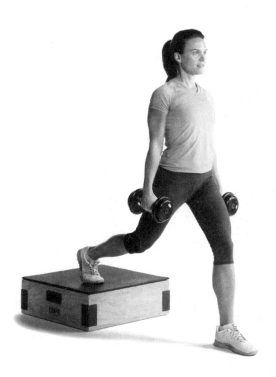
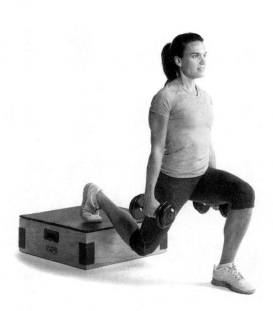

UNIVERSALLY DESPISED VARIATION

✳ Bulgarian split squat

This is the same exercise, only with your rear foot elevated on a bench or step that's at least 12 inches high, and with the instep of that foot resting on the bench, rather then the toes. You can use any of the loading variations described earlier: body weight, dumbbells, or goblet. Lifting your rear foot higher increases the range of motion, which means you're getting a much tougher workout. Just make sure that the discomfort you feel (and you will feel discomfort, guaranteed) is in the muscles rather than the knee joints. You'll hate the exercise but love the results. This may be the single best exercise in the program for developing the quadriceps.

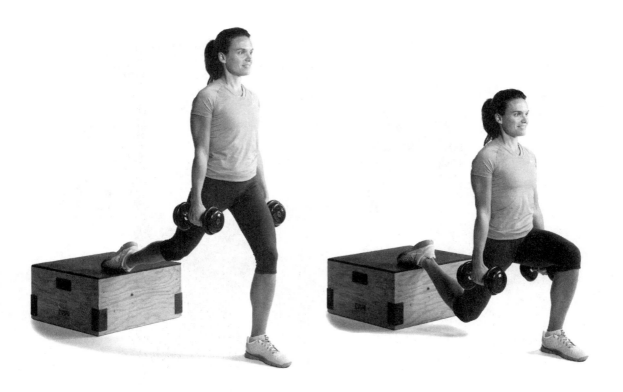

MUCH MORE ENJOYABLE VARIATION

✳ Suspended split squat

Attach the TRX (or any suspension-training system) to a chin-up bar or overhead support. With your back to the straps, put your right foot into a loop and hop forward with your left until you're in a comfortable position for split squats. Drop down into the lunge position and push back up. Do your reps, switch legs, and repeat.

You have a few options with your arms. At first you may want to hold them out to your sides for balance. When you're comfortable with the movement you can drive your arms up in a running motion. So when your left leg is forward, you drive your right arm up on the descent, and your left arm up as you rise. When your right leg is forward, you drive with your left arm on the descent.

Once you're comfortable with that, you can hold a pair of dumbbells as you do the lunge with the running motion. It's one of my favorite exercises for fat loss, and an option for Phase Three.

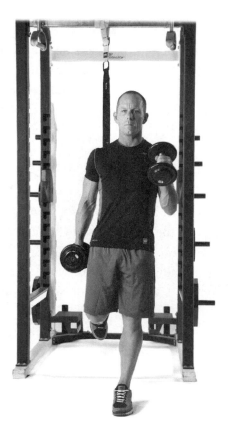
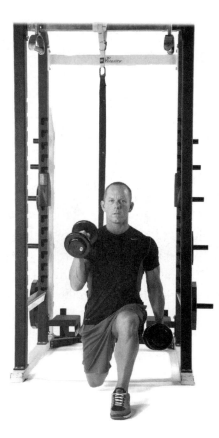

LEVEL 4

✳ Forward lunge

For many, this will be an easier exercise than the Level 3 split squat. But the fact that you find it easy doesn't mean you're qualified to do it. Go back to the in-line lunge test at the beginning of the chapter. Can you get 10 to 15 reps with each leg, holding the broomstick in place? If not, you have no business doing a forward lunge with somewhat heavy weights, and Alwyn doesn't want you doing this exercise without a challenging load (in addition to your body weight). You don't yet have the stability, balance, and mobility you need. Whatever problems you have in your lower body that keep you from doing the in-line lunge will only be exacerbated by doing this exercise before you're ready for it.

Conversely, it may be a surprisingly difficult exercise for some of us who have knee pain, even if we're otherwise fully qualified. Split squats and reverse lunges take some pressure off the kneecap of the forward leg, but when you step forward all the force goes right into that joint.

In *Advances in Functional Training*, Mike Boyle notes that knee pain is rarely a problem that originates in the knees. It could have a long list of causes beginning in the ankles or hips. Tightness or restricted mobility above or below can pull on the knee's tendons and produce pain that disguises its source. Alwyn's program, by itself, may take care of the problem, especially if you're diligent with your pre- and post-workout exercises. But if it doesn't, knee pain is your signal that you aren't yet ready for this exercise.

For those who are:

- Grab a pair of dumbbells and stand holding them at your sides with your feet hip-width apart. (If you can't use weights for all the repetitions in your current phase, you need to use a lower-level lunge variation.)
- Take a long step forward with your left leg, and lower yourself until the top of your left thigh is parallel to the floor. Your right knee should almost touch the floor while your torso remains upright.
- Push back to the starting position.
- Repeat with your right leg, and alternate until you've done all the repetitions with each leg.

<u>LEVEL 5</u>

✳ Walking lunge

I scratch my head when I see this exercise used in entry-level workout programs. I've always considered it an advanced lunge variation—one I rarely do in my own workouts—and Alwyn agrees. This is the first time he's included it in the NROL series, even though we've featured some extraordinarily challenging (dare I say "badass"?) exercises. But if you're ready for it, here it is:

- Grab a pair of dumbbells and stand holding them at your sides with your feet hip-width apart.
- Take a long step forward with your left leg, as described previously.
- Push off your right foot and step forward into a lunge with your right leg.
- Continue lunging forward, alternating legs, until you've done all the repetitions with each leg.

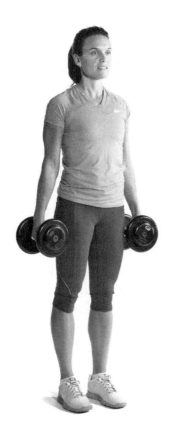
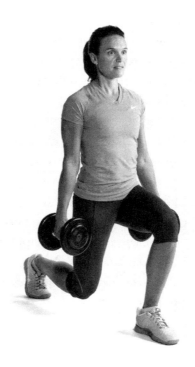

BEYOND LEVEL 5

✳ **Lunge-a-palooza**

The lunge is probably the most versatile exercise in the program. If we had more space and a bigger budget, I could include at least a dozen more lunge variations that I've used in my own workouts. I'm sure Alwyn knows five for each one I could come up with.

Here are some of the ways you can create a more advanced version of any of the exercises we've show in this chapter:

- **Change the angle**. You don't have to stop at forward or backward. You can lunge to the side or any angle in between.
- **Change the resistance**. We've shown you how to use three types of resistance: your body weight (which is never to be underestimated); dumbbells; and a single weight plate. You can also try kettlebells, a barbell held across the back of your shoulders, a sandbag, or even a small child who won't squirm too much.
- **Change the elevation**. You can step up or step down on any of the variations you see in this chapter. Technically, the exercise called "step-up" goes into the single-leg-stance classification, shown in the next chapter. But if you create your own step-up or step-down lunge, you can decide for yourself which category it fits. It's not like Alwyn is going to follow you around and scold you for the transgression. (Although it would be entertaining if he did. You haven't been scolded until you've heard it from a Scotsman.)
- **Change the stability**. I carry a set of Valslides with me to the gym, and from time to time I'll spice up my workouts by doing reverse lunges with the rear foot on a slide. It creates a balance challenge on the way down and extra work for the hip-flexor muscles on the way up. Plus, it's fun to move fast while staying under control.
- **Unbalance the load**. We've shown you one offset-loaded variation in this chapter, and in the next chapter we'll show you a bunch more. But you don't have to wait for us to describe every possible opportunity to use an offset form of resistance. Once you reach Level 5, you can create your own, using a dumbbell, kettlebell, band, cable machine, or anything else you can think of.
- **Mix and match**. One of my favorites is an offset-loaded reverse lunge, using a

kettlebell held overhead and a Valslide. I'm not brave enough to go all the way and do it with my front foot on a step, but I think it's kind of cool to combine three unique challenges—unstable surface, offset load, unconventional form of resistance—in one exercise.

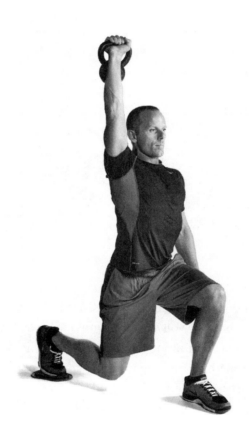

11

Single-Leg Stance

THESE EXERCISES ARE VARIATIONS on the squats, deadlifts, and lunges from the previous three chapters. But because you do them with one leg at a time, your balance and coordination are challenged in unique and useful ways. Single-leg balance is something we need, and something we lose rapidly with age and inactivity. Life is filled with situations in which we find ourselves suddenly teetering on one leg. Maybe one foot hits a patch of ice, oil, or mud. Maybe a foothold gives way. Maybe we're negotiating a narrow path, or climbing unusually steep steps. If you're an athlete in a sport like basketball or soccer, you may get very good at balancing and pushing off from the nondominant leg (the left if you're right-handed), but without corresponding balance and stability on the dominant leg.

Let's start with a very simple test of single-leg balance. Find a cone or something else that's about 12 inches high. Stand about 36 inches in front of it. Balancing first on your nondominant leg, reach forward and touch it with your dominant hand. Extend your dominant leg behind you for balance. Now, without touching the ground with your dominant foot, return to the starting position, and repeat for as many reps as you can without losing your balance. Do the same thing with the opposite leg.

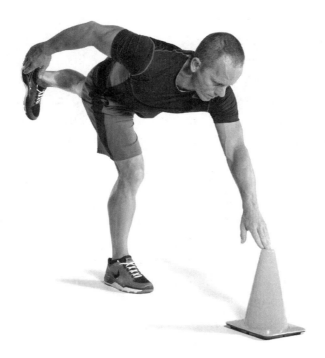

If you're able to touch the cone at least 10 times with each hand without touching the floor with the foot that's in motion, consider yourself qualified for Level 3. But even if you pass, you may want to start with the Level 1 exercise, as I'll explain.

LEVEL 1

✳ Step-up

Did you ever see the movie *Vision Quest*? It's about a high school wrestler who decides to drop several weight classes so he can take on Brian Shute, a three-time state champion. There's also some sex and stuff, and a trivia-question scene in which a then unknown Madonna sings "Crazy for You," a song that was way more successful than the movie back in 1985. I vaguely remember those things. The only part I remember *vividly* is when Brian Shute works out by climbing stadium stairs with a sawed-off telephone pole across his shoulders. You can keep your *Rocky III* and *G.I. Jane* workout montages. For me, that's the most startling workout scene ever filmed.

It also demonstrates that the step-up, Alwyn's Level 1 exercise, can be the hardest exercise in this chapter, if you make it so. I used to do my own version of Shute's Ladder with a barbell on my back, stepping up onto a 12-inch box. With enough weight, it was a brutally effective exercise.

But forget weight for now. Let's get the form right first:

- First you want to find a step, box, or bench to step up to. The higher the step, the harder the exercise. If you have any knee problems or balance issues, I recommend starting with a low step—12 inches or less—and working your way up if that's too easy.
- Grab a pair of dumbbells. If you have lifting experience, and you're working with a step that's lower than your knee, you can be aggressive with the weight. Whatever you choose, you have to be able to hold the weights long enough to complete the repetitions. In Phase One, that's up to 15 reps with each leg. All else being equal, some of you might do better with lighter weights and a higher step.
- Place your left foot flat on the step, with your right foot on the floor. (Do the opposite if you're left-handed.)

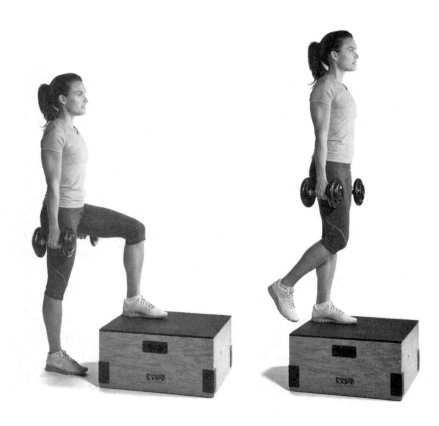

- Push down through the heel of your left foot and lift yourself up so your right leg is even with your left. The higher the step, the more you'll feel this in your glutes and hamstrings. The lower the step, the more you'll feel it in your quads and calves.
- Brush the step with your right foot to complete the repetition, but don't rest it on the step. You want to keep the tension on the working muscles of your left leg.
- Lower your right foot to the floor.
- Do all your reps with your left leg, then repeat with your right.

DIAL IT BACK? NO.

If you're at Level 1, just find a low enough step to complete the reps with each leg. Knee-challenged lifters who can use a low step pain-free should increase the weights as needed to make it challenging.

LEVEL 2

✳ Offset-loaded step-up

This was my go-to exercise for Phase Two. It adds a core challenge and also takes away one of the main drawbacks of the conventional step-up with two dumbbells, during which your gripping muscles may give out before your leg muscles have worked to a desired level of exhaustion. Execution is simple: Hold a single dumbbell or kettlebell at shoulder height on the side of your working leg—your left when you're stepping up with your left.

<u>LEVEL 3</u>

✳ Single-leg Romanian deadlift

- Grab a dumbbell with your right hand and hold it at arm's length at your side as you stand with your feet together.
- Hinge at the hip as you bend your torso toward the floor and extend your right leg behind you.
- Lower the weight toward the floor, with your right arm hanging straight down from your shoulder. Your right arm and left leg should be perpendicular to the floor. Do whatever you need with your left arm for balance.
- Your neck, torso, and right leg should form a straight line. If you have great balance and range of motion, that line will be parallel to the floor; don't worry if you can't get there right away. The key is to form that straight line.
- Return to the starting position, trying not to put weight on your right leg, and do all your reps. Remember that your left leg is working, even though your right leg is moving. You want to feel the contraction in your left glute.
- Repeat the set with your right leg, holding the weight in your left hand.

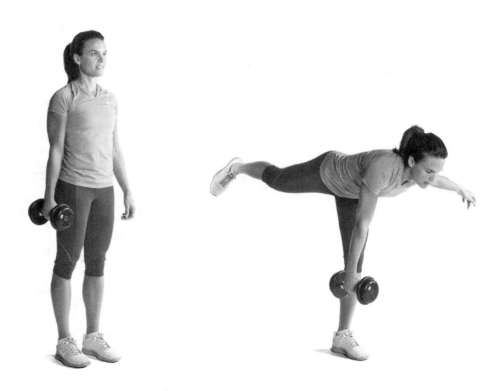

DIAL IT BACK? NO.

In my gym, a lot of the senior lifters do this exercise with support. I don't like it. I've never seen a senior advance to the unsupported version of the exercise. In fact, the tendency is to try to do it with heavier weight over time, which makes them *more* reliant on the support. If you qualified for the single-leg RDL by passing the balance test at the beginning of this chapter, you should have no problem doing it without support. Sure, you'll wobble a bit and land on your nonworking leg. It happens to everybody, and it's not a reason to rely on a support. The entire point of the exercise is to develop balance in a single-leg position.

LEVEL 4

✳ Single-leg squat

Not only do I suck at this exercise, I once injured my knee trying to get better at it. The problem isn't with the exercise. It's with the fact that I can do it pain-free to a certain range of motion, but risk injury when I go beyond that. So let's be clear about this: *On single-leg squats, there's no defined range of motion that is ideal or attainable for everyone.* Some people can go glute-to-heel with the working leg while the non-working leg extends straight out in front of them, a few inches off the floor. It's one of the most impressive-looking exercises I've seen, and I'd love to be able to do it, just as I'd love to be able to dunk a basketball or ski a black diamond. None of those things will happen in this lifetime, and I'm okay with that.

- Grab a light dumbbell and stand on your left foot near the side edge of a sturdy box or step that's at least 12 inches high. Your right foot will hang off the side of the box.
- Extend your arms in front of you as you push your hips back and lower yourself as far as you can go, allowing your left knee to bend naturally as your right foot goes below the edge of the box. (The weight in your hands should act as a counterbalance to the shift in your center of gravity.)

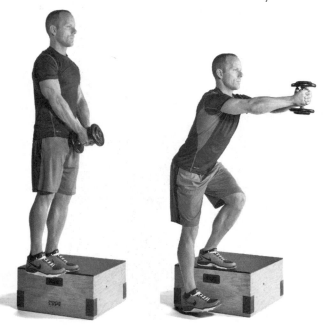

- Push back up to the starting position, finish your reps with your left leg, switch sides, and repeat the set.
- In subsequent workouts, the goal is to increase reps and range of motion, rather than add to the weight you're using as a counterbalance.

DIAL IT BACK

✳ Supported single-leg squat

- Attach the TRX (or any suspension-training system) to a chin-up bar or overhead support.
- Take a light grip on the handles and stand with your feet together. Start with as much or as little tension in the straps as you need. If you're doing this exercise for the first time, you'll probably start with a white-knuckle grip on the handles and full tension in the straps. But as you get more comfortable, try to leave a little slack in the straps so you're relying less on them for support.
- Lift one foot off the floor, and push your hips back. As you descend into the squat, allow your nonworking leg to extend out in front of you. Return to the starting position, do all your reps with that leg, and then repeat with the other leg.

Don't have a suspension-training system? Anything that supports your body weight will do, even if it's just a rope thrown over a tree limb.

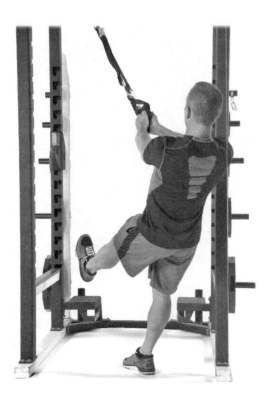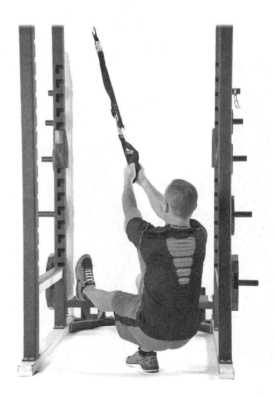

ADVANCED OPTION

✳ Kettlebell single-leg squat

If the single-leg squat off the step feels easy, then do the exercise standing on the floor, without the step. You can use dumbbells, but a single kettlebell, held with both hands, seems to allow better balance and range of motion. Again, you want to increase reps and squat depth before increasing the weight you use as a counterbalance.

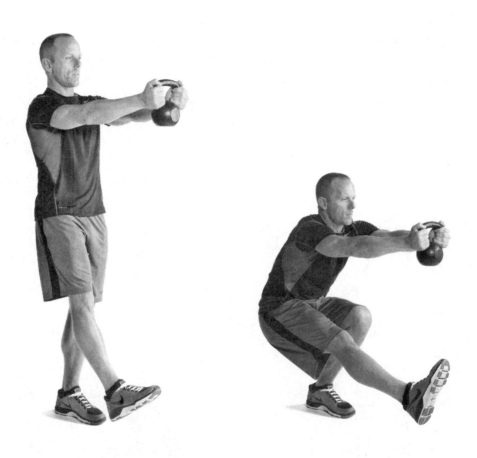

LEVEL 5

✳ Single-leg deadlift

For the single-leg squat, whatever weight you hold is a counterbalance to make the exercise easier, rather than a form of resistance to make it harder. Now, if you qualify for this level by mastering the single-leg squat, you're going to use weights to make it harder.

- Grab a pair of dumbbells and stand holding them at your sides.
- Lift your right foot off the floor behind you, bending your right knee about 90 degrees while keeping your thighs parallel to each other.
- Push your hips back and lower yourself as far as you can. Don't extend your non-working leg behind you; keep your thighs close to each other throughout the movement. Thus, when your hips go back and your left knee bends, your right leg should remain more or less perpendicular to the floor, with your knee bent just enough to keep your right foot from touching the floor.
- Push back up to the starting position, finish all your reps, and repeat with your right leg.

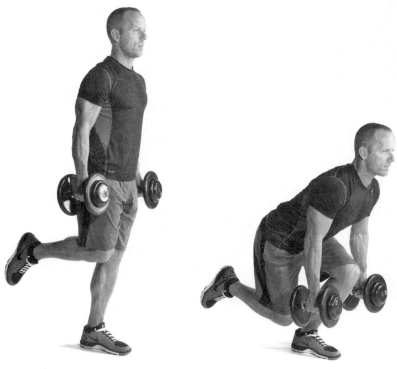

BEYOND LEVEL 5

✳ Higher steps

Earlier, I noted that the step-up can be the toughest exercise in the single-leg category. Here are three versions that add new challenges to a familiar movement.

✳ Crossover step-up

- Hold heavy dumbbells at your sides and stand next to a bench or step, with your left leg closer to the step and about 12 inches away. (Taller lifters should stand farther away, and shorter lifters may need to get closer.)
- Cross your right leg in front of your left and plant your right foot on the step.
- Push yourself up to the step, without touching it with your left foot.
- Step down with your left foot, followed by your right.
- Do all your reps, and then switch sides.
- After your first set, stand farther away from the step on subsequent sets. The exercise is advanced only if you create obstacles—the weights in your hand and the distance you have to step—that make it advanced.
- You can also create an asymmetrical balance challenge by using a single dumbbell. Hold it in your left hand when stepping up with your left foot.

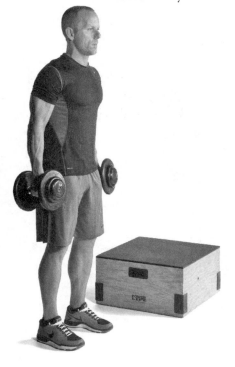
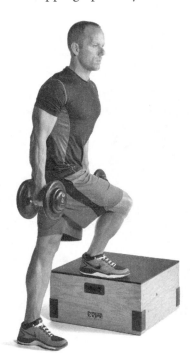

✴ Sprinter step-up

Set up as you would for a conventional step-up. Here, though, once you are up on the box, bring the knee of the nonworking leg up toward your chest. Once you get the hang of it, try to bring the knee up explosively. For advanced lifters this is a terrific Phase Three exercise. You develop power and create a high level of metabolic fatigue, which is the best tool we have for rapid fat loss.

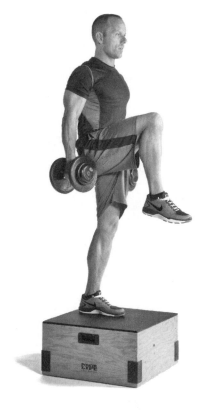

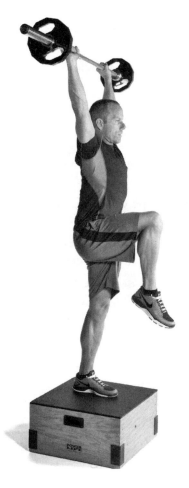

✴ Overhead sprinter step-up

Hold a light barbell overhead while doing the sprinter step-up described above. For advanced lifters with *really* good balance who want a challenge, this is the best step-up variation I've come across.

Push

THE DIRTY SECRET OF THE MUSCLE-BUILDING industry is that a lot of recreational lifters get hurt. A review study published in 2010 in the *Journal of Strength and Conditioning Research* dug up reports showing that as many as 60 percent of lifters experience shoulder pain in any given year. I'm one of them.

I could try to pretend that these injuries are mysterious, but they aren't. Talk to any serious, longtime lifter, and chances are good he'll tell you he hurt his shoulder doing either bench or shoulder presses, usually with a barbell. Indeed, the researchers found those two exercises show up frequently in studies of shoulder injuries. A few others include parallel-bar dips, behind-the-neck shoulder presses, chest flies, and, curiously, biceps curls.

Almost all of them fall into the push category, the subject of this chapter. These are the exercises that use your chest, shoulder, and triceps muscles. Pushing things away from you, either forward or overhead, is a natural movement pattern, and shouldn't be more dangerous than any other natural pattern. But we make it dangerous in three ways:

1. *We don't balance pushing and pulling.* Show me a male lifter who does a body-building "split" routine—working different muscles on different days—and I'll show you a guy who probably puts more time and effort into building his chest, shoulders, and arms. To my surprise, the review by Morey Kolber and colleagues at Nova Southeastern University showed that there's no data to link the amount of weight lifted to shoulder injuries. Heavy lifting doesn't necessarily produce more injuries, nor does lifting light weights for high reps prevent them. The problem comes when lifters, mostly male, overbuild chest and arm muscles at the expense of the back and shoulder muscles that perform the opposite movements.

2. *We do exercises in the "high five" position.* We've known for years that when the upper arms are pulled back and externally rotated, as they would for a behind-the-neck shoulder press, the shoulder is extraordinarily vulnerable. I'd never heard it called the "high five" position until I read this review, but I hope the name sticks. The position is great for celebrating life's best moments but really bad for lifting heavy weights.

3. *We extend the range of motion too far.* When you do exercises like parallel-bar dips and chest flies (the latter is typically done with dumbbells; you lie on a bench, lower the weights out to your sides, then pull them back over your chest), your upper arms probably go behind or beneath your torso. That strains the jumble of tendons and ligaments that converge around your shoulder joints.

The basic bench press is also a problem for lifters with a naturally narrow torso and long arms. Lowering a weight to your chest means your upper arms sink below your torso, potentially straining the biceps tendon. That tendon crosses your shoulder joint between the upper-arm bone and a bony structure called the acromion, the part of the shoulder blade that connects with the outside edge of your collarbone. It's also where a couple of rotator-cuff tendons converge, and it's all topped by a protective pad, called a bursa. The biceps tendon, stuck on the bottom of that dog pile between two bones, takes a hit when you overuse or misuse the biceps or the muscles surrounding it. That produces inflammation, and any swelling in that tiny space will produce pain.

Now that we've covered the things that hurt, let's talk about the exercises you'll actually do in this chapter. Or, rather, let's talk about the *exercise* you'll do. It's singular for a reason. The push-up and its many variations cover levels 1, 2, and 3.

I know what many readers are thinking: "Push-ups? *Me*? I want to lift weights!" Men reading this tend to assume the push-up is too easy. Women often assume it's too hard. Neither is true; this chapter includes both entry-level push-up variations and some that will humble advanced lifters.

Because you do so many push-up variations throughout Alwyn's program, it's really hard *not* to use lifts for variety, if nothing else. That's why Alwyn includes dumbbell bench presses (Level 4) and shoulder presses (Level 5), as well as the barbell bench press (Beyond Level 5), an exercise I can't even do anymore. As you'll see in Chapter 17, even beginners probably will need to do bench presses in Phase One. So you may wonder why Alwyn puts the "advanced" label on exercises that beginners have been doing since the dawn of the commercial fitness industry, and will most likely use throughout this program.

It's not that he hates chest and shoulder presses (although he doesn't think beginners have the strength and stability to do the latter with solid form). He just really likes push-ups. "It's such a superior exercise for metabolic purposes, time management, core stability, and shoulder health," he told me. That said, most male lifters, and some women, will get beyond the point at which they can increase strength and muscle size with push-ups alone. Alwyn and his trainers can load their clients up with weighted vests and chains, but you probably don't have access to either. Thus, bench presses are an important part of Alwyn's program for all lifters, even if push-ups are the more important and valuable exercise.

Here's how you decide which push-up level to start with:

Get down on the floor in the push-up position. Lower yourself to within an inch of the floor or until your upper arms are even with your shoulder blades, whichever happens first. (This protects the shoulders of those with longer arms and narrow frames, while allowing those with shorter arms or thicker frames to use a full range of motion.) Pause two seconds. Push back up and repeat.

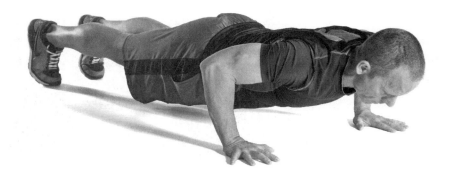

Those who can do at least 15 paused reps qualify for Level 2 or 3; it's really up to you which to start with. For the record, I made it to 15, but only barely, and I can't guarantee I paused for exactly two seconds at the bottom of the final three reps.

There's no particular test for shoulder presses (Level 5). Alwyn simply prefers that even advanced lifters wait until Phase Two or Three before using them.

LEVEL 1

✳ Push-up

- Get into push-up position: arms straight down from your shoulders and perpendicular to the floor, feet close together, weight resting on your hands and toes, and your body straight from neck to ankles.
- Lower your chest until it's within an inch of the floor or your upper arms are even with your shoulder blades, whichever happens first.
- Push back up to the starting position.

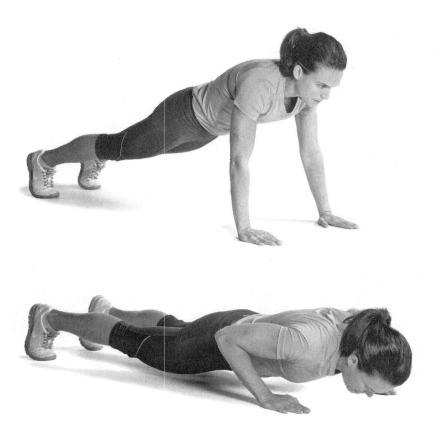

12 Ways to Make Push-Ups Tougher

When you can easily do sets of 15 push-ups the conventional way in Phase One, try one or more of these variations. For accounting purposes, each push-up counts as a single repetition, even if you're doing variations in which you're alternating from side to side. This is different from the way we count single-leg and split-stance exercises, when you do all the required repetitions with each leg.

- Stack your feet, resting one on top of the other.
- Elevate your feet on a step or bench.
- Raise one leg (do equal reps with each leg elevated).
- Elevate your feet with a TRX or similar suspension system.
- Put your hands on an unstable surface, like a foam pad or Bosu ball.
- Put your feet on an unstable object, like a Swiss ball.
- Put your hands on a Swiss ball.
- Put one hand on a medicine ball and the other on the floor (do equal reps with each hand on the ball).
- Put both hands on a medicine ball.
- Put each hand on a medicine ball of the same size.
- Lower your chest and shoulders toward one hand, then the other, alternating on each rep.
- Lift your right knee toward your right elbow, then your left knee toward your left elbow, alternating on each rep (this variation is usually called a Spiderman push-up).

DIAL IT BACK

✳ Push-up with hands elevated

Alwyn is no fan of the "girl" push-up, with knees on the floor. One of the main benefits of the push-up is the way it uses the core muscles to stabilize the spine and pelvis, and most of that benefit is lost when you cut your own body off at the knees.

Instead, do push-ups with your hands elevated as high as they need to go. If you're an absolute beginner, or recovering from something no one should ever have to recover from, you can even do wall push-ups: stand a few feet from a wall, lean forward, rest your hands on the wall, come up on your toes so your body forms a straight line, and do the exercise with whatever range of motion you can.

The point is, always do the hardest push-up variation you can manage for the required repetitions.

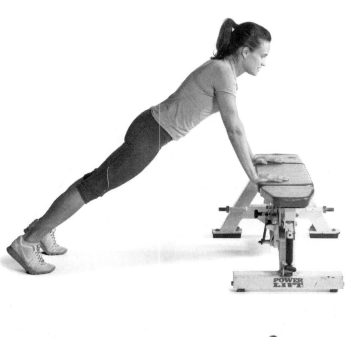

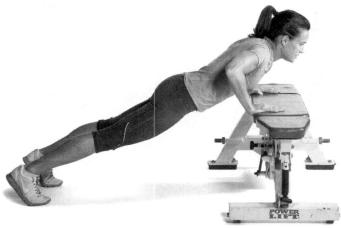

LEVEL 2

✳ Push-up with hands suspended

- Set up a TRX or similar suspension system so the handles are 12 to 24 inches above the floor. Higher is easier; lower is harder.
- Grab the handles and get into push-up position.
- Lower yourself until your upper arms are parallel to the floor, then push back to the starting position.
- When you can do all the required reps, make it harder by lowering the handles.

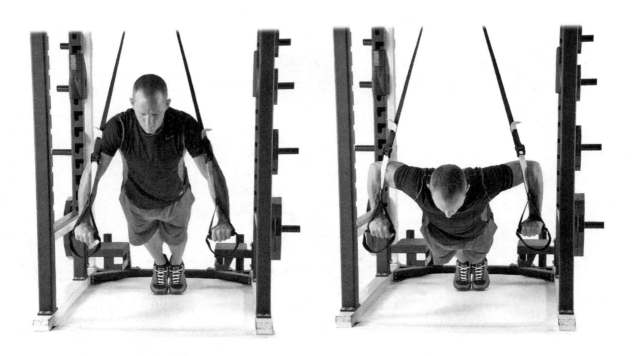

LEVEL 3

✳ T push-up

- Get into push-up position.
- Lower your chest toward the floor, and as you push back up, twist to your left so your left arm comes off the floor and finishes straight over your right arm. In this position your body will form a T.
- Twist back and immediately begin your next push-up.
- As you push back up, twist to the right, so your right arm ends up over your left.
- Remember that each T push-up counts as a repetition. So if the workout calls for 15 per set, you'll have to do either 14 or 16 to get the same number to each side. If you stop at an odd number, no problem; just start the next set to the opposite side.

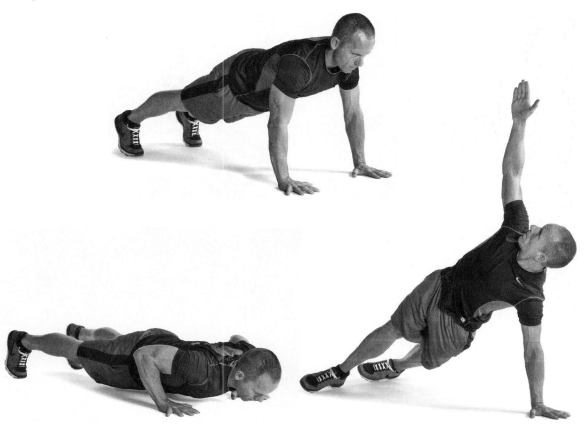

COOL VARIATION

✳ T push-up with weights

Grab a pair of hexagonal dumbbells and start with your hands on the weights, palms turned toward each other so the weights are parallel to your torso. Then do the exercise as described. If you don't have hex dumbbells, use a single round dumbbell. Hold it in one hand, do all your reps twisting to that side, then repeat the set with the dumbbell in the other hand.

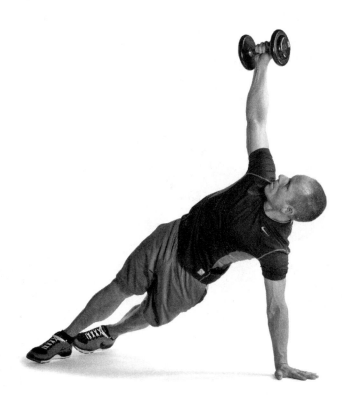

LEVEL 4

✳ **Dumbbell bench press**

- Grab a pair of dumbbells and lie on your back on a flat or incline bench. (I prefer the incline; it's *much* easier on my shoulders.)
- Hold the weights straight up over your shoulders, with your feet planted flat on the floor, shoulder-width apart. If your feet don't reach the floor when the bench is flat, either incline the bench, or better yet, skip this exercise altogether. The bench press, like the push-up, is a total-body exercise. With your feet on the bench, you lose half the muscles that would otherwise provide upper-torso stability. You absolutely must start with both feet flat on the floor.
- Lower the weights toward the edges of your shoulders, stopping when your upper arms are even with your shoulder blades.
- Press the weights straight up toward the ceiling, and repeat.

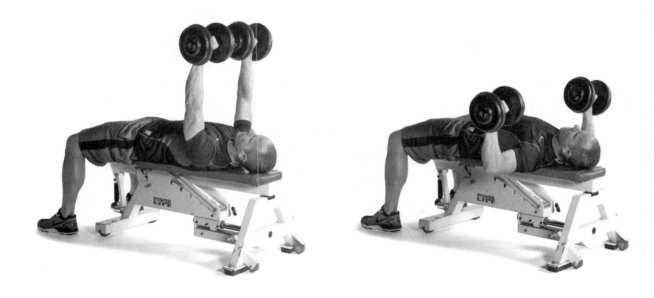

COOL VARIATION

✳ Dumbbell single-arm bench press

It's exactly like the conventional bench press, only with a dumbbell in one hand and your other hand resting on your stomach. You add a core-stability challenge when you unbalance the load like this. Again, you can use a flat or inclined bench.

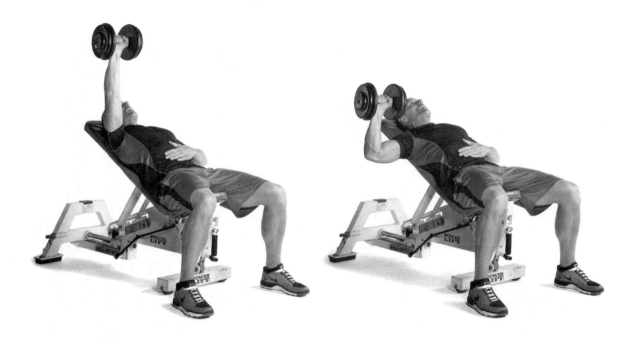

LEVEL 5

✳ Dumbbell shoulder press

- Grab a pair of dumbbells and stand holding them just above your shoulders, with your feet shoulder-width apart. You can turn your palms in if that's easier on your shoulders, or hold them the conventional way, with your palms forward.
- Press the weights straight up.
- Lower them to the starting position and repeat.

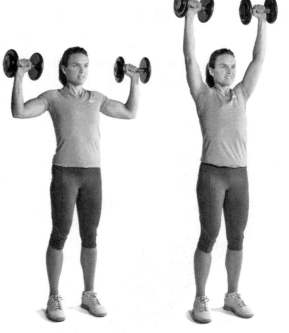

COOL VARIATION

✳ Dumbbell single-arm shoulder press

Same exercise, but press one weight at a time. It's a little more exhausting, and adds a bit more of a challenge to your core.

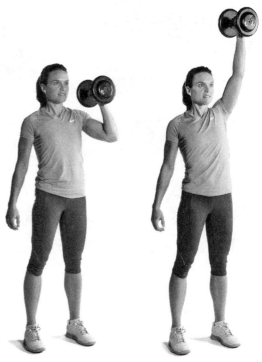

BEYOND LEVEL 5

✳ Barbell bench press

- Yeah, here it is. Flat or incline bench, your choice. Load a barbell and lie on your back with your feet shoulder-width apart and flat on the floor. Grab the bar overhand with your hands about one and a half times shoulder-width apart.

- Lift the bar off the supports and hold it straight over your chest. Tighten up everything, from your feet to your hands. You want your feet directly beneath your knees and angled out slightly. Your lower back is arched, your core is tight, and your shoulder blades are pulled together in back. Grab the bar like an iron dishrag you're trying to wring out.

- Lower the bar to your lower chest, keeping your upper arms close to your torso. Don't let your elbows flare out; you'll put more strain on your shoulders.

- Push the bar back up to the starting position, keeping your shoulder blades pulled together in back. You should feel your entire body pushing the weight, including your legs, as if you were standing up and pushing a car out of ditch.

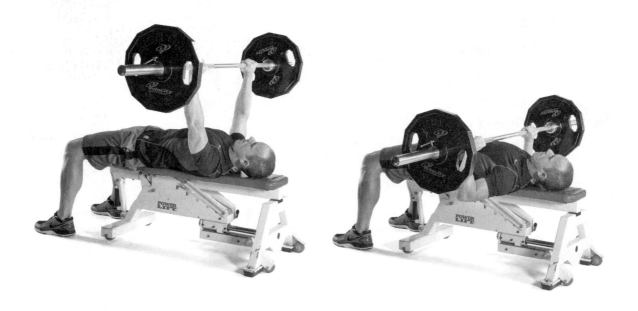

POSSIBLE SHOULDER-SAVING VARIATION

✳ Barbell board press

Same exercise, only with one or two pieces of 2-by-4 set flat on your sternum. If you use two, you can tape them together. A thick phone book works just as well. I'm supposed to recommend holding the boards in place with an elastic band, but to tell you the truth, I've never had a problem with the boards slipping off my chest. Power-lifters do this to shorten the range of motion so they can get used to lifting heavier weights and work on their lockout, which is more dependent on triceps strength. I like it because it doesn't hurt my shoulders as much as the conventional bench press.

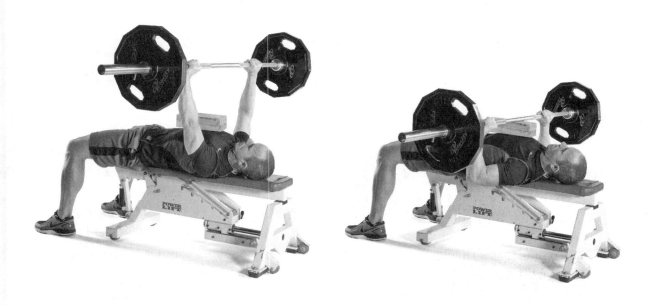

13

Pull

SITTING IS A PROBLEM for a lot of us. Or, put another way, *not moving* is a problem. We sit for longer hours each day than at any time in human history. As a result, we're fatter and schlumpier than any previous generation. So you'd think that sitting during your workout is a bad idea. If you're going to work out several times a week, you should spend that time on your feet, shouldn't you? Or at least in some posture that activates more muscles than you use when your butt's planted on a chair?

And yet, some of the most popular pulling exercises—the ones that activate the biggest muscles in your upper torso—involve sitting. You may think, "What does it hurt to sit on a bench for a cable row or a lat pulldown? After all, I'm working muscles while I'm sitting." True enough, except that many lifters also sit on the padded benches between sets. A minute of lifting might lead to three minutes of sitting.

One of the reasons Alwyn's clients typically get better-than-expected results is because he and his trainers don't let them sit down. The lat pulldown machine at Results Fitness doesn't even have a seat; you have to do pulling exercises standing or kneeling, keeping your core and postural muscles engaged throughout your workout. Alwyn brings that anti-sitting philosophy to this program. At most, you have to support yourself on a bench for a couple of the variations, but it's not a position that inspires comfortable rest between sets.

We can't claim that this simple modification will fix all the problems you want your training program to address. All it does is keep you on your feet, or at worst your knees. But it's something.

Let's talk about pulling exercises specifically. Traditionally, training programs focus on the lats, the muscles at the sides of the torso that pull your arms down and in. But those of us who measure our lifting experience in decades learn, sooner or later, that we look and feel better when we focus on the trapezius, the diamond-shaped muscle that connects the base of the neck with the shoulder blades and the middle part of the spine. In particular, the middle and lower traps, which pull your shoulder blades together and down, help improve posture. Better posture makes your shoulders look wider and, for guys at least, makes the chest muscles appear better developed.

All the exercises in this chapter work those muscles, along with the rear shoulders, in similar but slightly different ways. (See the sidebar "Gripped from the Headlines!" for more details.) Using a mix of pulls from different angles and with different hand positions ensures well-balanced muscle development.

Typically, a major goal of Alwyn's programs is to get you to the chin-up bar. The chin-up is the ultimate self-limiting exercise, as described in Chapter 8, and is one of the best measures we have of strength relative to your body's weight. It's also the most beneficial exercise I know of for developing your upper back and biceps.

Alas, it's also an exercise that very few readers will be able to do for the repetitions in Alwyn's program. You'd have to do 15 chin-ups per set in Phase One, a number I haven't hit since high school, when I weighed 40 pounds less. In Phase Two, you'd have to do multiple sets of 10. And Phase Three requires sets of 12 during highly fatiguing conditions.

That's why I recommend that everyone, beginner through advanced, start Phase One with the standing cable row, the Level 1 exercise. (If you don't have access to a cable setup, you have no choice but to start with one of the higher-level exercises.) Don't underestimate this exercise; it's fun and challenging, especially when you're doing sets of 15.

If you *can* do sets of 10, by all means use chin-ups in Phase Two, which is the most aggressive muscle-building part of Alwyn's program. Don't worry that you have to jump from Level 1 to Level 5. You've already qualified for all five levels. (You're awesome, too, in case you didn't already know.) For the rest of us, there's plenty to do in levels 1 through 4.

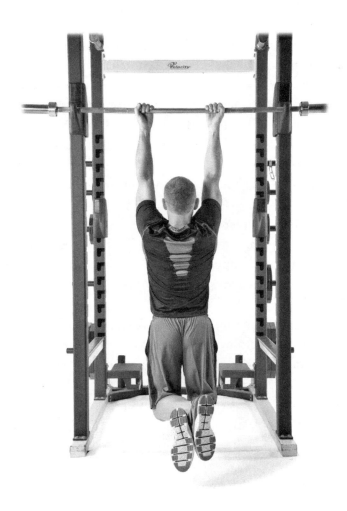

LEVEL 1

✳ Standing cable row

- Set the pulley of a cable machine to waist height, and attach a stirrup handle.
- Grab the handle in your nondominant hand (your left if you're right-handed) and step back from the machine until you have tension in the cable with your arm fully extended in front of you.
- Stand facing the machine with your feet shoulder-width apart, toes pointed forward, knees and hips bent slightly, chest up, shoulders back, and your working arm extended out in front of you. (You can rest your nonworking hand on your thigh or hip, or hold it behind your back, whichever you prefer.) Tighten your hip and torso muscles to brace your core.
- Pull the handle to the side of your torso, keeping your shoulders forward and minimizing rotation.
- Return to the starting position, do all your reps, switch arms, and repeat the set with your other arm.

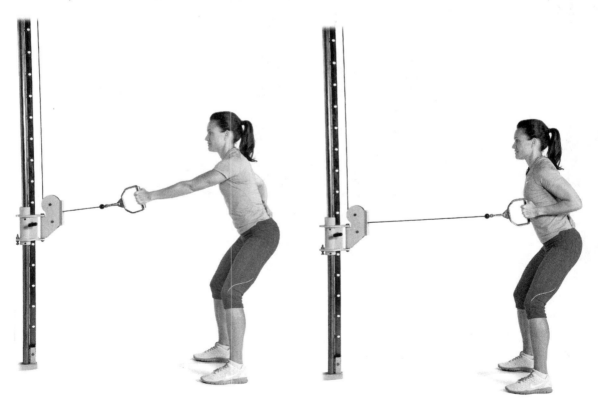

DIAL IT BACK

✳ Split-stance cable row

Same thing, only with one leg forward and the other back to give you a more stable platform. Put your right leg forward when you pull with your left hand, and vice versa. You still want to avoid rotation. Keep your shoulders square throughout the set.

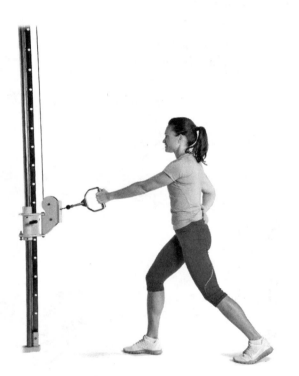
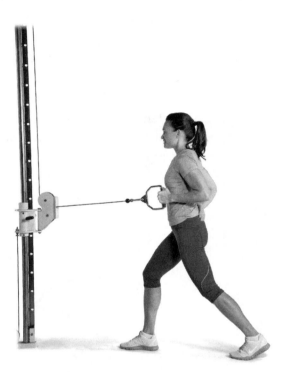

LEVEL 2

✳ Kneeling lat pulldown

- Attach a long bar to the overhead cable apparatus.
- Grab the bar overhand with a grip that's about one and a half times shoulder width (the same width you would use for a barbell bench press, if you do them).
- Kneel in front of the weight stack, pulling the bar down with you so your arms are fully extended overhead.
- Pull the bar down to your upper chest, while pushing your chest out to meet the bar. This will help you pull your shoulder blades down and back.
- After a few workouts with the wide overhand grip, you can switch to a shoulder-width underhand grip for more biceps work. Another option is the triangle handle, which gives you a narrow grip with your palms facing each other. It puts your arms in their strongest position, and allows you to use more weight than the other grips.

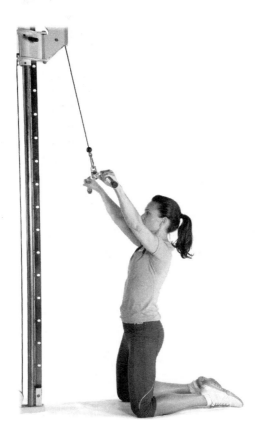 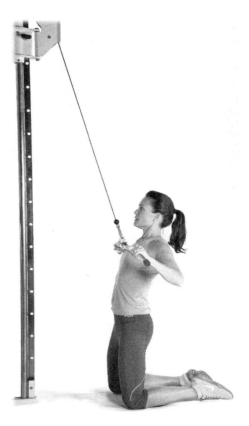

LOU'S FAVORITE VARIATION

✳ Standing lat pulldown

You can stand with your feet parallel to each other with lighter weights on high-rep sets, or with a split stance when you're getting more aggressive. You can use a wide overhand grip, a close grip, or anything in between. It turns the lat pulldown into one of the best core exercises you'll do.

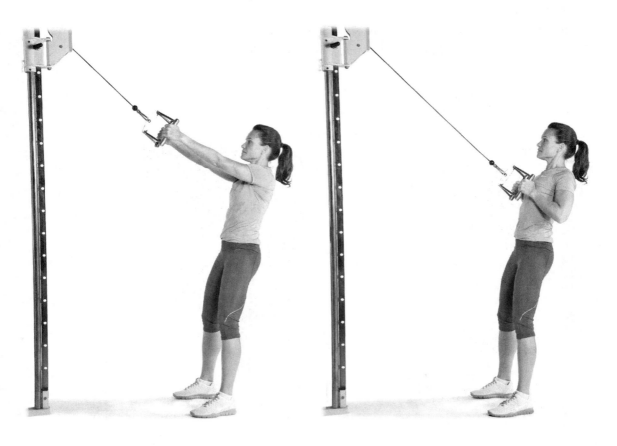

LEVEL 3, OPTION 1

✳ Dumbbell two-point row

- Grab a dumbbell with your nondominant hand. Stand with your feet shoulder-width apart and knees bent slightly.
- Push your hips back as you bend your torso forward.
- Hold the weight straight down from your shoulder with an overhand grip (palm facing back).
- Pull the weight straight up to the side of your abdomen. Lower it to the starting position, finish all your reps, then repeat the set with the other arm.

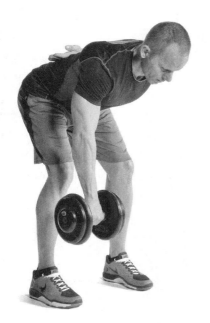 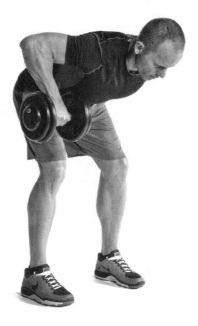

LEVEL 3, OPTION 2

✴ Dumbbell three-point row

Most lifters call the previous exercise a "bent-over" row. The most hardcore version is the barbell bent-over row, which I did often when I was younger. It allowed me to work with heavier weights than I could manage with a pair of dumbbells. But I avoided a variation that's usually called the dumbbell one-arm row. In that one, you rest your left hand and leg on a bench and set your right foot on the floor while you lift a dumbbell with your right hand. In fact, I disparaged it in *NROL* because it encourages bad habits: too much weight with poor form for one type of lifter, too little weight with too much attention to form for another.

Then I reached a point at which I could no longer do the traditional bent-over row variations. The barbell row put too much strain on my lower back, and I found it awkward and difficult to do the two-point row with a heavy weight for low reps. That's when I turned to the three-point row. It's the same as a two-point row, only with your nonworking hand resting on a bench. That extra support mechanism took all the unwanted pressure off my back and allowed me to work with the heaviest weights my back and arm muscles could lift.

My recommendation: Do the two-point row as long as you can increase weights from one workout to the next. When you hit a plateau, switch to the three-point version, and get aggressive with your weight selection. Push yourself to lift the heaviest weights possible without compromising form or falling way short of the required reps.

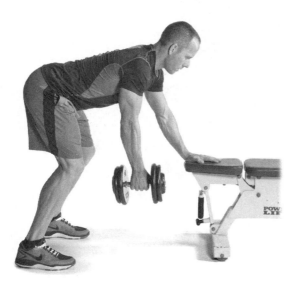
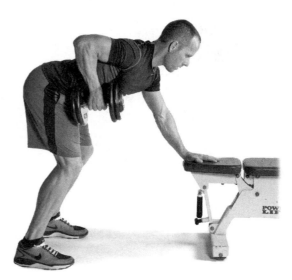

LEVEL 3, OPTION 3

✳ Dumbbell chest-supported row

- Set a bench to a 45-degree incline. Grab a pair of dumbbells and lie chest-down, with your head and shoulders beyond the top of the bench, your arms hanging straight down, and your toes on the floor.
- You can turn your palms so they face out (underhand), back (overhand), or toward each other (neutral). (See sidebar.)
- Pull the weights to the sides of your torso if you're using a neutral or underhand grip, or to the sides of your chest if you're using an overhand grip with your elbows out.

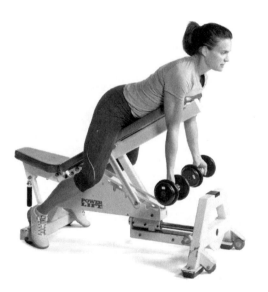 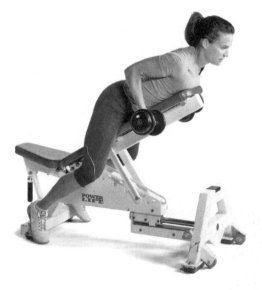

Gripped from the Headlines!

On all the pulling exercises in this chapter, your hand and elbow position can change the way you use your back, shoulder, and arm muscles. Using an underhand grip will put your biceps in their strongest position, and you'll probably feel them working harder. A neutral grip—palms facing in toward your torso—puts your arms in their strongest support position. It activates the biceps along with the brachialis (a thick muscle that lies between the biceps and your upper-arm bone) and brachioradialis (your biggest, strongest forearm muscle). An overhand grip puts the biceps in its weakest position, forcing the other muscles to do more of the work.

If you pull your elbows in close to your torso, as you would most often when using a neutral or underhand grip, you work your lats, which are responsible for pulling your upper arms in when they're extended above or in front of you. The middle part of your trapezius also contracts to pull your shoulder blades together.

When you keep your elbows out to your sides, as you typically do when using an overhand grip, you pull less with your lats and more with your rear deltoids, the muscles on the back of your shoulders. Your middle and upper traps also work hard in that position. The one drawback to the overhand grip, especially on a vertical exercise like the pull-up, is that you increase your risk of shoulder impingement. Your upper arms are close to that "high five" position described in Chapter 12, and things start to get crowded in and around your shoulder joints.

One more option: When you use a narrow grip—usually with your palms neutral or underhand—you get a bit of support from your chest muscles. I can't say how much they contribute, but I know I can always use more weight or get more reps with my body weight when I use a narrow grip.

LEVEL 4

✳ Inverted row

- Set up a barbell in a rack so it's somewhere between the height of your waist and hips. (You can also use a Smith machine for this, if you train in a gym that has one.)
- Slide under the bar and grab it overhand, with your hands just outside shoulder width. Set your body in a straight line from neck to ankles, and hang with your arms straight. Only your heels should touch the floor.
- Pull your chest to the bar, return to the starting position, and repeat.

- If you can't get all the reps in your current phase, raise the bar a few inches, which will make it a little easier.

- If you need to make it harder, you can lower the bar only so far before you lose the room you need to do the exercise with a full range of motion. You can raise your feet up on a bench or, if you're really advanced, you can put them on a Swiss ball. The unstable surface adds a serious core challenge to what's already a tough exercise for your upper-back muscles.

- For variety, and more direct biceps work, you can use an underhand grip.

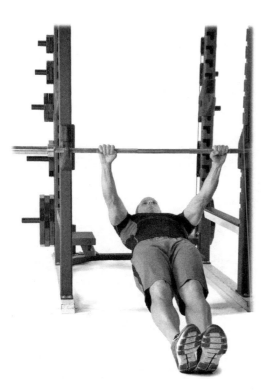 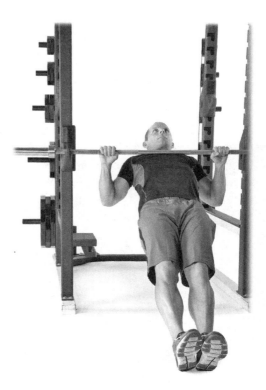

COOL VARIATION

✳ Suspended row

- Attach a suspension system—TRX or equivalent—to a chin-up bar.
- Grab the handles so you're facing the overhead support they're attached to and walk out until you have enough room to extend your arms without hitting the floor.
- Hang from the straps so your body forms a straight line from your neck to ankles. Only your heels should touch the floor.
- Pull yourself up until the handles reach the sides of your torso, lower yourself, and repeat.
- The beauty of a suspension system is that you can make the exercise easier by moving your heels closer to the point of attachment, thus increasing the angle of your body relative to the floor. Or you can make it harder by shifting your heels farther from the attachment, and lowering your body so it's closer to the floor. You can make this adjustment in the middle of a set if you need to.

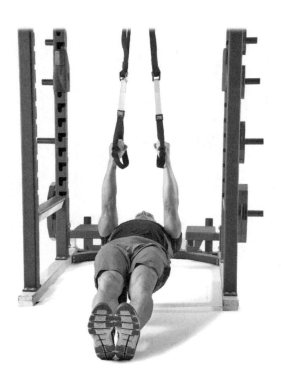 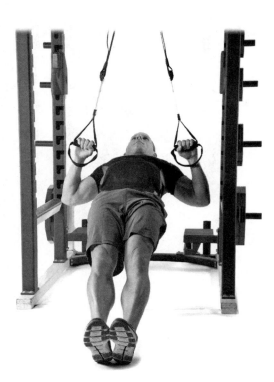

LEVEL 5
✳ **Chin-up**

- Grab the chin-up bar with a shoulder-width, underhand grip, and hang from the bar with your knees bent and ankles crossed behind you. Your body should form a straight line from neck to knees.
- Pull your chest up to the bar, lower yourself, and repeat.

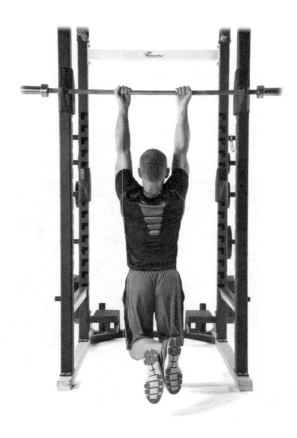

BEYOND LEVEL 5

✳ Pull-up

I never had a problem with this exercise when I was younger, but in middle age it just wrecks my shoulders. I assume that I've either worn out something in my joints that used to provide a cushion, or I've added bone or scar tissue that narrows the space. All I know for sure is that something rubs something the wrong way. I don't mind; I can do chin-ups without pain, and they offer as much challenge as I can handle. If you can do pull-ups without pain for sets of 10 or more, have at it.

- Grab the bar overhand, with your hands just outside shoulder width, and set your posture as described above.
- Pull your chest up to the bar, lower yourself, and repeat.

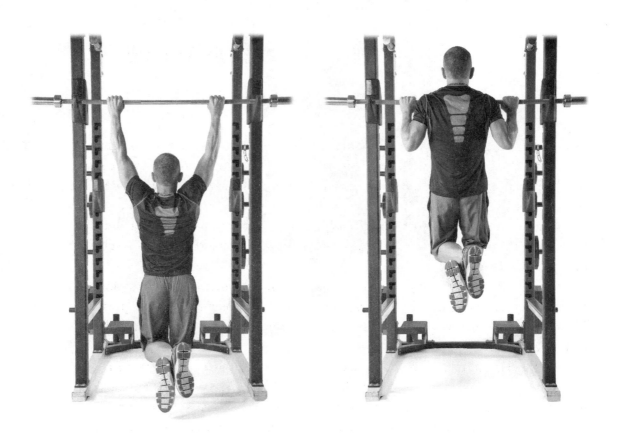

Combination
Exercises

14

THE EXERCISES IN THIS CHAPTER are here for two reasons: They use a lot of muscle, and they require a lot of effort. Picture yourself doing a lunge with a shoulder press. Already, the lunge is a complicated move, one that requires some balance and coordination as you lower and then raise your center of gravity. Add a shoulder press to the movement, and now you've created a bigger coordination challenge. You lower the center of gravity on the lunge, but also raise it as you simultaneously lift a weight over your shoulders.

There's nothing efficient about this movement. You're using all kinds of muscles to stabilize your body that you wouldn't need if you were doing a lunge or a press. The result is an acute oxygen deficit; it takes some time to catch your breath at the end of each set.

Another benefit of combination exercises: Like everything you do in the weight room, they pull glycogen from your working muscles. The more muscles you use, and the longer you use them, the more fuel you expend. You're also breaking down muscle tissue. Restoring that fuel, and rebuilding those muscles, is your body's highest priority in the hours following a workout. (This assumes you eat in a way that supports this process, which we'll cover in Chapter 18.) It's a metabolically expensive process all around:

- It takes more energy to do the complicated exercises.
- It takes more energy to recover from them afterward.

You'll work hard, breathe hard, and open the spigots to your sweat glands. When I was going through the program in the summer of 2011, I once walked out of the gym into a rain shower. I'd brought an umbrella but didn't bother putting it up because I was already soaked with my own perspiration. The rain helped me cool off, and I barely noticed the extra water on my clothes.

LEVEL 1

✳ Single-leg, single-arm cable row

The first combo exercise in the program is, admittedly, not really a combo exercise. Some of your lower-body muscles are moving, but they aren't truly challenged. For that matter, you won't be able to use much weight on the row, either. The demand for balance prevents an all-out effort by your upper back and arm muscles. But it's a hellacious challenge to your core, forcing your lats, lower back, glutes, and hamstrings to find a way to work with each other. That makes it a perfect choice to introduce your body to this category of exercise.

- Attach a D-shaped handle to an adjustable cable pulley and raise it to about mid-thigh height. (If your gym's cable machine doesn't adjust, use the low setting. And if you don't have a cable machine, a band will work.)
- Grab the handle with your nondominant hand and step back far enough to ensure tension in the cable throughout the range of motion.
- Facing the cable with your arm extended in front of you, lift your nondominant foot off the floor, so you're balancing on your dominant leg.
- Bend forward at the hips until your torso is at a 45-degree angle to the floor.
- Fire your hip muscles to straighten your body while at the same time pulling the handle to the side of your abdomen.
- Immediately bend forward and extend your arm to begin the next repetition. Do all your reps, then switch sides and repeat.

- Your first goal is to do all the reps with good form, which means you remain balanced on one leg throughout the set. Your second goal is to establish a rhythm with the movement, and then speed up the rhythm, so it's smooth and fast. Your third goal is to make the movement powerful; that is, really fire your hips forward and pull hard on the cable. The final goal is to move heavier weight with a smooth but powerful action.

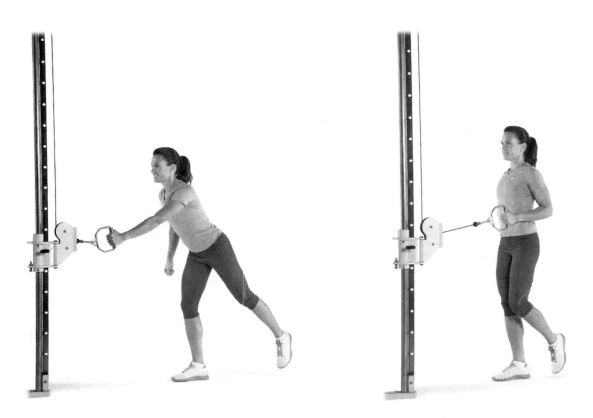

LEVEL 2

✳ Reverse lunge and cable row

- Set up the cable machine as described above, grab the attachment with your nondominant hand, and step back to create tension in the cable.
- Stand facing the machine with your arm extended and feet hip-width apart.
- Take a long step back into a reverse lunge with your nondominant leg, leaving your arm extended in front of you.
- As you return to the starting position, pull the handle to the side of your abdomen.
- Immediately step back and extend your arm to begin the next repetition. Do all your reps, then switch sides and repeat.
- This one will seem easy after the coordination challenges of the Level 1 exercise. Once you have the hang of it, you can increase weights quickly without compromising your form.

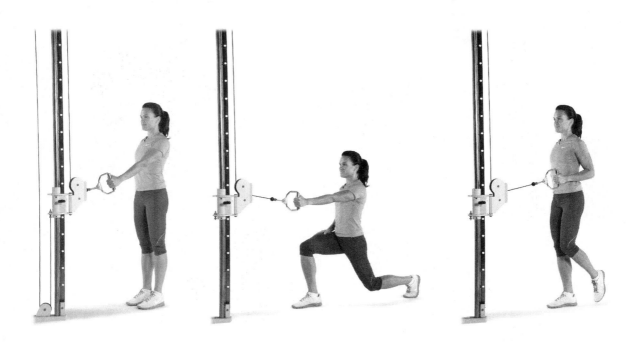

LEVEL 3

✳ Romanian deadlift and row

You can do this with dumbbells or a barbell. I recommend the barbell; the form is easier to learn when you're controlling one versus two moving objects. Another worry is that your upper-back and gripping muscles will get too fatigued when you're working with dumbbells. I'll describe it as if you're using a barbell, but of course it's your call which to use.

- Grab the barbell overhand, your hands just outside shoulder width. Stand holding it at arm's length against your front thighs, with your feet about shoulder-width apart.
- Push your hips back and lower the bar until it's just below your knees. Your knees will bend slightly.
- Pull the bar straight up to your lower abdomen without raising your torso.
- Lower the bar until your arms are fully extended again.
- Push your hips forward and return to the starting position. That's one rep.

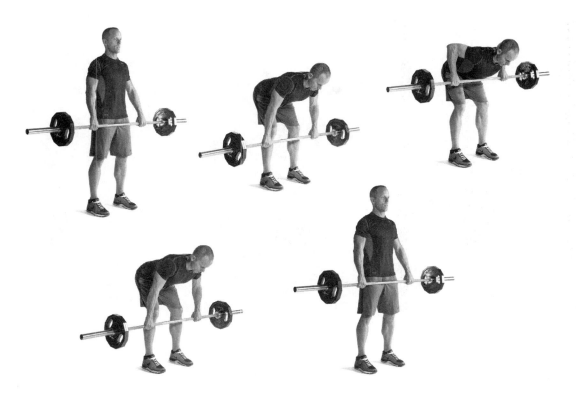

LEVEL 4

✳ Squat and press

- Stand holding a pair of dumbbells at the sides of your shoulders. You can turn your palms in or have them facing out, whichever is easier on your shoulder joints. Set your feet shoulder-width apart, toes pointed forward or angled out slightly.
- Push your hips back and lower yourself into a squat.
- As you return to the starting position, press the weights straight up over your shoulders. Lower them to the starting position, and immediately drop into a squat to begin the next repetition.

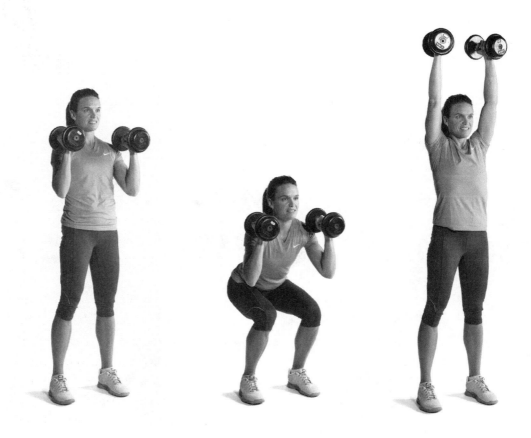

LEVEL 5

✳ Reverse lunge and single-arm press

- Stand holding a dumbbell just outside the shoulder on your non-dominant side. Your feet are hip-width apart.
- Take a long step back into a lunge position with your nondominant leg as you press the dumbbell straight up over your shoulder.
- Lower the weight as you step back to the starting position.
- Do all your reps, then switch sides and repeat.

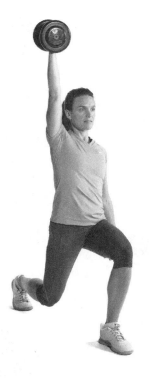

BEYOND LEVEL 5

✳ Use your imagination

- You can combine an overhead press with any of the lunge variations shown in Chapter 10, including the Beyond Level 5 suggestions at the end. You can do a reverse lunge from a step, or a forward lunge onto a step. The most hated exercise in the original *NROL* was the Bulgarian split squat with overhead press. So if you're feeling masochistic, try that one.
- If you're feeling blasphemous toward Alwyn, you can do biceps curls instead of presses or rows. On the Romanian deadlift and row, for example, you would hold the bar with an underhand grip. Push your hips back and lower the bar, as described, but instead of doing a bent-over row, fire your hips forward, curling the weight toward your shoulders as you return to the standing position. Lower the weight, then push your hips back to begin the next repetition.
- Finally, you can combine single- or double-arm shoulder presses to any of the step-up variations shown in Chapter 11. If you're doing a single-arm press, use your right arm if you're stepping up with your right leg, and your left with your left.

15

Take the
On-RAMP

I'VE DISCOVERED THE HARD WAY how important it is to prepare middle-aged muscles and joints for a good workout. The more thoroughly I warm up, the better my training sessions go, allowing me to get more done in less time. But when I skimp on my warm-up routines, I inevitably end up with knotted muscles and a compromised range of motion.

Alwyn's RAMP protocol is designed to help you avoid that. You'll start with simple range-of-motion exercises—the R in RAMP—and move on to faster movements that wake up your muscles and nervous system. That's the A, for "activation." The MP stands for "movement preparation," which you'll accomplish throughout the 10-minute routine.

Some of Alwyn's movements look different from what everyone else in the gym is doing. I include some modifications—noted as "social anxiety" options—for exercises that might draw unwanted attention. Other drills simply can't be performed in a crowded health club, where you can't move more than a step or two in any direction without bumping into another gridlocked exerciser. Those are the "no space" options.

You'll use this same protocol before every workout. As you get accustomed to the program, you may decide to add or change some things around, either from boredom or because of an injury that requires more focus in one particular area. You may find you train better when you use the recovery exercises in Chapter 18 as part of your warm-up. (It seems to work better for me.) The only rule is, do this as written until you have good reason to change it.

One other tip: Feel free to do more total work on one side than the other. Most of us have discrepancies in strength, balance, and mobility. That's why the strength chapters have you start single-limb exercises with your nondominant side. But when it comes to balance and mobility, the dominant side might be more restricted as a consequence of using it more. Whatever needs the most improvement should get the most attention, as long as you don't ignore the less-restricted side. That would just create new problems.

RAMP • Use at the start of each A and B workout	
Exercise	Reps/distance
Kneeling hip-flexor/lat stretch (page 174)	30 seconds each side
Single-leg hip raise (page 174)	8 each side
Open one-half kneeling adductor/ankle mobilization (page 175)	8 each side
Open one-half kneel with T reach (page 176)	8 each side
Squat to stand (page 177)	6
Wall slide (page 178)	10
Forward/backward jump (page 179)	20
Walking knee hug to forward lunge (page 179)	8 each leg
Side-to-side jump (page 180)	10 each direction
Walking lateral lunge (page 180)	8 each direction
Skipping (page 181)	2 runs of 10–20 yards
Carioca (page 182)	2 runs of 10–20 yards
Side shuffle (page 183)	2 runs of 10–20 yards

✳ Kneeling hip-flexor stretch

- Kneel on a pad on your right knee, with your left foot flat on the floor in front of you and your knee bent. You can put your hands wherever you prefer: on your left leg, on your hips, or in the prisoner grip behind your head.
  - Shift your weight forward, keeping your torso upright, until you feel a stretch on the right side of your pelvis.
  - Hold for 30 seconds, then switch sides and repeat.

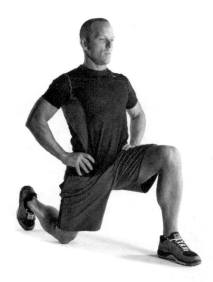

✳ Single-leg hip raise

- Lie on your back on the floor, with your knees bent, heels on the floor, and arms out to your sides. Lift your dominant leg a few inches off the floor.
- Push down through the heel of your nondominant foot and lift your hips off the floor as high as you can. You should feel it mostly in your glutes, partly in your hamstrings, and not at all in your back.
- Lower your hips close to the floor, and repeat.
- Do all your reps, then switch legs and repeat.

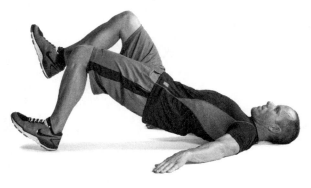

✳ Open one-half kneeling adductor/ankle mobilization

- Kneel on a pad on your right knee. Open your left leg to your side, perpendicular to your torso, with your knee bent 90 degrees and your foot flat on the floor, pointing the same direction as your left knee.
- Place the back of your left hand on the inside of your left knee, with your right hand on your right hip. Straighten your torso and pull your shoulders back.
- Keeping your torso upright, shift your weight to your left while pushing back on your knee with your left hand. Feel the stretch in your left inner thigh.
- Return to the starting position, do all your reps, and repeat with your right leg.

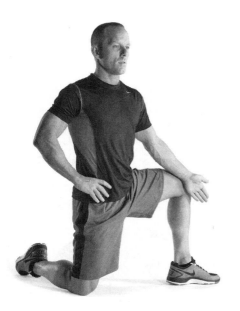
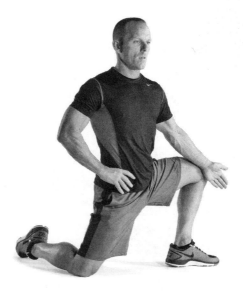

✳ Open one-half kneel with T reach

- Get into the open half-kneel position described above.
- Bend forward at the hips and place your left hand on the floor. Your torso is parallel to the floor, with your left hand directly beneath your shoulder.
- Turn your torso to the right and reach straight up with your right arm until your fingers point to the ceiling. Your arms should be in a straight line, perpendicular to the floor. Follow your hand with your eyes so your neck turns along with your torso.
- Turn your torso back toward the floor, bringing your arm back down, across, and slightly beyond your torso. That's one rep. Do all your reps, then switch sides and repeat.

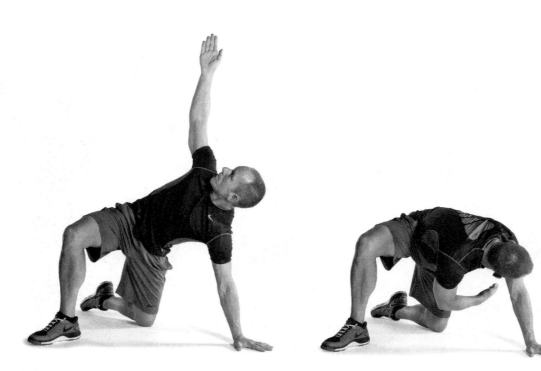

✳ Squat to stand

- Stand with your hands to your sides and your feet shoulder-width apart.
- Bend at the hips, keeping your legs straight, and reach toward your toes.
- Push your hips back, bend your knees, and descend into a squat, grabbing your toes whenever you can and pulling yourself down into the deepest squat you can manage. Keep your arms straight and just inside your knees, with your feet flat on the floor.
- Pull your shoulders and head back as you tighten your entire upper body.
- Raise your arms overhead and stand.
- Immediately start the next rep by bending at the hips and reaching toward the floor.

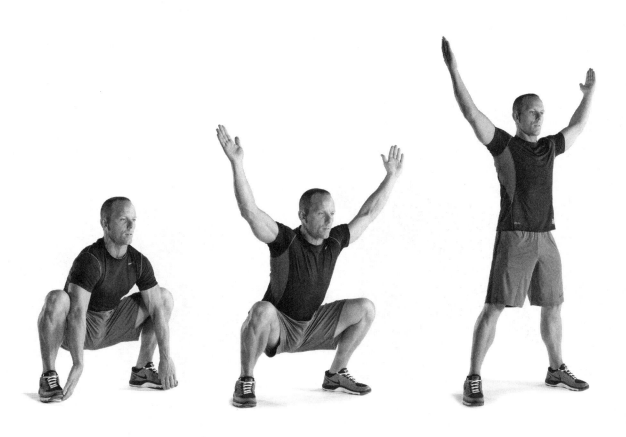

✳ Wall slide

Chapter 12 describes all the reasons you shouldn't lift with your arms in the "high five" position—upper arms out to your sides, elbows bent, fingers pointed toward the ceiling. This exercise uses that position to help alleviate shoulder problems by improving the mobility and stability of the complex and quirky joints and connective tissues of your upper back.

- Stand with your head, upper back, and glutes against a wall.
- Raise your arms in the high five position, with the back of your hands, wrists, and elbows touching the wall. Those three parts—along with your head, upper back, and glutes—must remain in contact with the wall throughout the exercise. Your range of motion is determined by how far you can go without losing one of those six points of contact.
- Pull your arms down toward your torso, keeping your elbows bent about 90 degrees. When you can't go any farther without losing contact, slide them back up the wall. Reach as high as you can. That's one rep. Repeat until you finish 10 reps.
- Work to expand your range of motion in subsequent workouts.

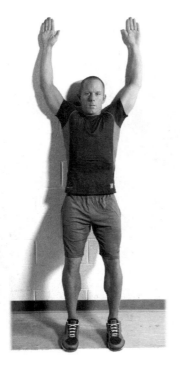
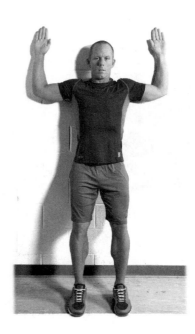

✳ Forward/backward jump

- Stand with your feet together, hands at your sides, and your knees, ankles, and hips all bent slightly.
- Jump forward a few inches, landing on the balls of your feet, and immediately jump back to the starting line. That counts as one jump; do a total of 20.

✳ Walking knee hug to forward lunge

- Stand with your feet hip-width apart, hands at your sides.
- Lift your right knee and pull it to your chest with both hands.
- Release your knee and take a long step forward with your right leg, lowering yourself into a lunge.
- As you come up from the lunge, step forward with your left leg and pull your left knee to your chest.
- Release your knee and start the next lunge by taking a long step forward with your right leg.
- That's one repetition; do a total of 8.

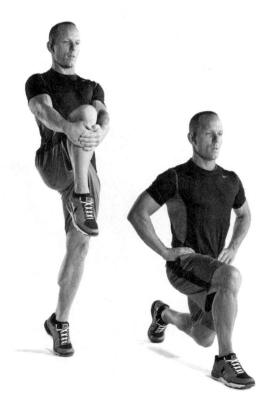

✳ Side-to-side jump

- Stand with your feet together and your hips, knees, and ankles bent slightly.
- Jump a few inches to your left, landing on your toes, then jump back to your right.
- Do 10 jumps in each direction; keep your landings soft, and get off the ground for your next jump as quickly as possible.

✳ Walking lateral lunge

- This drill, like the three that follow, requires a space where you can travel 10 to 20 yards without crashing into anyone or anything.
- Stand with your right side toward the open space, your feet hip-width apart, and your arms at your sides or in front of your chest.
- Take a long step to your right and drop into a side lunge, with your right knee bent 90 degrees, your left leg straight, and the toes of both feet pointed straight ahead. Your torso will lean forward, but you need to keep your shoulders square, not leaning or twisting to the side.
- As you rise up, bring your left foot over to your right, then take another long step to your right.
- Do 8 lunges to your right, then return to the starting point by doing 8 lunges to your left.

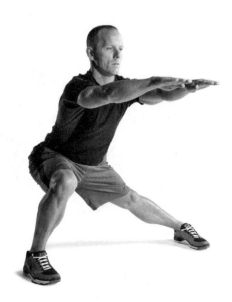

NO-SPACE OPTION

Lunge to your left, then lunge back to your right, and alternate until you've done 8 each direction.

✷ Skipping

Forgot how? Join the club. Boys of my generation didn't skip, and since I went to Catholic schools, where the girls had to wear skirts, they weren't real big on skipping either. You're going for an exaggerated running motion: Drive your right knee and left arm up and forward, lifting you off the floor. As your right toes touch the floor, drive your left knee and right arm up to start the next skip. You're going more for height than distance or speed. Do two runs of 10 to 20 yards.

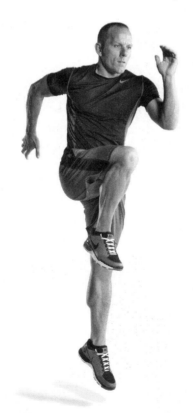

NO-SPACE/SOCIAL ANXIETY OPTION

Skip in place, driving each knee up with maximum acceleration.

✳ Carioca

This move may be unfamiliar to most readers. Even those of us who learned it for high school or college sports are probably rusty. It's a lateral-movement drill in which your trailing leg alternately crosses behind and in front of your lead leg. So let's say you're doing a carioca to your left. You start as you would for the walking lateral lunge shown above. Then:

- Swing your right foot behind and past your left foot.
- Take a long step to the left with your left foot.
- Swing your right foot in front of and past your left foot.
- Take a long step to the left with your left foot.
- Repeat until you've gone 10 to 20 yards, stop, catch your breath, and repeat, this time moving to your right.

It doesn't feel like much of an exercise when you do it slowly. That's why you need to speed it up as soon as you get the hang of it. When you go fast, your hips rotate rapidly, and your shoulders turn with your hips. Let your arms do whatever they want. It's fun to cut loose and let your body figure it out.

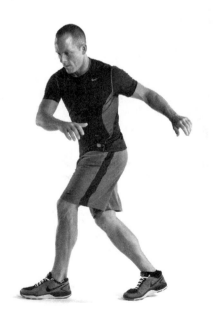
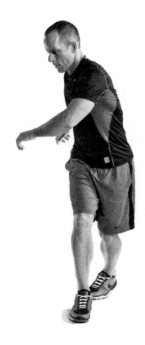

NO-SPACE/SOCIAL ANXIETY OPTION

There isn't really anything that replaces the carioca. But you can try a crossover jumping jack. Instead of bringing your feet together as your arms come down, cross them in front of and behind each other, alternating on each rep. You can also cross your arms in front instead of lifting them overhead.

✳ Side shuffle

- From the same starting point as the carioca and lateral lunge, get into an athletic position with your feet wider than your shoulders, knees bent slightly, torso leaning forward, arms out to your sides. It should look like you're guarding someone in basketball.
- Slide your right foot until it touches your left.
- Immediately step to the left with your left foot, and slide your right foot to meet it.
- Continue for 10 to 20 yards, stop, catch your breath, and repeat by sliding to your right.

NO-SPACE/SOCIAL ANXIETY OPTION

You can't really do this without some space. As for social anxiety, it's still going to look different from what everyone else is doing. But it's a good exercise, especially when you move fast.

- Shuffle twice to your left, then reach and touch the floor outside your left foot with your right hand.
- Shuffle twice to your right, reaching and touching the floor outside your right foot with your left hand. Do 10 to each side.

16

Metabolic Training

IMAGINE THAT YOU'RE JUST STARTING a fitness program, and you ask a trainer for advice. "Here's what I want you to do on the first day," he says. "Hop 750 times with your right leg. Then hop 750 times with your left leg."

"That's nuts!" you say, stating the obvious. What kind of dipstick would tell a beginner to perform a total of 1,500 high-impact plyometric movements, hitting two different sets of muscles and joints 750 times each?

"Okay," he says. "Do 750 hops, but alternate legs. And move forward while you do it."

So you try it, and you realize that it's a lot like running. In fact, Alwyn says, with only slight exaggeration, it *is* running, which he considers a high-impact exercise for a beginner, especially one who's overweight. A mile run is at least 750 joint-jarring steps for each leg. With a shorter stride, it could be a thousand or more.

And yet, on any given day, countless entry-level exercisers go out running. In Chapter 4 I mentioned two all-too-frequent consequences: They'll get hurt, and they'll gain weight. "What's the alternative?" you might ask.

"What's the goal?" Alwyn would say in reply. Is it to be a runner? Or is it to burn

184

calories, develop cardiovascular fitness, and in general feel like you have more energy and can go longer before getting winded?

If the goal is to be a runner, then of course you have to run. Same if you want to be a cyclist, swimmer, or any other type of endurance athlete. Alwyn has worked with athletes in all those sports. He's also been a champion martial artist, and trained fighters. In fact, he's worked with athletes in almost any individual and team sport you can name, from preteen gymnasts to superheavyweight powerlifters to one of the world's highest-paid soccer players. To my surprise, and probably yours, he says that actual cardio fitness plays less of a role than you would think.

Once you can run a mile, he says, you can probably walk 20 miles. Your feet would be sore afterward, but you wouldn't collapse before you got to the finish line. Cardio endurance wouldn't be a limiting factor at such low intensity. But if you tried to jog those 20 miles, without specifically training for that distance, you'd be in a world of pain and misery. You wouldn't come close to finishing. It would take years to develop enough muscular endurance, neuromuscular efficiency, joint stability, and pain tolerance. You would, in a way, have to reengineer your body: developing extensive capillary networks in the working muscles; increasing your muscles' ability to store glycogen while at the same time teaching your body to use more fat and less carbohydrate for energy; and repurposing muscle fibers for endurance at the expense of strength and power.

Alwyn offers this example: Lance Armstrong may be the most gifted endurance athlete in U.S. history. His VO2 max, the standard measure of aerobic performance, was an astounding 83 at the height of his cycling career. (The only time I had mine tested, in 2000, it was 41.6—half of Armstrong's.) When he decided to run the New York City Marathon in 2006, *Runner's World* magazine interviewed several experts on endurance training. No one suggested Armstrong would win, but one said that Armstrong's superhuman VO2 max is the equivalent of a 2:06 marathon. As it happened, the winner ran the 26.2-mile course in 2 hours, 9 minutes, and 58 seconds. Armstrong finished 50 minutes behind. It was still an amazing and gutsy performance; fewer than 900 runners finished in less than 3 hours, and more than 37,000 were slower (including then Arkansas governor Mike Huckabee, who had recently lost 110 pounds). But it also shows the specificity of each sport's demands on your body. Armstrong was quoted after the race as saying it was "without a doubt the hardest physical thing I've ever done."

You may wonder why we're talking about marathon training in a chapter that tells you what to do in the final 5 to 10 minutes of each workout. Alwyn's point: When the goal is to burn calories, or get a heart-rate response, or feel more "fit," however you define it, *the activity doesn't matter.* If you could get all that by doing calisthenics, or swinging a kettlebell, or carrying something heavy, would you feel cheated because you didn't get to run?

Now, if you *want* to run, don't let any of this stop you. It's certainly one of the options. Here are Alwyn's three rules for metabolic training:

- *It should be intermittent.* That is, it should be done as interval training: Go hard for 15 to 30 seconds, recover, and then go hard again.
- *It should be anaerobic.* You should breathe hard and get your heart rate up. The pace should be exhilarating, and at times you should feel as if you're doing something you didn't think you could do.
- *It should* not *cause any joint pain, during or after.* If something hurts your knees, ankles, hips, back, or shoulders, try something else.

Whatever you decide to try—we'll show you all the options next—you should do it in 1-minute rounds. Each workout in Alwyn's program calls for 5 to 10 minutes of metabolic training, which means 5 to 10 rounds.

Those who're new to training should start with a 3-to-1 ratio of recovery to work. If you work for 15 seconds, you would rest for 45. Most readers should shoot for a 2-to-1 ratio: go hard for 20 seconds, recover for 40. Advanced lifters can make it 1-to-1: 30 seconds on, 30 seconds off.

You can stick with one or two exercises for consecutive workouts, counting reps and working to improve your performance from week to week. Or you can do something different every week, with the goal of making your body train harder by doing unfamiliar activities.

Once you get the idea, you can try just about anything you want, as long as you follow the three rules, plus this one: Avoid exercises in which the working muscles fatigue before the end of your interval. For example, if you decided to do push-ups for the entire interval, after the first couple of rounds your chest, shoulder, and triceps muscles would burn out too soon. You'd end up with shorter work periods and longer recovery, which would compromise the program (although you'd certainly get better at doing push-ups).

Everything else is in the mix, including many of the exercises in the strength program. You can also use any toys at your disposal: barbell, dumbbells, kettlebells, battling ropes, dragging sleds, TRX-style suspension trainers, gymnastics rings, slides, sandbags.

Final tip from Nanny Lou: Make sure you do any high-impact exercises on a forgiving surface. If you can't work on carpet, at least find a wood floor that can absorb impact. I say this as someone who never had a knee problem until I played pick-up basketball on asphalt and concrete, and I've had nothing but knee problems since.

Now let's get to the fun stuff.

LEVEL 1 OPTIONS

✳ Body-weight squat

Go as fast as you can with good form (as described in Chapter 8) for 15 seconds, then rest for 45.

✳ Step-up

This is different from the exercise shown and described in Chapter 11. Start with both feet on the floor. Step up with your right, up with your left, down with your right, down with your left. Continue for 15 seconds, then rest for 45. Start the next round by stepping up first with your left foot. As soon as you get the hang of it, work to increase the pace of your steps in each round.

✳ Shadow boxing

Pick an imaginary opponent, and kick his or her imaginary butt. Just keep in mind that your opponent is also trying to hit you. So keep your guard up, move your feet, duck and twist to dodge punches, and throw combinations of jabs, crosses, uppercuts, and the occasional haymaker. Try for 20 seconds on, 40 seconds off.

LEVEL 2 AND 3 OPTIONS

✳ Burpee

Stand with your feet hip-width apart. Squat down and put your hands on the floor outside your feet. Kick your legs backward so you're in the push-up position. Pull them back in, and jump, throwing your arms overhead and coming all the way up off the floor. Land and go straight to the next rep.

✳ Kettlebell swing

Exactly as described in Chapter 7, only with a lighter weight and higher reps performed at a faster speed.

✳ Box jump

Again, it's the same exercise shown in Chapter 7. You probably want a lower box so you can work at a faster pace.

✳ Squat/push-up combo

Do body-weight squats (or jump squats, if you're more advanced) for half the interval, then switch to push-ups for the second half.

LEVEL 4 AND 5 OPTIONS

✳ Barbell matrix

Load a barbell with a weight you're sure you can use for all three exercises. Grab the bar with a shoulder-width, overhand grip and do 10 reps each of these:

- Bent-over row
- Front squat
- Shoulder press

After a few workouts with that matrix, try this variation:

- Pick up the barbell, bend forward at the hips, and do a bent-over row.
- Straighten your body, and "clean" the bar to your shoulders. Shrug your shoulders

to get the bar moving, then dip your knees and hips as you flip the bar up to your shoulders. It'll end up in what Olympic lifters call the "rack" position, which is the starting position for the front squat.

- Straighten your body again, and do a front squat.
- As you come up, roll the bar forward from your fingertips to your palms to get into the starting position for the shoulder press.
- Press the bar overhead.
- Lower it to your thighs to complete the first repetition, and repeat.
- Do as many as you can for 30 seconds, rest 30 seconds, and repeat for 5 to 10 rounds. (You may want to start with 20 seconds of work and 40 seconds of rest; it's a pretty tough drill.)

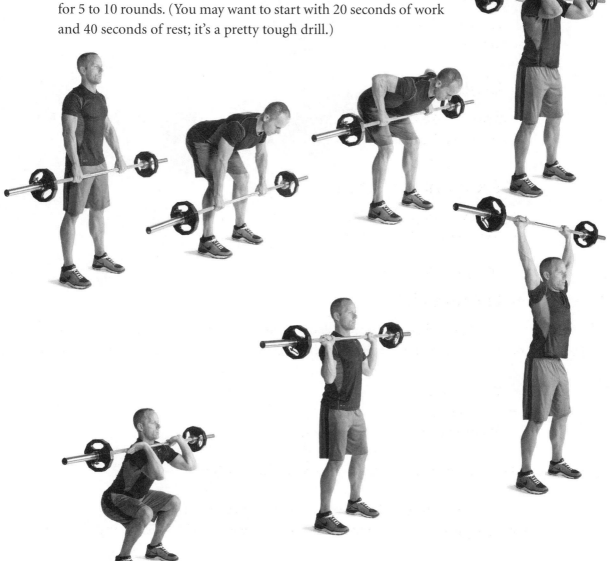

✳ Farmer's walk

Grab a pair of heavy dumbbells, walk for 30 seconds, set them down for 30 seconds, and repeat. You can also do this with a pair of barbells.

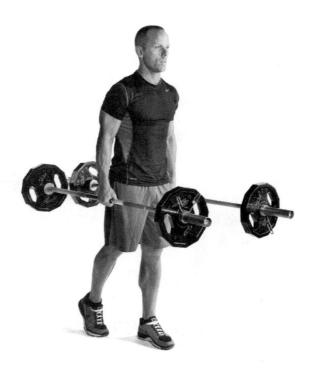

✳ Sprint

You really want to run? Outdoors or on an indoor track, run hard for 20 seconds, walk for 40 seconds, and repeat. Even better: Sprint up a hill, walk down, and repeat. You can do the same thing on a bicycle, either outdoors or inside on a stationary bike.

BEYOND LEVEL 5 OPTIONS

In no particular order:

✳ Jump rope

This is one of those things, like single-leg squats and skiing, that I've often wished I could do. But when I was younger I didn't have the coordination, and in middle age my joints can't take the impact. If you know how to jump rope and the impact isn't a problem, it's a great option.

✳ Take the stairs

At home or the gym (or anywhere, really), sprint up and down the steps, touching the floor at the top and bottom, for the duration of the interval. You can add push-ups at the bottom or top if you want to make it ever harder.

✳ Hit a heavy bag

If you have access to martial-arts equipment, you can kick or punch a heavy bag. Just make sure you wrap your hands or wear gloves.

✳ Turn your yard into a gym

You can chop wood, hit a tire with a sledgehammer (lots of private training studios now have tires and things to hit them with), or push a wheelbarrow filled with dirt or firewood. Another option is to push your car up and down the street, assuming you can find someone you trust to steer and not hit the brakes at random moments.

How to Build a Workout

BEFORE YOU BUILD YOUR OWN WORKOUT, let's review the basic parameters:

1. You're going to do two workouts—A and B—for each of the three phases.
2. Each workout starts with RAMP, which will be the same set of exercises for everyone. (You can modify it as you see fit, as I explained in Chapter 15, but for now let's assume you're going to do it as written.)
3. You'll need to select exercises for the next four parts of the workout: core, power, strength, and metabolic training.
4. Those are followed by recovery (Chapter 18). As with RAMP, we'll assume for now that you're going to use the recovery exercises as shown.
5. As you know from Chapter 5, the strength exercises you choose for Phase One are ones that you can do for one or two sets of 15 repetitions. If you're a beginner, you may not be able to do any of them 10 times, much less 15. Not a problem. You have to start somewhere, and you'll build strength and endurance quickly. For more advanced lifters, keep in mind that you have to be able to make progress from one

workout to the next. When you can do 15 reps for both sets, you have to add weight, increase the difficulty, or move up to the next level of that category.

6. The strength program in Phase Two calls for two to four sets of 10 reps. Pick exercises that allow you to increase both weight and volume. That will mean different types of choices in different exercise categories. You may need to go to a higher-level exercise in one category, and a lower-level exercise in another. The goal is to increase the amount of weight you lift as well as the volume of lifting you perform.

7. In Phase Three, pick exercises that allow you to perform two to three sets of 12 reps. You're adding a fifth exercise to each strength workout, and looking for improved conditioning. You want to breathe hard and get sweaty, if you haven't been doing that all along. (I know I did, starting with the first workout in Phase One.) This is where you go from grinding it out to *performing*. You should feel smoother, faster, lighter, more athletic. Alwyn calls this phase "Maximize" for a reason: You want to bring everything you have with the goal of emerging with more than you ever thought possible.

Realistically, there's only so much transforming, developing, and maximizing you can do in 12 weeks. That's why the program is set up to be repeatable. The second time through, you can do higher-level exercises, do the same ones with heavier loads, do more sets of each exercise, or some combination. Whatever you don't accomplish the second time through, you can try the third time. Or the fourth. An inexperienced lifter can do this program for a year and see improvements each time.

Advanced lifters can repeat the program using heavier weights for lower reps. The second time through, you can do two to three sets of 12 reps in Phase One, four sets of 8 reps in Phase Two, and two to three sets of 10 in Phase Three.

Once you get comfortable with the template, you can even fill in some of your own exercises. We could fill an entire book with push-up variations, or exercises you can do with a Swiss ball or TRX, or single-leg-stance exercises. This book has more exercises than any of its predecessors, and we've still just scratched the surface.

Advanced lifters can also vary sets and reps by movement pattern. You can stick with higher reps and lighter weights for exercises that require more balance and stability, but go heavier with the big-muscle exercises like squats, deadlifts, chin-ups, presses, and rows.

Now it's time to take a look at the workout templates. Remember that you can either start with these blank slates and fill in your own exercises, or use the done-for-you programs that we offer as examples. If you choose to fill in your own, you'll find lists of all the exercise options right after the templates. You can photocopy the templates in this book, download blank copies at thenewrulesoflifting.com, or get free training logs at werkit.com.

PHASE ONE: TRANSFORM

Workout A

Category/exercise	Sets/reps	Workout 1	Workout 2	Workout 3	Workout 4
Core					
Stability	2 x 30 seconds*				
Dynamic Stability	2 x 10				
Power					
Lower body	2 x 5				
Strength					
1a. Squat	1–2 x 15				
1b. Pull	1–2 x 15				
2a. Single-leg stance	1–2 x 15				
2b. Push	1–2 x 15				
Metabolic					
	5–10 minutes				

* You can hold for as long as 60 seconds if you find you've selected an exercise that you can easily hold beyond 30 seconds.

Workout B					
Category/exercise	Sets/reps	Workout 1	Workout 2	Workout 3	Workout 4
Core					
Stability	2 x 30 seconds				
Dynamic stability	2 x 10				
Power					
Upper body	2 x 5–8				
Strength					
1a. Hinge	1–2 x 15				
1b. Push	1–2 x 15				
2a. Lunge	1–2 x 15				
2b. Pull	1–2 x 15				
Metabolic					
	10 minutes				

Those who haven't done Alwyn's workouts may be confused by 1a and 1b and 2a and 2b in front of the strength exercises, which indicate *alternating sets*. You do the 1a exercise, rest long enough to catch your breath, do 1b, rest, and repeat until you've completed all your sets of both exercises. Then you move on to 2a and 2b. (There's also a "c" exercise in Phase Three, but the system is the same. Do a set of 1a, rest, 1b, rest, 1c, rest, and then repeat until you finish all your sets.)

One other difference for readers of previous NROL books: In the past Alwyn has given you specific rest periods, usually 30, 60, or 90 seconds. The only instruction this time is to stop long enough to catch your breath and regain your strength. How do you know if you've regained your strength? Trial and error. If you're noticeably weaker from one set to the next, you know you didn't rest long enough.

PHASE TWO: DEVELOP

Workout A					
Category/exercise	Sets/reps	Workout 1	Workout 2	Workout 3	Workout 4
Core					
Stability	2 x 30 seconds				
Combination					
	2 x 10				
Power					
Lower body	2 x 5				
Strength					
1a. Lunge	2–4 x 10				
1b. Pull	2–4 x 10				
2a. Hinge	2–4 x 10				
2b. Push	2–4 x 10				
Metabolic					
	5–10 minutes				

Workout B					
Category/exercise	Sets/reps	Workout 1	Workout 2	Workout 3	Workout 4
Core					
Dynamic stability	2 x 10				
Power					
Upper body	2 x 5–8				
Strength					
1a. Single-leg stance	2–4 x 10				
1b. Push	2–4 x 10				
2a. Squat	2–4 x 10				
2b. Pull	2–4 x 10				
Metabolic					
	10 minutes				

• PHASE THREE: MAXIMIZE

Workout A

Category/exercise	Sets/reps	Workout 1	Workout 2	Workout 3	Workout 4
Core					
Dynamic stability	2 x 10				
Power					
Lower body	2 x 5				
Strength					
1a. Hinge	2–3 x 12				
1b. Push	2–3 x 12				
1c. Lunge	2–3 x 12				
2a. Pull	2–3 x 12				
2b. Combination	2–3 x 12				
Metabolic					
	5–10 minutes				

Workout B

Category/exercise	Sets/reps	Workout 1	Workout 2	Workout 3	Workout 4
Core					
Dynamic stability	2 x 10				
Power					
Upper body	2 x 8–10				
Strength					
1a. Squat	2–3 x 12				
1b. Pull	2–3 x 12				
1c. Single-leg stance	2–3 x 12				
2a. Push	2–3 x 12				
2b. Combination	2–3 x 12				
Metabolic					
	10 minutes				

THE EXERCISES

Core: stabilization

Level	Exercise
Pre-Level 1	Torso-elevated plank (p. 54) Modified side plank (p. 55)
Level 1	Plank/side plank (pp. 54–55)
Level 2	Plank/side plank with reduced base of support (pp. 56–57)
Level 3	Feet-elevated plank/side plank (p. 58)
Level 4	Feet-elevated plank/side plank with reduced base of support (pp. 58–59)
Level 5	Feet-elevated plank/side plank with unstable point of contact (pp. 59–60)
Beyond Level 5	Feet-elevated plank/side plank with reduced base of support and unstable point of contact (pp. 60–61)

Core: dynamic stabilization

Level	Exercise
Level 1	Plank and pulldown (p. 61) Side plank and row (p. 62)
Level 2	Push-away (p. 63) Side plank and row with reduced base of support (p. 63)
Level 3	Spiderman plank (p. 64) Swiss-ball mountain climber (p. 65) (or) Mountain climber with slides (p. 65–66)
Level 4	Cable half-kneeling chop (p. 67)
Level 4 progression	Cable kneeling chop (p. 68)
Level 5	Cable split-stance chop (p. 69)
Level 5 progression	Cable horizontal chop (p. 70)

Power

Level	Exercise
Level 1, lower body	Box jump (p. 73)
Level 1, upper body	Elevated explosive push-up (p. 74) (or) Medicine-ball push pass from knees (p. 75)
Level 2, lower body	Body-weight jump squat (p. 75)
Level 2, upper body	Explosive push-up (p. 76) or levitating push-up (p. 76) (or) Medicine-ball push pass (p. 76)
Level 3, lower body	Kettlebell swing (p. 77)
Level 3, upper body	Dumbbell push press (p. 78)
Level 4, lower body	Dumbbell jump squat (p. 79)
Level 4, upper body	Explosive push-up from boxes (pp. 80–81)
Level 5	Dumbbell single-arm snatch (pp. 81–82)

Squat

Level	Exercise
Pre-Level 1	Supported body-weight squat (p. 86)
Level 1	Body-weight squat (pp. 84–85) (or) Suspended body-weight squat (p. 87)
Level 2	Goblet squat (p. 88)
Level 3	Front squat (p. 89)
Level 4	Back squat (pp. 92–93) (or) Hex-bar deadlift (p. 94)
Level 5	Overhead squat (p. 95)

Hinge

Level	Exercise
Level 1	Swiss-ball supine hip extension (p. 99)
Level 2	Cable pull-through (pp. 100–101) (or) Romanian deadlift (p. 102)
Level 3	Rack deadlift (p. 103)
Level 4	Deadlift (pp. 104–105)
Level 5	Wide-grip deadlift (pp. 106–107)
Beyond Level 5	Wide-grip deadlift from deficit (p. 108)

Lunge

Level	Exercise
Pre-Level 1	Supported split squat (p. 113)
Level 1	Split squat (p. 112)
Level 2	Dumbbell reverse lunge (p. 114) (or) Goblet reverse lunge (p. 115) (or) Reverse lunge from step (p. 115)
Level 3	Split squat, rear foot elevated (pp. 116–117) (or) Bulgarian split squat (p. 118) (or) Suspended split squat (p. 119)
Level 4	Forward lunge (pp. 120–121)
Level 5	Walking lunge (p. 121)
Beyond Level 5	Change angle, resistance, elevation, stability, balance (weight on one side of body), or any combination

Single-leg stance

Level	Exercise
Level 1	Step-up (pp. 125–127)
Level 2	Offset-loaded step-up (p. 127)
Level 3	Single-leg Romanian deadlift (p. 128)
Pre-Level 4	Supported single-leg squat (p. 131)
Level 4	Single-leg squat (p. 130) (or) Kettlebell single-leg squat (p. 132)
Level 5	Single-leg deadlift (p. 133)
Beyond Level 5	Crossover step-up (p. 134) (or) Sprinter step-up (p. 135) (or) Overhead sprinter step-up (p. 135)

Push

Level	Exercise
Pre-Level 1	Push-up with hands elevated (pp. 140–141)
Level 1	Push-up (p. 139)
Level 2	Push-up with hands suspended (p. 142)
Level 3	T push-up (p. 143) (or) T push-up with weights (p. 144)
Level 4	Dumbbell bench press (p. 145) (or) Dumbbell single-arm bench press (p. 146)
Level 5	Dumbbell shoulder press (p. 147) (or) Dumbbell single-arm shoulder press (p. 147)
Beyond Level 5	Barbell bench press (p. 148) (or) Barbell board press (p. 149)

Pull

Level	Exercise
Pre-Level 1	Split-stance cable row (p. 154)
Level 1	Standing cable row (p. 153)
Level 2	Kneeling lat pulldown (p. 155) (or) Standing lat pulldown (p. 156)
Level 3, option 1	Dumbbell two-point row (p. 157) (or) Dumbbell three-point row (p. 158) (or) Dumbbell chest-supported row (p. 159)
Level 4	Inverted row (pp. 160–161) (or) Suspended row (p. 162)
Level 5	Chin-up (p. 163)
Beyond Level 5	Pull-up (p. 164)

Combination

Level	Exercise	Notes
Level 1	Single-leg, single-arm cable row (pp. 166–167)	
Level 2	Reverse lunge and cable row (p. 168)	
Level 3	Romanian deadlift and row (p. 169)	
Level 4	Squat and press (p. 170)	
Level 5	Reverse lunge and single-arm press (p. 171)	
Beyond Level 5	Create your own combo	

RAMP

Exercise
Kneeling hip-flexor stretch (p. 174)
Single-leg hip raise (p. 174)
Open one-half kneeling adductor/ankle mobilization (p. 175)
Open one-half kneel with T reach (p. 176)
Squat to stand (p. 177)
Wall slide (p. 178)
Forward/backward jump (p. 179)
Walking knee hug to forward lunge (p. 179)
Side-to-side jump (p. 180)
Walking lateral lunge (p. 180)
Skipping (p. 181)
Carioca (p. 182)
Side shuffle (p. 183)

Metabolic Training

Level	Exercise
Level 1	Body-weight squat (p. 187) (or) Step-up (p. 187) (or) Shadow boxing (p. 187)
Levels 2 and 3	Burpee (p. 188) (or) Kettlebell swing (p. 188) (or) Box jump (p. 188) (or) Squat/push-up combo (p. 188)
Levels 4 and 5	Barbell matrix (bent-over row, front squat, shoulder press) (pp. 188–189) (or) Farmer's walk (p. 190) (or) Sprint (p. 190)
Beyond Level 5	Jump rope (p. 191) (or) Take the stairs (with or without push-ups) (p. 191) (or) Hit a heavy bag (p. 191) (or) Turn your yard into a gym (chop wood, sledgehammer, wheelbarrow pushes or pulls) (p. 191) (or) Push your car (p. 191)

Now we'll fill them in. Let's suppose you're a novice lifter, or someone who's new to NROL-type training. I start with these assumptions:

- You're healthy, with no back pain or limitations in your knees, hips, or shoulders. I know it seems odd to write a book for people with limitations and then assume the sample lifter has no issues. I do it this way because I don't know what your individual problems may be.
- You have access to a gym with all the standard equipment, like cable machines and Swiss balls.
- You're a sometimes-active person who can walk around the block a couple of times without stopping to rest.
- Here's how you might select exercises for your first time through the program.

PHASE ONE: TRANSFORM

Workout A (beginner)					
Category/exercise	Sets/reps	Workout 1	Workout 2	Workout 3	Workout 4
Core					
Stability: *Plank* (p. 54)	2 x 30 seconds				
Dynamic stability: *Side plank and row* (p. 62)	2 x 10				
Power					
Lower body: *Box jump* (p. 73)	2 x 5				
Strength					
1a. Squat: *Goblet squat* (p. 88)	1–2 x 15				
1b. Pull: *Standing cable row* (p. 153)	1–2 x 15				
2a. Single-leg stance: *Dumbbell step-up* (pp. 125–127)	1–2 x 15				
2b. Push: *Push-up* (p. 139)	1–2 x 15				
Metabolic					
	5–10 minutes				

Workout B (beginner)					
Category/exercise	Sets/reps	Workout 1	Workout 2	Workout 3	Workout 4
Core					
Stability: *Side plank* (p. 55)	2 x 30 seconds				
Dynamic stability: *Plank with pulldown* (p. 61)	2 x 10				
Power					
Upper body: *Elevated explosive push-up* (p. 74)	2 x 5–8				
Strength					
1a. Hinge: *Swiss-ball supine hip extension* (p. 99)	1–2 x 15				
1b. Push: *Dumbbell bench press* (p. 145)	1–2 x 15				
2a. Lunge: *Dumbbell split squat* (p. 112)	1–2 x 15				
2b. Pull: *Kneeling lat pulldown* (p. 155)	1–2 x 15				
Metabolic					
	10 minutes				

PHASE TWO: DEVELOP

Workout A (beginner)

Category/exercise	Sets/reps	Workout 1	Workout 2	Workout 3	Workout 4
Core					
Stability: *Plank with reduced base of support* (p. 56)	2 x 30 seconds				
Combination					
Single-leg, single-arm cable row (pp. 166–167)	2 x 10				
Power					
Lower body: *Jump squat* (p. 75)	2 x 5				
Strength					
1a. Lunge: *Dumbbell reverse lunge* (p. 114)	2–4 x 10				
1b. Pull: *Kneeling lat pulldown* (p. 155)	2–4 x 10				
2a. Hinge: *Romanian deadlift* (p. 102)	2–4 x 10				
2b. Push: *Push-up with feet elevated* (p. 140)	2–4 x 10				
Metabolic					
	5–10 minutes				

Workout B (beginner)

Category/exercise	Sets/reps	Workout 1	Workout 2	Workout 3	Workout 4
Core					
Dynamic stability: *Push-away* (p. 63)	2 x 10				
Power					
Upper body: *Explosive push-up* (p. 76)	2 x 5–8				
Strength					
1a. Single-leg stance: *Offset-loaded step-up* (p. 127)	2–4 x 10				
1b. Push: *Dumbbell bench press* (p. 145)	2–4 x 10				
2a. Squat: *Front squat* (p. 89)	2–4 x 10				
2b. Pull: *Dumbbell two-point row* (p. 157)	2–4 x 10				
Metabolic					
	10 minutes				

PHASE THREE: MAXIMIZE

Workout A (beginner)

Category/exercise	Sets/reps	Workout 1	Workout 2	Workout 3	Workout 4
Core					
Dynamic stability: *Cable half-kneeling chop* (p. 67)	2 x 10				
Power					
Lower body: *Kettlebell swing* (p. 77)	2 x 6–8				
Strength					
1a. Hinge: *Rack deadlift* (p. 103)	2–3 x 12				
1b. Push: *Push-up with hands suspended* (p. 142)	2–3 x 12				
1c. Lunge: *Split squat, rear foot elevated* (pp. 116–117)	2–3 x 12				
2a. Pull: *Dumbbell chest-supported row* (p. 159)	2–3 x 12				
2b. Combination: *Squat and press* (p. 170)	2–3 x 12				
Metabolic					
	5–10 minutes				

Workout B (beginner)

Category/exercise	Sets/reps	Workout 1	Workout 2	Workout 3	Workout 4
Core					
Dynamic stability: *Swiss-ball mountain climber* (p. 65)	2 x 10				
Power					
Upper body: *Push press* (p. 78)	2 x 8–10				
Strength					
1a. Squat: *Back squat* (pp. 92–93)	2–3 x 12				
1b. Pull: *Dumbbell three-point row* (p. 158)	2–3 x 12				
1c. Single-leg stance: *Single-leg Romanian deadlift* (p. 128)	2–3 x 12				
2a. Push: *Dumbbell single-arm bench press* (p. 146)	2–3 x 12				
2b. Combination: *Reverse lunge and cable row* (p. 168)	2–3 x 12				
Metabolic					
	10 minutes				

I could go on all day about why I selected each exercise from the available options. But what it comes down to is this: There really are no right or wrong answers. Nor are there any *permanent* answers. That's the beauty of Alwyn's template system. You can adjust anything you want on the fly. Alwyn's only hard-and-fast rule is that you stick to the category of exercise. You can jump to higher levels or back to lower levels if those exercises make the most sense in the context in which you're doing them.

Or you can just choose all Level 1 exercises for Phase One, Level 2 for Phase Two, and Level 3 for Phase Three. Yes, you'll get some redundancies. You may get tired of certain exercises, and on others you'll have to move up to the next level before you've gotten all you can out of them.

But those are minor problems, which may not apply to you. And even if they do, what's the worst outcome? That you get 90 percent of the potential benefits of Alwyn's program, rather than 95 percent? Believe me, you'd be happy with that.

Now it's time to look at something a bit more complex: the choices I made in my own NROL for Life workouts. I annotated some of my decisions, so you can either follow along with my thought process, or ignore it entirely. It's a good workout either way.

PHASE ONE: TRANSFORM

Workout A (advanced)

Category/exercise	Sets/reps	Workout 1	Workout 2	Workout 3	Workout 4
Core					
Stability: *Plank* (p. 54)*	2 x 30 seconds				
Dynamic Stability: *Swiss-ball mountain climber* (p. 65)	2 x 10				
Power					
Lower body: *Box jump* (p. 73)†	2 x 5				
Strength					
1a. Squat: *Goblet squat* (p. 88)‡	1–2 x 15				
1b. Pull: *Standing cable row* (p. 153)	1–2 x 15				
2a. Single-leg stance: *Single-leg Romanian deadlift* (p. 128)	1–2 x 15				
2b. Push: *Push-up* (p. 139)**	1–2 x 15				
Metabolic					
	5–10 minutes				

Workout B (advanced)

Category/exercise	Sets/reps	Workout 1	Workout 2	Workout 3	Workout 4
Core					
Stability: *Side plank* (p. 55) *	2 x 30 seconds				
Dynamic stability: *Spiderman plank* (p. 64)	2 x 10				
Power					
Upper body: *Explosive push-up* (p. 74)	2 x 5–8				
Strength					
1a. Hinge: *Deadlift* (pp. 104–105) ^	1–2 x 15				
1b. Push: *Dumbbell incline bench press* (p. 145)	1–2 x 15				
2a. Lunge: *Reverse lunge from step* (p. 115) ^^	1–2 x 15				
2b. Pull: *Suspended row* (p. 162)	1–2 x 15				
Metabolic					
	10 minutes				

* As explained in Chapter 6, I ran through all five core-stabilization levels in Phase One, doing different plank and side plank variations every workout. That included some we didn't have room to show in this book. My goal was to do something that was harder each workout, and when I ran out, I at least tried to do something different.

† I hadn't done box jumps in ages. It was a blast, until I ran out of higher boxes. (Some of the young athletes at my gym stack boxes on top of each other, but I'm not that brave.)

‡ For the first couple of workouts, I did a hybrid goblet/front squat holding two kettlebells against my chest. I had to switch to the conventional barbell front squat when I maxed out the paired kettlebells in my gym.

** I did a different push-up variation every workout, all from the "12 Ways to Make Push-Ups Tougher" sidebar in Chapter 12. I'll be honest: I couldn't come close to 15 reps on some of them.

^ It was surprisingly fun to do 15-rep sets of deadlifts. When I experimented with heavier weights I couldn't get all the reps. The exercise felt best when I used 135 or 155 pounds and went for speed (with good form).

^^ I used light dumbbells for the reverse lunge from a step, but really, after all those deadlifts, my body weight would've been tough enough to use for 15 deep lunges with each leg.

PHASE TWO: DEVELOP

Workout A (advanced)					
Category/exercise	Sets/reps	Workout 1	Workout 2	Workout 3	Workout 4
Core					
Stability: *Level 5 plank variations* (pp. 59–60)	2 x 30 seconds				
Combination					
Reverse lunge and cable row (p. 168)	2 x 10				
Power					
Lower body: *Kettlebell swing* (p. 77)	2 x 8–10				
Strength					
1a. Lunge: *Suspended split squat* (p. 119)	2–4 x 10				
1b. Pull: *Suspended row* (p. 162) *	2–4 x 10				
2a. Hinge: *Deadlift* (pp. 104–105)†	2–4 x 10				
2b. Push: *Push-up with hands suspended* (p. 142)	2–4 x 10				
Metabolic					
	5–10 minutes				

Workout B (advanced)					
Category/exercise	Sets/reps	Workout 1	Workout 2	Workout 3	Workout 4
Core					
Dynamic stability: *Mountain climber variations* (pp. 65–66)‡	2 x 10				
Power					
Upper body: *Dumbbell push press* (p. 78)	2 x 5–8				
Strength					
1a. Single-leg stance: *Offset-loaded step-up* (p. 127)	2–4 x 10				
1b. Push: *Dumbbell incline bench press* (p. 145) **	2–4 x 10				
2a. Squat: *Front squat* (p. 89) ^	2–4 x 10				
2b. Pull: *Dumbbell three-point row* (p. 158) ^^	2–4 x 10				
Metabolic					
	10 minutes				

* In Phase One I did a fairly easy version of the suspended row, with my body at a 45-degree angle to the floor. But in Phase Two I made it much harder, with my body close to parallel to the floor. (For the record, I *really* don't like the harder version, which is how I knew I needed to do it.)

† I repeated the deadlift here, but used heavier weights for slower reps.

‡ I can't imagine a good workout program that doesn't include a hip-flexion exercise—raising your leg up in front of your torso. Mountain climbers are great for core strength, hip mobility, and all-around conditioning and athleticism.

** I use the incline press because my shoulders won't tolerate a flat bench press. If you can use challenging weights on a flat bench without discomfort, feel free to substitute.

^ The front squat is another repeated exercise from Phase One. But with heavier weights, it feels more like a progression than a redundancy. As long as you're training with slightly heavier weights from one workout to the next, the exercise is doing what it's supposed to do.

^^ As an experiment, I tried doing the two-point row (aka standing bent-over row) and the three-point row (feet on the floor, nonworking hand resting on a bench) back to back. I could use twice as much weight on the three-point row. The two-point row is a terrific exercise for core training, but eventually the lower back becomes the weak link. Putting your hand down on the bench removes the weak link and puts your body in a strong position for lifting heavy stuff.

PHASE THREE: MAXIMIZE

Workout A (advanced)					
Category/exercise	Sets/reps	Workout 1	Workout 2	Workout 3	Workout 4
Core					
Dynamic stability: *Cable horizontal chop* (p. 70)*	2 x 10				
Power					
Lower body: *Dumbbell single-arm snatch* (pp. 81–82)†	2 x 6–8				
Strength					
1a. Hinge: *Wide-grip deadlift* (p. 106)	2–3 x 12				
1b. Push: *T push-up* (p. 143)‡	2–3 x 12				
1c. Lunge: *Walking lunge* (p. 121)**	2–3 x 12				
2a. Pull: *Kneeling lat pulldown* (p. 155)^	2–3 x 12				
2b. Combination: *Squat and press* (p. 170)^^	2–3 x 12				
Metabolic					
	5–10 minutes				

Workout B (advanced)					
Category/exercise	Sets/reps	Workout 1	Workout 2	Workout 3	Workout 4
Core					
Dynamic stability: *More mountain climber variations* (pp. 65–66)	2 x 10–20				
Power					
Upper body: *Explosive push-up from boxes* (pp. 80–81)	2 x 6–8				
Strength					
1a. Squat: *Hex-bar deadlift* (p. 94)	2–3 x 12				
1b. Pull: *Chin-up* (p. 163)#	2–3 x 12				
1c. Single-leg stance: *Crossover step-up* (p. 134)##	2–3 x 12				
2a. Push: *Dumbbell alternating shoulder press* (p. 147)###	2–3 x 12				
2b. Combination: *Reverse lunge and cable row* (p. 168)	2–3 x 12				
Metabolic					
	10 minutes				

*   I chose horizontal chops because I've never gotten a good feel for the diagonal version. I set my feet wide when I do the horizontal chop, giving me an extremely stable base, and use aggressive weights.

†   I skipped over loaded jump squats, which are very tough on my knees, to get to the single-arm snatch. I still jump on this exercise, but for whatever reason it has less of a jarring effect when I land.

‡   I'm going for a metabolic benefit with T push-ups, rather than strength or size.

**   I can't tell you why, but the basic forward lunge hurts my knees, while the walking lunge creates no discomfort.

^   I'll be honest: After alternating sets of wide-grip deadlifts, T push-ups, and walking lunges, I needed a technically easy exercise here. The kneeling lat pulldown is as simple as it gets.

^^   The entire workout builds up to the squat and press. I've kept stress off my knees and shoulders so I can impose stress here.

\#   I can't do chin-ups for 12 reps, but I still want to do them here because they're the best exercise.

\#\#   Single-leg squats and deadlifts are nonstarters with my wounded knees. The crossover step-up (and the sprinter step-up, which I'll sometimes swap in) gives me similar benefits without pain.

\#\#\#   Once more, for exercise 2b I picked the movement that best complements the rest of the exercises in the workout. Since I used a push-up variation for a power exercise, bench presses would be redundant (not to mention tough on my shoulders). It also pairs up well with the combination exercise I selected, the reverse lunge and row.

Recovery

I FIRST REALIZED THE IMPORTANCE OF post-workout nutrition when I was a young and broke musclehead whose job required early-morning workouts. When I got home from the gym I was hungry enough to eat almost anything. I say "almost" because no amount of hunger or vanity could stifle my gag reflex when I tried to choke down the protein supplements of the mid-1980s. They looked like chalk and tasted like mulch. Instead, I made a post-workout meal with three eggs and three egg whites, scrambled, with a couple of English muffins. I chased it with a glass of skim milk, maybe two. (Over the course of a day I would sometimes drink a half-gallon.) I'm pretty sure it worked. The more consistent I was with my eggs and milk, the better I looked. I also noticed that the harder I worked out, the more consistent I was with nutrition. When my workouts got stale or erratic, so did my meals.

The next time I gave the subject any thought was 1992. I had just started working as a part-time copy editor at *Muscle & Fitness* magazine. An editor there told me that the "window of opportunity" for building muscle after a workout was extremely short. Could be an hour, could be half that. Just to be on the safe side, you should really have something before you leave the gym.

That's been my working model ever since. Eventually I found protein supplements that taste good (my favorite, Biotest's Metabolic Drive, is *seriously* good), and I've never really wavered from the soon-as-possible paradigm. There was plenty of research to confirm what I was already inclined to believe.

But in May 2011, I was forced to reconsider. Alan Aragon, a nutrition consultant based in Southern California, presented a talk called "What Really Matters" at The Fitness Summit in Kansas City. Aragon showed new research suggesting that the "windows of opportunity" aren't as narrow as gym rats imagine. "They're more like bay windows of a mansion," he said. "Our physiology basically has the universe mapped out, and we're thinking it needs to be taught addition and subtraction."

It's not that post-workout nutrition isn't important. Everyone agrees that your muscle protein breaks down rapidly after a workout, and if it has a ready supply of dietary protein to work with, it'll build up new tissue even faster. Without protein, you'll get a net breakdown of muscle tissue, at least in the short term. Aragon's point is that your body can use protein you've eaten before the workout just as easily as it uses post-workout protein. (It takes protein up to six hours to work its way through your system.) A well-nourished adult training later in the day can eat a normal meal an hour or two after a workout and not miss out on any potential post-workout muscle growth or recovery. Even better: Your muscles remain in an anabolic state—that is, receptive to protein above and beyond what they need for maintenance—for up to twenty-four hours after you lift.

And yet, knowing that our bodies allow us more leeway doesn't really change what most of us do. "I have no research to back this up, but I'm 100 percent convinced there is a difference with the timing," Alwyn told me. His clients get better results when they have a protein shake immediately post-workout. I suspect I do as well. That's why I rarely wait more than a half-hour after training for my protein fix. It's partly habit, and partly because the shake tastes so good. But it's also because I've never forgotten the lesson I learned back in the 1980s: The harder I train, the better I eat; the better I eat, the faster I can see the results of my workouts. Seeing results, in turn, increases my motivation to train.

I can't prove this, but I think it's entirely possible that many of the habits we associate with successful weight management don't work because of any significant, substantial, or even measurable effect on our physiology. I think they work mainly because they help us remember that we're trying to manage our weight, and secondarily because we do them instead of other habits that would take us further from our goal.

The nice thing about this theory is that it doesn't matter if I'm right or wrong. Either way, we end up looking better, eating better, and feeling better.

If you're going to have a post-workout shake, there's pretty wide agreement that milk-based proteins—whey and casein—are your best choice. Perhaps most important for older lifters is the high concentration of the amino acid leucine. Milk proteins have 10 to 12 percent leucine, compared with 8 to 9 percent for the protein in meat and eggs, and less than that for non-animal proteins. Twenty to 40 grams of whey or a whey-casein blend should be plenty.

You can also find a wide range of nondairy protein supplements, made from soy, pea, or even hemp protein. I assume the taste varies widely, as would the quality of the amino acids and leucine concentration.

RECOVERY EXERCISES

There's no fixed protocol for post-workout recovery. The following exercises are a sample of those Alwyn might have his clients use before they go home. You can use all or some of them, combine them with your own favorites, or do something else altogether. I do some of them at the beginning of my workout (kind of a pre-RAMP) rather than the end. As with other aspects of Alwyn's program, it's best to try the protocol as it's presented here before adding, subtracting, or modifying.

Just make sure you do something to restore the quality of your muscle and connective tissue. Stretches address the length and tension of those tissues, which can shorten and tighten during a workout. Foam-rolling exercises address tissue quality by smoothing out the knots and adhesions that affect performance.

If you work out at home, or your gym doesn't have a 6-inch-thick foam roller like the one shown in these photos, you can pick up your own at a sporting-goods store or online at performbetter.com.

General guidelines:

- On foam-rolling exercises, Alwyn recommends spending 10 to 20 seconds if nothing is particularly tender when you apply pressure. Give those areas extra attention. (This doesn't apply to actual injuries, which we cover in Chapter 3. We're just talking about surprisingly sensitive spots in otherwise functional tissue.)
- Hold stretches about 30 seconds. You can do more work on one side if it's shorter or tighter than the other.
- Although it's not shown here, you will probably benefit from rolling a tennis ball

around the bottom of your feet. It loosens up the fascia and improves range of motion throughout your lower body.

- There's no perfect time or place for mild stretches and tissue-manipulating exercises. A lot of older lifters I know do them every day, separate from their strength workouts. The only time you don't want to do stretches is first thing in the morning, when you have excess fluid in your spinal discs, which makes them more vulnerable.

- For a more aggressive stretching program, you want to make sure you're thoroughly warmed up. It's probably best to do that at the end of your workout, when your core temperature is elevated.

✳ Back Roll

- Lie on the floor with the roll under the middle of your back, perpendicular to your torso.
- With your heels on the floor, pull and push your body over the roll, hitting your lower and middle back.

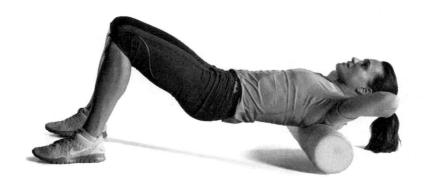

✳ Glute roll

- Since the fibers of the gluteus maximus run east and west, rather than north and south, you're going to start with the roll parallel to your torso.
- Sit on the roll with one cheek, with your targeted leg crossed over your nonworking leg, and roll sideways.
- You can also try rolling the other way, with the roll perpendicular to your torso.

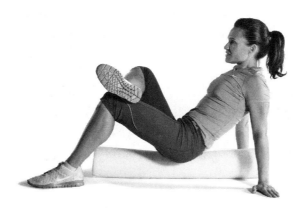

✳ Calf roll

- Set the roll under one calf, and cross the ankle of your nonworking leg over that shin to increase the pressure.
- Lift your hips up, supporting your weight on your hands, and pull and push your calf muscles over the roll from ankle to knee.
- Switch legs and repeat.

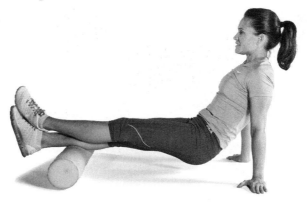

✳ Ham roll

- Same technique as the calf roll, except now you roll from the bottom of your knee to the gluteal crease.
- With this and the next two exercises, feel free to work one leg at a time, and spend more time on one side than the other, if one leg is more problematic.

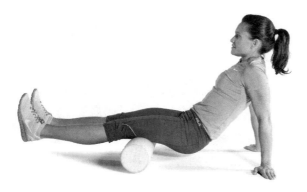

✳ Quad roll

- Lie facedown, with your front thighs on the roll and your weight on your forearms.
- Pull yourself over the roll, hitting everything from the top of your knee to your groin.

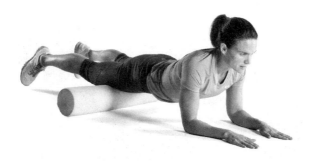

✳ IT-band roll

- Lie on your side, with the outside of your thigh on the roll and your weight on one hand.
- Pull and push yourself over the roll from your hip to the top of your knee.
- To take some pressure off, you can place the foot of your non-rolling leg on the floor.

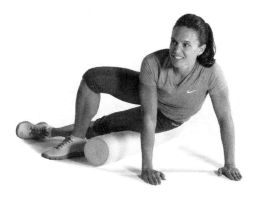

✳ Adductor stretch

- From a kneeling position, lean forward and place both hands on the floor. Extend your right foot as far as you can to your side, with your right foot flat on the floor.
- Push your hips back, feeling the stretch along your right inner thigh.
- Hold for 30 seconds, switch sides, and repeat.

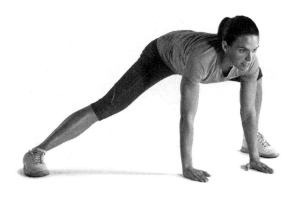

✳ Hip flexor/lat stretch

- Get into lunge position, with your left foot forward and your right knee on or near the floor. Raise your right arm over your head.
- Shift your weight forward as you lean to your left, feeling the stretch in your right lat and on the right side of your pelvis.
- Hold for 30 seconds, switch sides, and repeat.

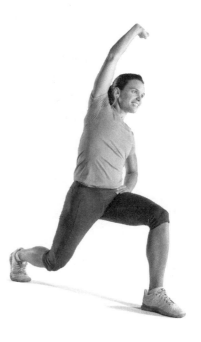

✳ Figure-four stretch

- Lie on your back with your knees bent and the outside of your left ankle against your lower right quadriceps, just above your knee.
- Grab the back of your right leg just behind the knee.
- Pull your right thigh toward you until you feel a stretch in your left glute.
- Hold for 30 seconds, switch sides, and repeat.

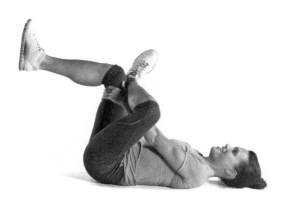

PART 3

THE WIDE ALBUM

Flabby Road

I SHOULD FEEL GOOD ABOUT MYSELF. According an article in *USA Today*, the average American man in his fifties weighs 199 pounds. Me, I'm usually 185 when I weigh myself first thing in the morning. I'd always thought I was average for my height, gender, and age, but here was proof that I'm 14 pounds lighter. The article piqued my curiosity, leading me to wonder if I'm any lighter now, compared with my peer group, than I was at earlier ages.

Using data from the National Center for Health Statistics, I put together the following chart. The vertical axis shows the years in which data was collected, and the horizontal axis shows mean weights for American adults by age. (For the statisticians: I refer to "average" weight above, which is how *USA Today* described the data, while the studies actually show "mean" weight, meaning equal numbers of people weigh more or less than the figures shown.)

Mean weight for adult women and men in the United States (shown as women/men)							
	20s	**30s**	**40s**	**50s**	**60–74**	**75+**	
1960–62	128/164	139/170	143/169	147/168	147/160		
1971–74	134/170	144/178	149/177	148/173	146/166		
1976–80	136/168	146/176	149/180	150/176	147/168		
1988–94	142/173	154/182	158/187	163/189	154/181	139/166	
1999–2002	157/183	163/189	168/196	169/192	165/192	147/173	
					60s	**70s**	**80s**
2003–06	156/188	165/194	171/202	172/199	171/198	156/187	142/168

Source: National Center for Health Statistics.

What I discovered isn't particularly impressive. My current weight is 93 percent of the mean for men in their fifties. Over my lifetime I've typically been between 91 and 94 percent of the mean for my age at the time of each survey, although I bulked up to 104 percent at one point in my late thirties. This was during my late-to-the-party attempt at bodybuilding, at which I failed pretty spectacularly. But aside from that blip, a lifetime of serious exercise has kept me in more or less the same place, relative to my peers.

I encourage you to run your own numbers; just divide your weight by the mean for your age and gender at each time point. It gives each of us a baseline to keep in mind when we talk about how and why Americans have gotten so freakin' big in such a short period of time.

TELL ME WHY YOU FRY

That we've gotten massive is beyond dispute. That we eat more than we used to is beyond dispute. But in the past few years I've seen all of these additional hypotheses suggested as reasons for the girth of our nation:

- *We move less.* In *NROL for Abs* I noted a Mayo Clinic study that pinpointed one aspect of modern life—the fact that few of us walk to work anymore—and suggested this alone could account for the surplus energy we're storing instead of burning.
- *We're wired to store fat.* This was the conclusion of *Rethinking Thin*, a deeply researched 2007 book by *New York Times* fitness reporter Gina Kolata. While self-

discipline matters, people who are fat are genetically destined to eat more food when it's available, and gain more weight.

- *Capitalism is making us fat.* The book *The End of Overeating*, by David A. Kessler, M.D., shows how the food industry has mimicked the tobacco industry in the way it manipulated food with sugar, fat, and salt to make it more palatable and harder to stop eating once you start.

- *It's all about the corn.* This is a corollary to the indictment of the food industry. Nixon-era subsidies for corn farmers eventually led to the presence of high-fructose corn syrup in everything from soft drinks to salad dressing. Food became cheaper than ever to produce, leading to the ubiquitous presence of fast-food restaurants on every corner. Even the poorest people in the United States have easy access to affordable, high-calorie meals.

- *Your friends make you fat.* Obesity as a social disease, spreading through networks of friends, has gotten much play in the media. The idea is that you eat like the people you eat with, and if you're all overweight there's an implied acceptance.

- *We simply make bad food choices.* And we should know better, according to a 2011 study in the *New England Journal of Medicine.* Looking at a sample of more than 120,000 American men and women, with data going back to 1986, Harvard researchers came up with incredibly precise figures. Consumption of potato chips increased subjects' weight by 1.69 pounds over four years; sugar-sweetened drinks added 1 pound; unprocessed red meat, 0.95 pounds. A couple of foods were associated with lower weight, including yogurt (which reduced weight by 0.82 pounds) and nuts (0.57 pounds).

- *Our lifestyles are a mess.* In the same study, the data showed that sleeping less than six hours or more than eight hours a day was correlated with weight gain, as was smoking, drinking, and watching TV.

Those are the big ones. They're all "true," in the sense that we can find data to back them up. They all make sense. Most of us have sedentary jobs. We all know the food chain makes the worst stuff cheap and the best stuff expensive. And no one with a mind open to science and reason denies the genetic roots of both behaviors and outcomes. You can't take a body that's thick by design—the loving creation of a human life by two people whose DNA tilts toward XXL—and make it thin. Not only is it physiologically impossible to do such a thing without surgery or powerful drugs, it's stupid and immoral to suggest that all of us should have matching silhouettes.

I have a thin mom and a fat dad, and somehow ended up with a narrow frame. Most of my siblings struggle with their weight. Same deck, different cards.

Still, I can't help but lean toward the "bad choices" hypothesis. It comes closest to matching my experiences and observations. If you'll indulge yet another of my rambling stories:

I went to a Catholic high school in a semirural part of Missouri. The suburban-sprawl kids like me were a minority. Most of my classmates had deep roots in small towns. Some were farmers. As much as I observed anything beyond girls and sports, I noticed an odd type of couple: a solidly built man married to an obese woman. I can't recall seeing that in the suburbs; if you saw a mismatch, it tended to be more like my parents, where the male was soft and pot-bellied and the female more concerned with her figure.

Something else I noticed: The farm boys were the biggest and strongest in the school. My football coaches and teammates were anti–strength training but pro-farming. Some of the biggest kids spent their summers throwing hay bales onto flat-bed trailers. Some of the skinniest kids (like me) lifted weights. So almost everyone assumed that it took a lot of repetitive work each day to get big and strong, something you couldn't possibly achieve in a few hours a week in the weight room.

But it wasn't simply exercise that made the farm kids bigger and stronger. It was the way they ate before and after they worked the fields. Farm kids consumed far more calories than the rest of us, as did their parents. That explains why male adult farmers so often seemed half the size of their spouses; they ate the same way, but the men burned most of it off outdoors while the women (who were hardly sedentary) spent more time indoors. It also explains why I was still skinny despite my work in the weight room. I went home and ate like everyone else in the suburbs. We had our meat, potatoes, and dessert, while my farming peers were eating all that plus biscuits, corn, and butter. Given my age, metabolism, and activity level, I was probably undereating by hundreds of calories a day.

I've fallen out of touch with my classmates, but I still get the alumni newsletter, and what I saw in one issue just shocked me. It was a picture of a group of alumnae, most from my era, who'd volunteered for something or other. They were absolutely huge. I doubt if a single one was an actual farm wife, but they'd all managed to grow to that size, if not beyond. These weren't strangers riding electric carts in Walmart, people we look right past without wondering how they got that way. These were people I once knew, whose potential adiposity wasn't at all apparent in the 1970s.

I get that humans have the ability to store calories; it's an evolutionary trait that helped our species survive when food was scarce. In past generations, when it was fashionable to stuff themselves, the upper classes did exactly that. According to Bill Bryson in *At Home* (a terrific history of how we came to live and eat the way we do), this was a recommended menu for a six-person dinner party in the mid-nineteenth century: mock turtle soup, fillets of turbot in cream, fried sole with anchovy sauce, rabbit, veal, stewed beef, roasted fowl, and boiled ham, followed by a long list of desserts.

While gluttony wasn't an option for most people, those who could afford the food (along with the household personnel to cook and serve it) ate fantastical quantities. And of course they grew to fantastical sizes. America's heftiest presidents, ranked by our best guess at their body-mass index, all served consecutively in the late nineteenth and early twentieth centuries: Grover Cleveland, William McKinley, Theodore Roosevelt (who was also our most physically active president), and William Howard Taft, who weighed an estimated 340 pounds when he left office in 1913.

This was decades before the invention of fast food.

History shows that people who want to consume massive volumes of food have always done so, as long as they have motive, means, and opportunity. The open question is why people of our generation, who don't want to eat to excess and desperately want to avoid storing fat, get big anyway. Let's explore.

NEW RULE #17 • It's actually kind of hard to gain weight.

There's a pernicious myth, propagated by health and nutrition professionals who should know better, that weight gain and weight loss are linear processes. Add a single cookie to your daily diet, the public is told, and over time it adds up to dozens, if not hundreds, of pounds. It's not true. As two Dutch researchers explained in a commentary in the *Journal of the American Medical Association*, over time your body will adjust to the extra calories, along with whatever weight you gain initially. That amount of food—your previous diet plus the cookie—becomes exactly what your body requires to maintain its new, higher weight. You have a long list of hormones and metabolic processes to stabilize your weight . . . as long as you don't add any more cookies to your daily diet.

Even then, it's kind of hard to supersize. Your body upregulates your metabolism and downregulates your appetite to compensate for any new infusion of calories. The researchers used the example of a twenty-five-year-old male who has a body-mass index of 25, the edge of what we consider overweight. Let's make him five-foot-ten,

174 pounds. If he kept his activity level exactly the same over the next twenty-five years, he would need to eat an extra 680 calories a day to reach a BMI of 35, the mid-point between "obese" and "Holy crap, is that guy fat." He would weigh 244 pounds.

You could argue that no one would actually maintain the same activity level while gaining 70 pounds, and I'd agree. But at a higher weight he'd burn more calories with every step, so he could move a lot less and burn the same number of calories he did at 174 pounds.

How much he moves is really beside the point, which is this: We've been told for eons that a pound of fat is 3,500 calories, and an extra 500 calories a day should increase your weight by a pound a week. That would be 52 pounds a year, and after twenty-five years we'd be looking at a man who weighed close to 1,500 pounds—three-quarters of a ton.

Do you know someone who weighs more than a thousand pounds? I doubt if I've ever met anyone over 500. And yet, all of us know people who weigh at least 70 pounds more than they did a quarter-century ago. Some of you reading this have gained that much, and more.

Which brings us back to the original problem: How did something that should be really hard become the signal feature of our generation?

NEW RULE #18 • We don't really move less.

Along with the myth that weight gain and weight loss are linear and easily quantifiable is the notion that all of us move a lot less than we used to. I've always believed this to be true, despite the fact that I grew up at a time when adults hardly moved at all. My father and the other men of his generation had grown up in the Depression and served in the military. They reveled in their suburban leisure. In my neighborhood you rarely saw a middle-aged man do anything more strenuous than mow a lawn or trim a hedge on a Saturday. Even then, the work was done by mid-afternoon, and the drinking started soon after.

Women certainly moved more than their husbands. *Someone* had to shop and prepare food for all of us baby boomers, and those ranch houses didn't clean them-selves. But it's not like they were taking daily Pilates classes.

Research now shows that our generation probably doesn't move less than our parents'. A 2009 study in the *American Journal of Clinical Nutrition* calculated how much food we had available in the 1970s versus the 2000s, subtracted the amount that's thrown out or wasted, and showed that weight gain correlates pretty well with the higher volume of food we eat. If anything, their data suggest that we probably move more now; otherwise, the average American adult would be about five pounds heavier.

Moreover, it takes a *lot* of movement to counteract all that food. Harvard researchers reported in the *Journal of the American Medical Association* that middle-aged women who gained fewer than five pounds over a thirteen-year period averaged about sixty minutes a day of exercise.

That leaves us with one remaining suspect in the fattening of our generation.

NEW RULE #19 • Tasty food makes it too easy to gain weight, and too hard to lose it.

Weight-loss researchers long ago gave up on the idea that all members of a species react to food in the same way. When they study mice or rats, they genetically modify them to make them more or less susceptible to whatever stimulus they plan to administer. They can't modify humans, but that doesn't mean we're all the same to begin with. An exercise study I quoted in Chapter 4 divided subjects into "responders" and "nonresponders." It works the same way with nutrition. Researchers know that some people simply respond to food with less inhibition or satiety than others. They're hungrier, and they eat more before their appetite-control mechanisms kick in.

So which are you? Come on, you know. If you sometimes lose control of yourself when eating, gain weight easily, and hang on to everything you've gained, then you're the human equivalent of one of those obesity-prone lab animals. It's what you are, and it's what you'll always be. Someone who's obesity resistant, like me, will still gain weight when we eat highly palatable food without restraint. But we'll also lose it when we stop eating the things that made us fat. I know it's not fair. As Denis Leary said, "Life sucks, get a helmet."

NEW RULE #20 • Every pound you don't gain is one you don't have to worry about losing.

Ask a weight-loss researcher what works for people genetically susceptible to weight gain, and if she's honest, she'll say something like this: "Don't gain weight in the first place." If it's too late for that, then you're stuck with the same old advice you've always gotten from people like me: Burn as much energy as you can with your training program, and modify your diet to take care of the rest.

You know what not to eat. You know that highly palatable foods—those engineered to contain unnatural amounts of sugar, fat, and salt—are both irresistible and unsatisfying. You can't stop eating them once you start. (Most of us are old enough to remember the Lay's potato chip ads, which used their inability to satiate *as a selling point*.) That's true for everyone. Whether we're talking about snack foods, Big Gulps, movie-theater popcorn, big-chain pizzas, or french fries, we know we can't stop once we start. The only strategy that works is to avoid those things entirely.

Slightly less obvious is the need to avoid foods that are your personal triggers. A trainer I interviewed for a magazine article advises his clients to "know your Kryptonite." For me it's pancakes, donuts, and all the other stuff that falls under the "dessert for breakfast" rubric. I wake up hungry, and if sweets are an option, I'll eat far more than I can burn off with any amount of activity, including Alwyn's workouts. For someone else, it might be a couple of drinks. Alcohol is only mildly associated with weight gain, if at all, but its reputation for lowering your inhibitions is well deserved. If your night of drinking typically concludes at the nearest White Castle, the problem isn't really the sliders and cheese fries. You wouldn't end the evening there if you hadn't started at the pub.

Two more ways to control your environment:

- *Use smaller plates, bowls, glasses, and cutlery.* If you're lucky enough to inherit your great-grandmother's china and silverware (the kind made from actual silver), you can't help noticing how small it is, compared with the stuff you bought last year at Pottery Barn. It was designed for smaller people to use for smaller servings. Brian Wansink, Ph.D., a professor of marketing and applied economics at Cornell, has shown in numerous studies that you eat more when you're served a larger portion, even if you don't like the food. Flipping that around, the smaller the plate you use, the bigger any portion looks.
- *Don't leave food where you can see it.* Wansink's studies have also shown that you eat less when food is kept out of sight, even if you know exactly where you put it.

My big points are these:

1. You can't change your appetite, or your propensity to store excess calories. That's in your DNA. But even the biggest appetite has brakes, including a complex sys-

tem of hormones that produce feelings of fullness and satiety. Your job is to avoid the things that have been engineered to override those appetite-control mechanisms.

2. Increasing your physical activity can certainly be part of the solution, even if lack of movement isn't necessarily the problem. It's not your only tool for weight management, but everyone agrees that it's an important one.

3. The biggest wild card is your behavior, especially your ability to avoid the situations in which you know you'll overeat. This is so important, and the subject of such intriguing new research, that it deserves its own chapter.

Your Enemy, Yourself

IF YOU HAVE WEIGHT TO LOSE, I assume you've made multiple attempts to lose it. You've tried at least one or two structured diets, but most often your goal was simply to eat less while exercising more. Each attempt, though, was tripped up by the fact you got too hungry to remain on the diet. Your body demanded more food. Appetite is the steroid-enhanced bully of physiological functions. It's the New York Yankees, Manchester United, GE, and Apple all rolled into one. No amount of self-control can keep hunger at bay forever. It wins almost every time.

Eating is what social-science researchers call an "automatic behavior." You can choose not to smoke or hang out in meth labs, but you can't choose not to eat. Almost all the eating we do is habitual, a product of both routine and necessity. Some of us are better or worse at forming new habits and routines, or at breaking the old ones. But for anybody, breaking one habit to establish another is a stressful process, and each of us has a limit to the amount of stress we can tolerate.

It's one thing if the habit is as simple as exchanging one breakfast cereal for another that has less sugar and more fiber, especially if it's an even swap in terms of calories or satiety. Making the change involves nothing more taxing than getting rid of the old one and remembering to buy the new one instead.

Dieting is something else entirely. The goal is to eat fewer calories, which is tremendously stressful all by itself, especially as the calorie deficits accumulate and your body responds by adjusting your metabolism. On top of that, you're simultaneously changing a series of eating behaviors: more meals, less food at each meal, different food, more prep time. You can't just *eat* anymore. You have to stop, think, plan, prepare.

At the same time, you're probably changing your workout routine—another form of stress. I try to be as clear as possible about how challenging Alwyn's routines are. That's by design. These are *training* programs. The entire point is to get your body to do something it doesn't currently do, or do something better, or at minimum do something differently. If it's a singular stress, something you impose on yourself three times a week with plenty of time to recover in between, I predict you'll be happy with the results. If the workouts are part of a series of stressful changes to your normal routine, you may not last long enough to see the payoff for all your work.

Which bring us to the next two rules.

NEW RULE #21 • Self-control, like muscle strength, can improve with training.

That's the good news. Unfortunately . . .

NEW RULE #22 • Weight management has little to do with self-control.

That's the surprise finding of a 2011 research review in *Personality and Social Psychology Review*. One of the coauthors is Roy F. Baumeister, Ph.D., a psychology professor at Florida State University, whose groundbreaking studies into self-control have shown just how important it is. People with the best self-control, the review notes, enjoy life the most, and have the most successful lives. Flipping it around, the people with the least self-control have the most problems. They're more prone to drink, smoke, commit fraud, drive without using a seat belt, and go online to post negative reviews of books they haven't read. (I just made up the last one. I'm sure it's true, but I can't back it up with data.)

So, given all these commonsensical implications of having versus not having com-

mand over your thoughts and behaviors, you'd assume that there's a strong correlation between self-control and weight management. There isn't. The correlation is
just 17 percent. That's still something, but it's not close to what most of us expect.
By contrast, there's a 36 percent correlation with success in school and work, and a
33 percent correlation with personal well-being. This appears to be the bottom line:
People with high self-control are more likely to do well in school, have successful
careers, and feel good about their place in the world than people who lack self-control.
But those successful people have the same struggles with their weight as everyone else.

Why? Because eating, again, is an automatic behavior most of the time. We get
hungry at predictable times, and the less attention we can pay to what and how we
eat, the more we can focus on the parts of life that bring us the biggest rewards. Are
you going to jeopardize your job performance so you can spend more time shopping
for and preparing food? Are you going to compromise your most important relationships? Or, if you're financially stressed, are you going to spend limited funds on wild
salmon when you could get hamburger for a fraction of the cost?

Of course the choices aren't so dire for most of us. One of the benefits of reaching
middle age is gaining some stability in work and relationships. You've put in the long
hours at the office. You've survived turbulence at home. And let's say you're now ready
for another go at a serious weight-loss plan. You understand that your only shot at
long-term success is to make permanent changes to your automatic eating behaviors,
and you're willing to do that. What now?

NEW RULE #23   •   A weight-loss plan is good for six months, max.

Through many years of reading and puzzling over weight-loss research, one trend
shows up in all the long-term studies I can recall. The best results occur in the first
six months. After that, study subjects inevitably start to regain their weight. It's not because they aren't trying hard enough. They're just hungry. Or they're sick of whatever
the diet forces them to eat. Or they want their old life back. Or some combination.

Six months is also long enough for *adaptive thermogenesis* to kick in. This is
a well-known physiological mechanism that I've described several times without
naming. Your metabolism, in response to a prolonged calorie deficit, slows down.
Your body uses less energy throughout the day. Exercise becomes more efficient, meaning your muscles use fewer calories to accomplish the same thing. Everything is
primed to prevent further weight loss and to regain what you've already shed. If you've

lost a significant amount—10 percent of your initial body weight—your metabolism has probably declined 15 percent.

It may not even take six months. Here are two more signs that you've gone as far as you can with a diet:

- *Weight loss has stopped, or slowed dramatically.* If you've lost only a pound or two in a month, after experiencing substantial success in previous months, that's your sign to call it quits. Your body is starting to fight back.
- *Your workouts have stopped working.* You aren't getting stronger or leaner, and you might even feel weaker. The problem could be with the program, especially if you haven't changed things up in four weeks or more. But nutrition is a likely culprit, hindering recovery and perhaps causing a loss of muscle tissue.

Any or all of these signs tell you it's time to shift your focus from weight loss to weight maintenance. After all, what was the point of losing it if it doesn't stay lost?

NEW RULE #24 • Weight maintenance requires new strategies and a different skill set.

Weight loss is an outcome goal. You go out of your comfort zone and willingly sacrifice comfort for a specific result. For some, it's easier to cut calories and begin exercising at the same time, as one set of outcome-focused behaviors will reinforce the other. The exercise itself, as noted in previous chapters, doesn't contribute substantially to weight loss. That's almost all diet. Exercise works because you feel good about what you're doing, and by extension you feel good about yourself.

But if you went into your weight-loss program with an all-out focus on the outcome—measured in pounds, inches, and/or sizes—you may be tempted to quit training just as your body has recalibrated itself to regain all of it, plus some. You couldn't possibly make a bigger mistake.

Exercise becomes the main event when a diet ends and you start eating in a more normal, sustainable way. It shows up in every study as a bulwark against regaining lost weight. Workouts like Alwyn's override the metabolic efficiency of your new, lighter body. Intense weight workouts, combined with a higher-calorie diet, allow you to gain strength and increase muscle tissue. *This is exactly what you want to happen.*

Weight maintenance involves process goals, rather than outcome goals. You may, for example, set a goal of twenty workouts per month, which is one of Alwyn's favorite tactics. Twelve would be strength workouts, and eight would be something else—Spinning classes, hiking, yoga, sports. Whatever your process goal is, focus on hitting that number of workouts without fail.

The following process goals linked to successful weight-loss maintenance have shown up in research from Penn State Hershey Medical Center, as well as the National Weight Control Registry:

- *Weigh yourself regularly*. It doesn't have to be every day, but it has to be something you monitor frequently. Your instinct is to stop weighing yourself once you realize you're no longer losing weight. Adjust your expectations, and celebrate each day that the scale hits the same number. If it shows something slightly higher, tighten up your diet until it goes back down. It's a lot easier to lose one pound than ten.
- *Drink lots of water*. Whatever effect water has on weight or metabolism is mild, if it's even measurable. But as a habit, drinking water throughout the day reminds you that you're still focused on the process of weight control.
- *Eat the same number of meals each day*. There's no magic number of meals. It could be four, five, or six—whatever works best for you. You just have to be consistent.
- *Question, quantify, qualify*. Data from the National Weight Control Registry is kind of depressing. People who successfully maintain a reduced weight typically eat low-fat, low-calorie, and low-sugar food. What does that even leave, besides chicken breasts and broccoli? But I'm not sure those factors matter as much as the fact that they stop to think about what they eat, which seems counterintuitive: If eating is an automatic behavior, how can you quantify everything you eat? You can't, unless quantification itself becomes automatic. And really, you have to worry only about stuff you haven't eaten before. Even then, you don't have to deprive yourself of everything. You just have to slow down long enough to understand what you're about to eat, and ask why you're eating it. The answer might be, "Because it looks good and I really want it." Great. Just make sure you ask yourself the question, and give yourself an honest response.

When the Going Gets Weird, the Weird Turn to Protein

BACK IN 2009, the PBS show *Nova* debuted a brilliant three-part series called *Becoming Human*. In part three, "Last Human Standing," the show explained why our species, Homo sapiens, outlasted the Neanderthals. Neanderthals had all of Europe to themselves for hundreds of thousands of years, with all the big game they could hunt down and kill. Their fossilized teeth and bones show that our Neanderthal cousins ate meat, and pretty much nothing else. Granted, there wasn't a lot of vegetation during the many ice ages they endured. But even when things thawed out, there's no evidence they had interest in anything that grew from the ground or swam in the rivers and seas. In a way, it's hard to blame them. They needed an estimated 5,000 calories a day to sustain their heavily muscled bodies and full-contact hunting style. (They got right up on their prey and took them down with spears; as a consequence, most Neanderthal skeletons show traces of multiple fractures.)

Back in Africa, meanwhile, early Homo sapiens were pushed close to extinction by a drought that turned most of the continent to desert. Small, isolated bands of humans made a last stand on the coasts, where a remarkable change occurred some 70,000 years ago. Humans adapted, but not just to their immediate circumstances.

They adapted to change itself. They learned to gather and cook shellfish, which required not just new tools but also a more sophisticated understanding of their environment. They hunted small game, which required new weapons and strategies. They gathered and ate a wide variety of roots and berries.

When the drought ended, these newly empowered humans worked their way back across the continent. Some migrated to Europe, others to Asia. Wherever they went, other human species quickly became extinct. Our ancestors could reproduce faster and more successfully (presaging our own baby boom by several dozen millennia), and they could find ways to thrive in almost any environment.

Moreover, humans learned to manipulate those environments, even to the point of self-destruction. For reasons unknown, our big human brains have from time to time proven incapable of thinking far enough ahead to avoid deforesting our habitats or hunting our prey to extinction. Today we have a food chain manipulated to give us fewer foods produced in larger quantities, at clear cost to human health.

So how do we resist? One increasingly compelling and popular answer is to look back to our cave-dwelling forebears, who saved our species from extinction by adapting to a lean but nutritious diet: meat, fish, eggs, fruits, seeds, and vegetables, along with some grains and tubers. It's relatively low in carbohydrates, but not religiously so. If we've learned anything from the unrelenting expansion of American waistlines during our own lifetime, it's that there's no simple explanation for how we got here, and no simple path back to a normal-sized population.

Low-fat and low-carb diets fail for most people because they're too restrictive. Low-calorie diets don't work for long because few of us can voluntarily deprive ourselves of the feeling of fullness that comes with a hearty meal. As explained in Chapter 20, it's really hard to make anything work beyond the first six months.

Moreover, as our friend John Berardi, Ph.D., has noted, most people don't have the time or interest to sort out the food fights that get played up in the media day after day. Berardi's company, Precision Nutrition, counsels a broad spectrum of dieters (including people who're trying to *gain* weight). Everyone has too much information, and few of us know what to do with it, which is why he estimates 60 percent of his clients struggle to follow any diet plan. For their benefit—and for ours—he simplifies every good weight-loss plan down to five simple concepts:

1. *You must eat less.* Don't believe anyone who says you can eat all you want as long as you avoid one type of food. You have to find a way to eat fewer total calories without triggering your body's anti-starvation mechanisms.

2. *You need more protein.* Your body can thrive with relatively little protein, as long as it has plenty of everything else. When you reduce everything else, you need more protein. Protein fills two enormously important roles during weight loss: It increases satiety, so you feel full longer between meals, and it takes much more energy to process than carbs or fat. Your body burns as much as a quarter of its dietary protein during digestion. Finally, since much of your body is made of protein (about 20 percent of your muscles, heart, and liver, and 10 percent of your brain), a higher-protein diet puts your body into an anabolic mode, one that builds tissues rather than breaking them down.

3. *Decrease carbs.* It's not that every carb is bad. We can thrive on a wide range of fruits, vegetables, seeds, grains, and roots, as well as the carbs found in dairy products. But we all eat more than we need because there's so friggin' much food available. If it's cheap to produce, our food chain gives us too much of it, and we fill up on bread, pasta, rice, corn, and potatoes instead of the things that would help us achieve and maintain a healthier weight.

4. *Increase vegetables.* Vegetables like broccoli, lettuce, carrots, and asparagus provide relatively few calories per unit of volume or weight, compared with energy-dense foods like bread or potatoes. Plus, they provide fiber, which not only contributes to your digestive health (the importance of which we certainly appreciate by middle age), but also works like protein to slow your appetite between meals.

5. *Replace unhealthy fats with healthy ones.* This is a complicated subject, but it really comes down to a fairly basic guideline: Naturally occurring fats in meat, dairy, eggs, fish, and plants are, on balance, good for you in moderate amounts. When possible, we should choose the leaner, lower-fat versions of those foods, and minimize our use of vegetable oils for cooking and flavoring. It's not because the fats are bad; we just don't need the calories. The fats you want to limit, like soybean oil, are mostly found in prepared foods. The fats found in fish and fish-oil supplements are worth going out of your way to obtain. They were once plentiful in our food chain, and are associated with a long list of cardiovascular, orthopedic, and mood-related benefits. (If you don't eat a lot of fish, taking three to six fish-oil capsules a day is probably a good idea.)

It sounds like five separate pieces of advice—add this, take away that, and mix and match all this other stuff. But really it's one huge yet surprisingly simple concept: The more food you eat that's close to its natural state, the more protein, fiber, and healthy fat you'll have in your diet, with fewer overall calories and a steep drop in carbs and unhealthy fats. You'll also, to the extent it's possible, feel more satisfied with less food.

Easier said than done? Keep reading.

FREE FUEL FOR YOUR METABOLIC FIRE

Billy Beck III, owner of BB3 Personal Training and Performance Center in Weston, Florida, has the most straightforward meal-planning system I've ever come across. I won't pretend it's easy to execute, but at the very least it's easy to remember. More important, it gives you a foolproof template to follow Berardi's five nutrition principles. Beck has his clients narrow all food choices down to three types of meals:

* Fire
* Fuel
* Free

A fire meal is a plate that's 50 percent lean protein and 50 percent vegetables (or fruit, or a combination of the two). A fuel meal is one-third lean protein, one-third vegetables, and one-third high-energy carbs. Lean protein can be meat, poultry, fish, or eggs. Vegetables, for this discussion, include all the colorful stuff (plus cauliflower), but not potatoes and other tubers. Those fall into the category of high-energy carbs, along with grains, including rice and corn.

A free meal is something you eat because you really want to. There are no rules, except that it applies only to that one meal. If a free meal turns into a day of unrestrained eating, or a weekend, the plan won't work.

Here's how simple it is:

Grill a steak and some asparagus, and it's a fire meal. The steak can be bigger or smaller to suit your appetite. Add a baked potato or a grilled ear of corn and it's a fuel meal.

You don't have to grill the steak. Broil it, bake it, boil it—it's still a steak. (Unless you dip it in batter and fry it. At that point it's a mutant blend of nutrition and antinutrition, and a threat to life as we know it.) Of course it doesn't have to be a steak. It can be a piece of fish, a chicken breast, a turkey burger.

The vegetables can be whatever you like, prepared however you like.

You can use the system dining out. At Ruby Tuesday, just to pick one, you can get a substantial fuel meal by ordering grilled salmon with broccoli and mashed potatoes. The company's website says it's 664 calories, with 46 grams of protein, 35 grams of carbs (including 8 grams of fiber), and 39 grams of fat.

But I mentioned the dreaded C word: calories. How do you manage those? Let's tackle that first, and then I'll show you a basic template for balancing fire, fuel, and free meals, followed by some tasty, easy-to-prepare fire and fuel meals.

CALORIE SLAVES

This is the part of the book where, in the past, I would do two things: First I'd give you a formula for estimating how many calories you need each day. Then I'd tell you to write down everything you eat for three days, go to an online calculator (such as fitday.com), enter each morsel of food, and emerge with an estimate of your average daily calorie intake. If the first number is smaller than the second, I would tell you to calculate the difference and deduct that many calories from your daily meals.

The first number suggests that a formula based on height, weight, and age can guess how much energy you burn with exercise, digestion, fidgeting, or getting up to use the bathroom. With the second number, you hope that you wrote down everything you ate, that you ate the things you would typically eat (resisting the instinct to clean up your diet to feel better about yourself), and, most important, that you correctly estimated serving sizes of everything you logged and reported. For that matter, you hope that the calorie counts used by the website are accurate, even though different sources report different values for the same foods.

Both numbers tell you something. But I'm no longer confident they're meaningful or helpful. Energy balance is too dynamic, with too many variables.

I think there's a simpler equation, one that requires nothing more complicated than a scale, a tape measure, and some brutal honesty: Are you getting fatter? Has your weight increased in the past year? Two years? Three? Has your waistline, or any other circumference you care about, gotten thicker? How long has it been since you bought new clothes because something you like no longer fits?

Now you have a data point that matters. If you're getting fatter, you have an energy surplus—a mismatch between what you eat and what you burn. If your weight and everything else has been stable—regardless of *where* it stabilized—then you're in energy balance. Lost weight recently? You have (or had) an energy deficit.

Each situation requires a different strategy.

If you're in energy balance: I recommend doing Alwyn's workouts for a month before making any major changes to your diet. Clean it up where you can, but don't deliberately eat a lot less. See what the workouts do without a diet overhaul. You won't lose a lot of weight from a ramped-up exercise program, but if you lose some, get stronger, and feel better without feeling hungrier, then you know your body responds to training. You don't need to cut a lot of calories to see results.

If you're gaining weight: I recommend starting a reduced-calorie diet along with the workouts. The workouts alone may stabilize your weight, but they're unlikely to create a negative energy balance unless you get control of your diet. You need to eat less, which, unfortunately, may affect your performance in the weight room. But you need both interventions to reverse your energy surplus.

If you're losing weight: In the early stages of a successful weight-loss program, the last thing you want to do is pivot away and try something else. You're already changing your exercise routine (assuming you were doing something else before you switched to NROL). The key for you is to monitor your workout performance along with your mood, energy level, and anything else that could be related to nutrition. A lack of steady, measurable progress from week to week, despite your best effort in the gym, suggests you aren't recovering enough between workouts. That, in turn, suggests you aren't eating enough. Alwyn designs every element of his training system with the idea that his clients or readers will work hard and then recover adequately. You won't get the results you want from an NROL program if your diet has left you depleted.

Beck's fire-and-fuel meal-planning system offers solutions for all three situations.

BURN NOTICE

In a moment I'll show you some easy ways to create fire and fuel meals. You'll see how a fire meal can easily become a fuel meal, and how you can expand the portions of any meal to accommodate a bigger body and a more robust appetite.

How you balance each type of meal depends on your goals, but we'll start with two givens: You plan to eat four meals a day (even if you eat just three, or as many as six, go along with the example for now), and you won't go more than four hours between meals. We'll say breakfast at eight a.m., lunch at noon, a mid-afternoon meal at three or four p.m., and dinner at six or seven. Some will be bigger or smaller; it doesn't really matter at the moment.

Your current state: energy surplus

You've been gaining weight, and need to reverse it. On the days you do one of Alwyn's workouts, you might have two fire and two fuel meals. Ideally you'll have the fuel meals before and after your workout. When you train matters, of course. Those who work out first thing in the morning aren't going to get up two hours early to prepare a fuel meal and give it time to digest. A fuel meal right after your workout is the best choice. Have the second fuel meal whenever it works for you.

On non-workout days, you might choose to have three fire meals and one fuel. You'd have the fuel meal whenever you're most likely to need it—breakfast, lunch, or dinner.

Starting out with more fire than fuel meals is aggressive, and it might end up being a lot less food than you're used to having. That's where the free meals come in handy. Beck has his clients eat three free meals a week, which is a good starting point for us. It's probably best to plan one or two of them, especially when you have a party or special night out on the calendar. At the same time, it's good to keep at least one in reserve for the times when you just need to break the rules and fill up on something you really miss when you're adherent. Pizza. Pasta. Chicken wings. Chocolate cake. Whatever it is, have it, enjoy it, brush your teeth, and return to the plan.

Your current state: energy balance

I suggest an equal balance of fire and fuel meals, with three free meals each week. It probably won't be more food than you currently eat, but it could be less. Monitor your hunger and energy levels. If you feel so hungry you're tempted to have a free meal every day, adjust portion sizes until it feels like a normal amount.

After a month of Alwyn's workouts, reassess. If you're losing weight and/or inches (or at least centimeters), and you feel good, stay the course. If you feel good but aren't losing anything you can see or measure (assuming this is your goal), switch to three fire and one fuel meal on non-workout days. Look for strategic ways to cut back slightly on portions in your fuel meals.

Your current state: energy deficit

As I mentioned earlier, you don't want to change anything when your current diet is working. The fire-and-fuel plan may fit that diet, but it may not. If it doesn't, you can always switch when your diet quits working, or when you hit the six-month mark, as discussed in Chapter 20.

For the moment, let's suppose that you're using fire and fuel meals, and you're losing weight steadily. But you aren't getting the results you want from your workouts. You need more food to recover, but not so much that you stop losing weight.

Try adding an extra meal on the days you work out. It could be as simple as a protein shake immediately after your workout, followed by a fuel meal an hour or two later. If the workouts don't get better, and you feel a general fatigue more often than not, you probably need to add more total food to your diet. Start with bigger meals on workout days, which give you more energy to train and a more robust recovery.

FIVE EASY PIECES

I can't cook worth a darn. I've never asked Alwyn about his culinary skills, but given how often he jokes about nutrition quality in his native Scotland (considered the worst in Europe), I suspect they aren't a lot better than mine. That's why I turned to my friend Galya Ivanova Denzel, a trainer and weight-loss coach based in Southern California, who also happens to be a very good cook. The following five recipes are entirely hers.

Remember, these are just examples of what you can do with fire and fuel meals if you have some time and feel like cooking something special. You can use the system with any foods you like, no matter how basic and unadorned, as long as they match the criteria: lean protein and vegetables and/or fruit for a fire meal, with each taking up half the space on your plate; lean protein, vegetables, and high-octane carbs for a fuel meal, with each filling a third of the plate.

BREAKFAST

Coconut Omelet

1 tablespoon coconut oil
4 egg whites

1 whole egg
4 drops natural vanilla extract
1 tablespoon unsweetened coconut flakes
½ cup strawberries

- Heat the oil in a medium skillet over medium heat.
- In a medium bowl, beat the egg whites and whole egg with the vanilla and coconut flakes. Pour into the skillet and cook until lightly browned on both sides. Serve with the strawberries.

  337 calories; 21 grams protein; 9 grams carbs (3 grams fiber); 24 grams fat

- For a bigger appetite, make the omelet using 4 whole eggs instead of 1 whole egg and 4 whites.

  510 calories; 25 grams protein; 10 grams carbs (3 grams fiber); 41 grams fat

- To make either of these a fuel meal, add a cup of blueberries, which gives you 82 more calories, with 4 grams of fiber.

LUNCH

Lebanese Salad

5 ounces lean lamb or 6 ounces chicken breast
Sea salt
1 teaspoon ground cumin
¼ teaspoon ground cinnamon
1 medium tomato
1 small cucumber
¼ cup cooked chickpeas
½ ounce walnuts (about 7 pieces)
1 teaspoon olive oil
1 tablespoon chopped parsley

- Preheat the oven to 375°F.
- Season the lamb or chicken with salt and the spices, place in a roasting pan, and roast for 20 minutes. (You can also grill it if you prefer.) Remove from the oven and slice the meat.

- While the lamb is roasting, cut the tomatoes and cucumber however you like (sliced, cubed, chopped). Place in a salad bowl and add the chickpeas and walnuts. Toss with the olive oil and parsley. Place the sliced meat on top of the salad.

  490 calories; 38 grams protein; 19 grams carbs (5 grams fiber); 28 grams fat

- The calories and fat will vary tremendously, depending on whether you use lamb or chicken. Different cuts of lamb will also vary quite a bit. These numbers are an average of the range between chicken breast (which has very little fat after you remove the skin) and a lean cut of lamb. If you make it heartier, with a bigger piece of lamb or chicken, the range will be even greater.
- To turn it into a fuel meal, add another half cup of chickpeas. That gives you 142 more calories, with 8 grams of protein, 23 grams of carbs (including 7 grams of fiber), and 2 grams of fat.

California-Style Turkey Burger

1 slice bacon
One 4-ounce turkey burger patty
2 cups salad greens
½ cup sugar snap peas
4 or 5 olives
1 teaspoon olive oil
Sea salt
¼ orange
Mustard and/or ketchup (optional)
¼ avocado
2 large lettuce leaves

- Cook the bacon in a medium skillet over medium heat until crisp. Set the cooked bacon on a paper towel, drain the oil from the pan, and cook the burger in the pan. (Or you can grill it if that's easier.)
- While the bacon and burger are cooking, make a salad by combining the salad greens, sugar snap peas, and olives in a salad bowl. Toss with the olive oil and a pinch of salt. Squeeze the juice from the orange over the salad. When the burger's cooked, throw on mustard or ketchup if you like, top with the avocado and bacon, and wrap it all in the lettuce leaves in place of a bun.

  582 calories; 39 grams protein; 13 grams carbs (8 grams fiber); 41 grams fat

● You can turn the burger into a fuel meal by serving it in a whole-grain bun. An Oroweat bun (other brands will be different) adds 170 calories, with 7 grams of protein, 32 grams of carbs (including 7 grams of fiber), and 2.5 grams of fat.

DINNER

Peppery Salmon and Greens

Lemon pepper
6 ounces boneless wild-caught salmon
1 cup broccoli florets
½ cup baby carrots
2 cups baby greens
1 ounce slivered almonds
Balsamic vinegar
Sea salt

● Heat a medium skillet over medium heat. Rub lemon pepper to taste into the salmon and cook on both sides until lightly browned and cooked through.
● Meanwhile, steam the broccoli and carrots for 10 minutes. Place in a salad bowl and cool. Add the greens and almonds, then toss with vinegar and salt to taste.

474 calories; 46 grams protein; 18 grams carbs (8 grams fiber); 25 grams fat

● You can make this dish more substantial by starting with 10 ounces of salmon. That adds 66 calories, 24 grams of protein, 5 grams of fat, and no more carbs.
● It becomes a fuel meal with a medium baked potato. That adds 168 calories, with 4.5 grams of protein, 37 grams of carbs (including 4 grams of fiber), and no more fat. (Obviously, a smaller potato has less of everything.)

Shrimp Stir-Fry

1 tablespoon coconut oil
½ cup sugar snap peas
½ cup bell pepper strips (multiple colors if possible)
½ cup broccoli florets
½ cup bamboo shoots
1 cup peeled and deveined shrimp
Sea salt or soy sauce

● Heat the coconut oil in a thin pan or wok, then toss in the vegetables and let them cook for a few minutes, stirring constantly. (Less cooking time leaves them crunchier.) Add the shrimp and salt or soy sauce to taste and cook for 2 to 3 minutes, stirring constantly, until the shrimp are firm and no longer pink.

445 calories; 47 grams protein; 21 grams carbs (including 8 grams of fiber); 20 grams fat

● You can make this a fuel meal by serving the stir-fry over a cup of cooked wild rice (made from ⅓ cup uncooked). To cook wild rice, first soak it in water for 20 minutes, rinse well, then boil with 1½ cups water for 40 minutes. The nutty flavor makes it worth the extra time it takes compared with white or brown rice. It adds 65 calories, with 7 grams of protein, 35 grams of carbs (including 3 grams of fiber), and no fat.

PART 4

THOSE THINGS YOU DO

Wherever You Train, There You Are

Before I try to answer some of the questions that come up with each book in the series, let's review the elements of Alwyn's NROL for Life program:

1. *RAMP,* which combines range-of-motion exercises (improving flexibility and mobility) with agility and overall conditioning.
2. *Core training,* which improves the strength, stability, and endurance of the muscles supporting your lower back and pelvis.
3. *Power training,* which improves your ability to generate force rapidly, and is probably the most overlooked aspect of fitness for those of us who remember watching the 1960s on TV. (I don't know about you, but that was as close as I got to the fun stuff.)
4. *Strength training,* which in addition to building strength helps you develop all the aforementioned fitness qualities: mobility, coordination, core strength, power, and overall conditioning.
5. *Metabolic training,* which develops cardiovascular fitness, burns a lot of calories

in a very short time, and, depending on the exercises you choose, can also improve power, strength, and muscular endurance.

6. *Recovery*, a combination of exercises to improve tissue length and quality, along with nutrition to put your body in an anabolic state, and keep it there as long as possible. You'll build up your muscles and connective tissues after your workout has broken them down.

The most unique feature of this book—the freedom to choose your own exercises—may also be the most confusing. That's why we provided two complete programs, one each for beginner and advanced lifters, with sample exercises selected.

One of our goals was to head off the question we hear more than any other: "Is it okay if I do X instead of Y?" In the three previous *NROL* books, the answer was "Yes, but only if you understand what you're doing and have a really good reason to make the change." Here the answer is "Hell yes," with just these caveats:

1. **Stick to the category.** If you need a different squat variation, we've provided a comprehensive list. Just don't replace a squat with a pull. Remember Alwyn's Chinese-menu analogy. Don't combine chicken with pork, or rice with noodles, or for that matter white rice with brown.

2. **Qualify for the level.** Alwyn gives you five levels for each exercise category. Make sure you qualify for each level by mastering the one that precedes it. Don't squat with a barbell on your back (Level 4) before you've perfected your form with the body-weight squat (Level 1).

3. **Treat each category as its own challenge.** In theory, it's possible for a beginner to do all Level 1 exercises in Phase One, Level 2 exercises in Phase Two, and Level 3 exercises in Phase Three. But I'd be very surprised if anyone does it that way. Alwyn and I started this book with the idea that each reader has unique challenges. Some advanced lifters may be ready for Level 5 in one category but struggle to get past Level 3 in another. Healthy beginners may rocket past Level 1 exercises in some categories, but stay at Level 1 for a while in others.

4. **Challenge yourself.** Each workout should be *hard*, for lack of a better word. It's okay to breeze through one or two training sessions while you sort out which exercises are best for you. I guarantee no one can figure it out on paper; you have to get into the gym and decide if the exercises you choose actually work the way you think they will. You'll tinker constantly. Just keep in mind that these are still *training* sessions. You're training your body to be stronger, faster, leaner, more

athletic, more durable, more mobile. You can't do that if you take it easy on yourself. You have the power to change your body, but only if you're willing to use that power.

Now let's turn to the other frequently asked questions.

"I don't understand the workouts."

What about them is confusing, other than "everything"? A quick review of the system:

- The program has three phases. You do only one at a time—Phase One, followed by Phase Two, followed by Phase Three.
- Each phase has two workouts, A and B. This trips up a lot of people, but it's simple. You start each new phase with Workout A. Two or three days later, you do Workout B. Then you alternate A and B until you finish the phase. You'll never do both A and B on the same day, or even on consecutive days. (You should need 48 to 72 hours between workouts for recovery.) Most of you will do A and B four to six times each before you finish that phase and move to the next phase. You'll have a different Workout A and Workout B in the new phase, but the idea is exactly the same.
- Each workout starts with RAMP (the warm-up routine shown in Chapter 15) and ends with recovery (Chapter 18). In between you'll have a series of program components (core, power, strength, etc.), which you'll perform in the order shown in the workout templates in Chapter 17.
- Most of those components are broken down further into exercise categories. In core training, for example, you have stabilization and dynamic stabilization categories. In strength training, you have squat, hinge, lunge, single-leg stance, push, pull, and combination exercises. In power training, you have movements that primarily use upper- or lower-body muscles. But you'll do only one exercise per category per workout. All you need to focus on is that one exercise. Work to get better and stronger each time you do it. When it's time to advance to another exercise in that category, focus on the new one until it's time to change again.
- The exercise categories are further divided into levels. Each category has exercises listed from Level 1 to Level 5. Some go beyond Level 5, but that's the last thing you need to worry about if you're just starting. Sometimes you have options within a level. But you're still focusing on one exercise at a time. Pick one and do it until you're ready to move up to the next.

● Some exercises appear in pairs: 1a and 1b, 2a and 2b. This is a standard feature of workouts in books, magazines, and websites; it's an efficient and effective way to train: Do a set of exercise 1a. Rest. Do a set of 1b. Rest. Do your second set of 1a. Rest. Do your second set of 1b. Rest. If you need to do third or fourth sets of each, do it. Then move on to 2a and 2b.

If you're still confused, or just want some advice on which exercise to choose, go to forums.jpfitness.com. There you'll find forums for each book in the NROL series. Some of the forum veterans—a mix of trainers and enthusiasts—will have advance copies of *NROL for Life*, and will be able to help you with your questions.

"What's with all the negativity about cardio exercise? Are you telling me I should quit running?"

No. Or, as Darth Vader memorably emoted, "Nooooooooooo!" Alwyn and I aren't runners, but lots of *NROL* readers are. In fact, both of this book's models are runners (Dan is a triathlete), as are the book's editor and our agent. Rachel Cosgrove, Alwyn's wife, has done an Ironman, and was on a national triathlon team. Their gym, Results Fitness, has a running team that participates in local distance races.

Human survival depended on the ability to travel long distances on foot, while also performing feats of strength, power, and athleticism. We all want to have a mix of endurance and strength.

Alwyn and I make three big points about endurance training:

1. Running is not an entry-level activity for someone who's currently sedentary. The heavier you are, the more stressful it is. As Alwyn has often said over the years, you don't run to get fit. You get fit, then run.

2. Endurance activities are more specialized than most people understand. It takes years to develop a cardiovascular system capable of delivering oxygen and nutrients to your working muscles for hours at a time during a moderate-intensity activity like running. It takes years to develop the muscular endurance and neural efficiency to cover long distances. But we live in a world in which running a marathon is considered the pinnacle of athletic achievement, and that convinces a lot of people to push their bodies past the breaking point.

3. Traditional, steady-pace endurance exercise isn't a necessity for health, fitness, or weight control. You can achieve all those things with the NROL for Life training program.

Running, in other words, is great for runners. We don't want to talk anyone out of doing something they enjoy and consider beneficial. Alwyn's program is ideal for those (like me) who want to focus on lifting and have no interest in running farther than the mailbox. But it's also terrific for those who enjoy both strength and endurance exercise.

Final word: We're fitness professionals, and we're pro-fitness. We're in favor of everyone doing physical activities that they love. If all you love is lifting, Alwyn's programs give you a way to develop every important fitness quality without leaving your primary workout space. But the bigger goal is to provide you with a program that enhances every aspect of your life, helping you do more inside and outside the weight room, and do it better.

"How do I incorporate other activities with these workouts? Can I do two things on the same day?"

We all have to make choices. The older we get, the harder it is to pursue multiple fitness goals with similar intensity. Recovery becomes an ever-more-pressing concern. However, some types of exercise work better as complements to strength training than others. Anything that involves low-intensity, low-impact movement seems to help with recovery. An ideal training schedule might be three days a week of NROL for Life workouts with something else in between—yoga, Spinning, swimming, cycling, sports practice. If it gets blood into your muscles, and puts your joints through a range of motion, it'll probably help.

Conversely, a high-stress workout—competitive sports, interval training, long-distance running or cycling, full-contact martial arts—requires its own period of recovery. Not only are your muscles and joints stressed, your brain is fried.

As for two types of exercise on the same day, sure, it can work, as long as the two things don't compete in terms of the energy systems they use. Alwyn's workouts will push your anaerobic systems, the ones that require short bursts of hard work followed by a period of recovery to catch your breath. You can probably combine that with exercise that relies on your aerobic energy system, in which you don't push yourself to exhaustion. If you do them back to back, it's best to do the strength workout first, since that requires the most energy and focus.

"How come there aren't any arm exercises in the program?"

There's nothing wrong with biceps curls and triceps extensions. They obviously work your arm muscles. But so do the pushing and pulling exercises, which use your biceps, triceps, and forearms in conjunction with the rest of your upper-body muscles. If you want to target them more directly, you can use an underhand grip on most pulling exercises, which will give your biceps direct stimulation, and move your hands closer together on push-ups and presses, which makes your triceps work somewhat harder. I don't think there's any need (beyond a medical or therapeutic reason) to do specific exercises for your forearms. The gripping muscles will be tested early and often with deadlifts, pulls, and some of the lunges and single-leg exercises. The core, power, and combination exercises offer even more chances to use them.

Would your arms get a little bigger if you added some curls and extensions to the program? Probably. The open question is whether they're worth the time. In a 50-minute workout, will you be better off using 10 minutes for arm exercises, targeting small muscles you've already used in multiple exercises? Or would you get better results by doing drills that make you stronger, leaner, and more athletic?

Let's be honest: A middle-aged guy in a gym wants to feel good about himself, and he's more likely to get that with pumped-up biceps than with quads turned to Jell-O by front squats and reverse lunges. An overweight woman wants to attack the pockets of fat that make it embarrassing or uncomfortable to wear her favorite outfits. She may understand, on an intellectual level, that no volume of triceps kickbacks will spot-reduce arm fat, just as she understands that crunches won't really make her belly smaller. But she does them anyway, because if we're going to work on a problem, we want to attack it directly.

This is one time when the indirect approach will be far more effective for most readers. An overweight lifter with a 40-inch waist will probably have bigger arms than a lean lifter, but whose arms look better? A woman looking to drop a size or two will get there faster with total-body training that employs her biggest muscles, the ones that use the most calories and push the metabolism as far as it can go.

"What do I do when I finish the program?"

Repeat it. Go back to Phase One, and start over again with one or more of these changes:

- Do more advanced exercises.
- Use heavier weights.
- Increase the volume. If you did one set of 15 reps in Phase One, make it two sets of 15. If you did two sets of 10 in Phase Two, try three sets of 10.

- Go faster. Once you're comfortable with your form on an exercise, try to increase your repetition speed.

Advanced lifters can also adjust the reps to allow more aggressive strength and size development. You can try it like this:

	Phase One: Transform	Phase Two: Develop	Phase Three: Maximize
First time	1–2 sets, 15 reps	2–4 sets, 10 reps	2–3 sets, 12 reps
Second time	2–3 sets, 12 reps	3–4 sets, 8 reps	2–3 sets, 10 reps
Third time	2–3 sets, 10 reps	4–5 sets, 5–6 reps	2–3 sets, 8–10 reps

If you go through the program a fourth time, you can adjust the sets and reps within each phase, so you do more sets with heavier weights on squats, deadlifts, presses, and pulls, and fewer sets with lighter weights on lunges and single-leg-stance exercises. As long as you hit all the movement patterns and improve something from one week to the next, the workouts should continue working for you.

"What about nutritional supplements? Should I use them?"

I use:

- protein supplements following my workouts (about 40 grams of protein mixed with water), and occasionally on non-workout days
- fish oil (3 to 6 pills per day is a standard recommendation)
- creatine

Since this is the first time I've mentioned creatine, I should explain my backstory: I used it off and on in the early 2000s, when I was training for maximum strength. I always got a boost when I used it, but eventually my supply would run out and I'd go on with my training without giving it any thought. In early 2011, I was struggling to regain strength following hernia surgery a few months before. I started using creatine again, putting 5 grams into my post-workout shakes. Within a couple of weeks I was making extraordinary gains, which continued for two or three months before things leveled off.

It wasn't like I was unaware of the benefits. I've written and edited articles about creatine and seen the results. If anything stopped me (other than using up my supply and being too cheap or lazy to get more), it was the one side effect: weight gain. You can expect to gain a couple of pounds. It was worth it to me to regain some of the strength and muscle size I'd lost with the string of injuries that started around my fiftieth birthday.

I don't think there's a final word on whether the lifelong use of creatine will lead to better muscular fitness than you could obtain by lifting and following a sensible diet. Studies in all age groups tend to show short-term effects (although some don't), and as always, individual results are all over the place.

If you want to try it, stick with a basic creatine monohydrate powder. Take 3 to 6 grams a day, mixed in water or in a post-workout shake. More isn't better. Once your muscles are saturated, there's no additional benefit.

Nutritionists often suggest a multivitamin for insurance against deficiencies. I'm not quite sure what deficiencies a typical adult would have with a non-extreme diet (other than EPA and DHA, the two polyunsaturated fats you get in fish and fish oil). We get the most important vitamins and minerals from fruit, vegetables, dairy, eggs, meat, beans, and fortified breads and cereals. (Even though it's best to avoid the highly processed foods in that last category, most of us end up eating some.) If a doctor or nutritionist recommends that you supplement something else—calcium, iron, vitamin D—by all means follow his or her advice.

"I bought your book for my Kindle, and I can't read the charts. What do I do?"

Go to werkit.com. Otto and Aoife Hammersmith design training logs for all the NROL books. You can download blank logs for each workout, print them out, and take them to the gym with you.

"What should I do on the days I'm just not motivated to work out? Work out anyway?"

The key question is, why aren't you motivated? Some possibilities:

ILLNESS, CURRENT OR IMPENDING

A few years ago, I noticed that when I worked out despite feeling off my game, with less energy and focus than usual, two things happened: I'd have a mediocre workout, and by the next day I'd have cold or flu symptoms. My body tends to be pretty good at fighting things off. But if I pile training stress on top of a pathogen assault, the illness wins. If I listen to my body and take it easy for a day, I give my immune system a chance to work its magic.

That, of course, is a judgment call, and it's going to work differently for each of us. I've heard lots of people say that a workout is exactly what they need to get the juices flowing on the days they feel sluggish.

If you have an illness, it's a much easier decision. Don't go to the gym when you're sick. Forget that old "it's okay if the symptoms are above the shoulders" advice. Even if you work out at home, with no risk of infecting others, you still have a body under stress. Adding more stress just delays your recovery.

TOO MUCH GOING ON IN YOUR LIFE

Someone starting a new program often has a black-and-white perception of training: miss a workout, ruin the program. It's not that way at all. There's no harm in putting a workout off here or there. You don't have to go back to the starting line. At worst you'll need more time to get the results you want. You don't lose everything you've worked to that point to attain.

Even if you need to put the program on hold for a week or two, it won't take long to get your groove back. Yes, that first post-layoff workout may be ugly. Get through it however you can, and then pick up where you left off.

We all have personal business we have to take care of. Some of us can structure our lives so they rarely interfere with our training, but most of us can't. Keep in mind that this is a lifelong pursuit. You don't forget how to read if you go a week without a book, and you don't forget how to lift when life keeps you out of the gym.

BURNOUT OR POOR RESULTS

From time to time I'll hear from somebody who's been doing the exact same thing for years. They write to me because they haven't been getting much in the way of results lately. Lately? I get bored with a workout in four weeks or less. And yet my correspondents wonder why year four of a program isn't as successful as years one, two, and three.

If you're feeling burned out or unsatisfied, you need to change something. Alwyn and I have done our best to provide you with alternatives. More than that, our goal in *NROL for Life* is to give you the knowledge to come up with your own solutions when the need arises. You now know far more about selecting the right exercises for your body and your goals than the average lifter in your local health club. (You may even be ahead of some of the trainers.)

Whatever your problem is, however it may originate, you owe it to yourself to figure out the solution. Nobody can tell you exactly what it might be. It's like any other part of your life: work, family, friends, leisure. You have to figure out what turns your own gears.

All we know for sure is that we have gears. We have physical mechanisms that need to move. They also need fuel, maintenance, and the occasional replacement part. Point is, they're *your* gears. Maybe they need to move faster than mine. Or slower. Or spend more time turning. Or less. You won't know until you put them into motion and figure out what does and doesn't work.

I'm flattered that you've decided to give these programs a shot. Of course we're confident that they'll work for most people who try them; Alwyn wouldn't risk his reputation on anything less, and I wouldn't risk my livelihood. But that doesn't mean the system is perfect for everybody, or will solve every problem you have. It's a system that works well for Alwyn's clients, and for his coauthor. For you, there's a full spectrum of possibilities, from "this is the Holy Grail of training programs" to "I think I'll try Zumba next."

Just keep this in mind: A system works only if you use it systematically. Again, it's like those other parts of your life—work, family, friends, leisure. You don't keep a job if you show up whenever it's convenient and your effort is random and unpredictable. You can't stay in a relationship if your partner never knows when or even if you'll be home for dinner. Your friends would back away if you suddenly started calling them every day, and then three months later stopped calling altogether. Even your book club would kick you out if you forced them to read *Pride and Prejudice* one turn and *Jackass: 10 Years of Stupid* the next.

Your body won't fire you or file for divorce or stop returning your texts or change the location of its meeting with other bodies without telling you where it is. Still, those gears of yours perform best with consistent challenges imposed in a predictable pattern. The trick for each of us is to find the right mix of variety, to keep our workouts interesting and productive, and predictable, which ensures we're ready for new challenges when they arise. If it's too easy, you get nothing out of it, and if you hit your body with challenges for which it's completely unprepared . . . well, maybe you *should* read *10 Years of Stupid*.

A great training experience sometimes feels like a miracle. It's not. It's a proven system you've chosen to use while adjusting it to address your own abilities, limitations, and goals. That said, if this system works beyond your expectations, feel free to describe it as miraculous to your colleagues, family, friends, and book club, and accept our gratitude when you do.

Appendix

The Rules

These are the rules from all three NROL books, starting with the basic rules of exercise:

1. Do something.
2. Do something you like.
3. The rest is just details.

These are the original New Rules of Lifting:

1. The best muscle-building exercises are the ones that use your muscles the way they're designed to work.
2. Exercises that use lots of muscles in coordinated action are better than those that force muscles to work in isolation.
3. To build size, you must build strength.
4. To build size and strength, you must train hard but infrequently, with plenty of recovery time between workouts.
5. The goal of each workout is to set a record.
6. The weight you lift is a tool to reach your goals. It is not a goal by itself.

7. Don't "do the machines."
8. A workout is only as good as the adaptations it produces.
9. There is no magic system of exercises, sets, and reps.
10. Don't judge a system by the physique of the person promoting it.
11. You'll get better results working your ass off on a bad program than you will loafing through a good program.
12. Fast lifting is not more dangerous than slow lifting.
13. A good warm-up doesn't have to make your body warm.
14. Stretching is not a warm-up.
15. You don't need to warm up to stretch.
16. Lifting by itself may increase your flexibility.
17. Aerobic fitness is not a matter of life and death.
18. You don't need to do endurance exercise to burn fat.
19. When you combine serious strength training with serious endurance exercise, your body will probably choose endurance over muscle and strength.
20. If it's not fun, you're doing something wrong.

These are the New Rules of Lifting for Women:
1. The purpose of lifting weights is to build muscle.
2. Muscle is hard to build.
3. Results come from hard work.
4. Hard work includes lifting heavier weights.
5. From time to time, you have to break some of the old rules.
6. No workout will make you taller.
7. Muscles in men and women are essentially identical.
8. Muscle strength is a matter of life and death.
9. A muscle's "pump" is not the same as muscle growth.
10. Endurance exercise is an option, not a necessity, for fat loss.
11. "Aerobics" doesn't mean what you think it means.
12. Calorie restriction is the worst idea ever.
13. Traditional weight-loss advice is fatally flawed.
14. To reach your goals, you may need to eat more.
15. On balance, a balanced-macro diet is best.
16. Protein is the queen of macronutrients.
17. More meals are better than fewer.
18. Don't do programs designed for someone else's needs.

19. You don't need to isolate small muscles to make them bigger and stronger.
20. Every exercise is a "core" exercise.
21. The biggest blocks to your success could be the ones you've erected.

These are the New Rules of Lifting for Abs:
1. The most important role of the abdominal muscles is to protect your spine.
2. You can't protect your spine by doing exercises that damage it.
3. The size of your abdominal muscles doesn't matter.
4. The appearance of your abs doesn't matter either.
5. The core includes all the muscles that attach to your hips, pelvis, and lower back.
6. The lats are part of the core.
7. The crunch is not a core exercise.
8. Your spine is already flexed, and flexing it more just makes it worse.
9. Stability in your lower back depends on mobility in the joints above and below it.
10. You can't out-exercise a hunger-inducing lifestyle.
11. Your computer is the enemy of your abs.
12. TV and video games are almost as bad as your computer.
13. You can sleep your way to a better body . . . or not sleep your way to a bigger belly.
14. "Convenience" food is designed to make you eat more convenience food.
15. Processed food makes you stupid and depressed.
16. All that said, calories still matter more than anything else.
17. Don't do a complicated intervention unless you've tried all the simple ones.

Finally, these are the New Rules of Lifting for Life:
1. The older you are, the more important it is to train.
2. The goal of training is to change something.
3. Your body won't change without consistent hard work.
4. Hard work doesn't mean beating the crap out of yourself every time you train.
5. You're not a kid anymore. Don't train like one.
6. Decline is inevitable.
7. How fast you decline is up to you.
8. You are not a rural Okinawan.
9. Everyone is injured. But not every injury hurts.
10. If an activity hurts, stop doing it.
11. If it hurts after you do it, it may or may not be a problem.
12. Never try to fix an acute injury by stretching it.

13. When in doubt, refer out.
14. Exercise burns calories. Sometimes that's a problem.
15. "Fat-burning" exercise doesn't always burn fat.
16. Alwyn figured this out a long time ago.
17. It's actually kind of hard to gain weight.
18. We don't really move less.
19. Tasty food makes it too easy to gain weight, and too hard to lose it.
20. Every pound you don't gain is one you don't have to worry about losing.
21. Self-control, like muscle strength, can improve with training.
22. Weight management has little to do with self-control.
23. A weight-loss plan is good for six months, max.
24. Weight maintenance requires new strategies and a different skill set.

Notes

Chapter 1

Year of my birth: 1957 is generally acknowledged as the height of the post–World War II baby boom. The 4.3 million recorded births in 1957 were a U.S. record until 2007, when 4.317 million were born.

Decline with age: I got this from countless sources—individual studies as well as textbooks. I probably referred to these two more than any others: Melov et al., "Resistance exercise reverses aging in human skeletal muscle," *PLoS ONE* 2007; 2 (5): e465; and "Strategies for Aging Well," by Christina Geithner and Diane McKenney, in the October 2010 issue of *Strength and Conditioning Journal.*

Pet peeves: In order of annoyance, my personal list would go something like this:

1. *Blocking the dumbbell rack to do shrugs, curls, or worst of all, lateral raises.* I have no idea why people do this when they could just as easily step back a few feet and not block the rack. I also have no idea why the worst offenders are advanced male lifters who should know better.

2. *Squeezing me out of my implied exercise space.* I absolutely hate it when I'm warm-

ing up or doing core exercises on the floor and someone comes along and drops their foam mat right in front of me. In my gym they do it so they can see the clock or the nearby TV on the wall. It prevents me from doing any exercise that involves taking a step forward, which usually means I have to go somewhere else to finish that part of my routine, even though I was using the space first.

3. *Turning iPod music up so high I can hear it ten feet away.* I'm one of the last hold-outs against plugging your ears in the gym. I hit on the reasons why it could be dangerous for newbies in Chapter 1. For people who aren't a danger to themselves or others, my only issue with personal music is that it should stay personal. I shouldn't have to listen to it. I know I sound like a cranky old fart when I complain about this. So I'll also note that when I've asked people to turn down their music, they're always surprised to learn that I can hear it, and no one has ever taken my request the wrong way.

I could list one more annoyance—talking on cell phones in the weight room—but it's everyone's pet peeve, and I'm sure I don't need to explain why.

Chapter 2

Strength decline in elite weightlifters: "Aging Alibis," by James Krieger and Dan Wagman, *Pure Power*, March 2003.

Looking older: Gunn et al., "Why some women look young for their age," *PLoS ONE* 2009; 4 (12): e8021. (This study included a brief overview of aging and appearance for both genders, which is where I got the data about balding and graying.) Guyuron et al., "Factors contributing to the aging of identical twins," *Plastic and Reconstructive Surgery* 2009; 123 (4): 1321–1331.

Rural Okinawans: You can find a good overview of what we know from longevity research at bluezones.com, which is based on *The Blue Zones: Lessons for Living Longer from the People Who've Lived Longest*, by Dan Buettner (National Geographic Books, 2008).

Jack LaLanne: I wrote at length about LaLanne on my blog: louschuler.com/blog/jack-lalanne-and-the-limits-of-human-mortality. If you go there, you'll find links to several articles and posts I wrote over the years. In a follow-up post (louschuler.com/blog/sports-spelling-and-genes), I have links to news reports about Jack and his brother.

Muscle Beach: I've read so much about Muscle Beach over the years that it's hard to remember what I know from which source. Here are a couple of books that I keep on my shelves: *Remembering Muscle Beach*, by Harold Zinkin with Bonnie Hearn (Angel City Press, 1999); and *Muscle Beach: Where the Best Bodies in the World Started a Fitness Revolution*, by Marla Matzer Rose (L.A. Weekly Books, 2001).

Health-club chains: The company now known as Bally Total Fitness bought up both Vic Tanny's and Jack LaLanne's health-club chains, as well as the old Nautilus chain and others. Interestingly, Bally started as a company that made pinball and slot machines and then branched out into the casino business. From there it began buying up health clubs in the 1980s. The first gym I belonged to, in 1980, was still called Vic Tanny, although by then Tanny himself was long gone from the business.

There's a direct line from Tanny—who expanded his clubs on a pyramid-scheme model that depended on the fees from members of existing clubs to fund construction of new ones—to Bally, which has gotten into trouble multiple times for its rough and deceptive business practices. If you belong to a gym that's part of a chain, and you're frustrated with the way it does business, it's probably not reassuring to know that aggressive marketing and poor customer service aren't an aberration. They're pretty much the traditional business model.

Jeanne Louise Calment: I admit I got this from Wikipedia.

Aging and human performance: This information comes from too many sources to record, including the aforementioned studies cited for Chapter 1. So let me throw a plug in here for a book that was tremendously helpful and that I thoroughly enjoyed reading: *The Athlete's Clock*, by Thomas Rowland, M.D. (Human Kinetics, 2011). I also interviewed Dr. Rowland for a feature in *Men's Health* magazine (September 2011), although I don't think I used any information from the interview in this book.

Mitochondria and telomeres: I mostly used this study: Lanza and Nair, "Mitochondrial function as a determinant of life span," *European Journal of Physiology* 2010; 459: 277–289.

Lifters rarely use appropriate weights: Although this section refers to a bunch of studies published between 2004 and 2008, these three were the most noteworthy: Ratamess et al., "Self-selected resistance training intensity in healthy women: the influence of a personal trainer," *Journal of Strength and Conditioning Research* 2008; 22 (1): 103–111; Glass and Stanton, "Self-selected resistance training intensity in novice weightlifters," *Journal of Strength and Conditioning Research* 2004;

18 (2): 324–327; Glass, "Effect of a learning trial on self-selected resistance training load," *Journal of Strength and Conditioning Research* 2008; 22 (3): 1025–1029.
The first study showed that even women who worked out with a personal
trainer tended to choose weights that were too light to elicit strength gains. The
third study, a follow-up to the second, showed that when entry-level lifters were
given detailed instructions on how to lift, they still chose weights that were too
light. They also stopped their sets well short of the point of muscular fatigue.

Dr. Mark Tarnopolsky: I specifically refer to the study previously cited as Melov et al.
I also refer to two terrific articles from *The New York Times Magazine*: "The In-
credible Flying Nonagenarian," by Bruce Grierson, published in the November 28,
2010, issue, and "Can Exercise Keep You Young?" by Gretchen Reynolds, from
March 2, 2011. Dr. Tarnopolsky is quoted in both.

Senior lifters compared with young non-lifters: Candow et al., "Short-term heavy resistance training eliminates age-related deficits in muscle mass and strength in
healthy older males," *Journal of Strength and Conditioning Research* 2011; 25 (2):
326–333. I've quoted similar studies in previous NROL books, which arrived at
similar conclusions: If you take seniors who are healthy and active but not currently lifting, a strenuous program will give them strength equal to healthy young
people who aren't currently lifting. Old lifters can become good lifters, but they
can't become young lifters. The best they can do is match young non-lifters.

Chapter 3

Controversies: In early drafts of this chapter, I included more information about the
Squat Wars of 2009 and 2010, which began with an article by Mike Boyle called
"Build Bigger Legs, One at a Time." It was first posted at T-nation.com on August 3, 2009 (I edited the article), and advocates the exercise we call the Bulgarian
split squat instead of the traditional barbell back squat. Mike later released a series
of DVDs called *Functional Strength Coach 3.0*, which, despite its innocuous title,
was marketed aggressively with a focus on Mike's aversion to back squats.

NSCA v. Boyle: For details on the battle, go to strengthcoachblog.com and search for
posts tagged "NSCA." As far as I know, the NSCA hasn't offered its side of the
story, so it remains unclear if the revoked speaking invitation was entirely, partly,
or not at all a result of the Squat Wars.

Back injury without back pain: Jensen et al., "Magnetic resonance imaging of the lumbar spine in people without back pain," *New England Journal of Medicine* 1994; 331: 69–73. I chose this one, to be honest, because it was the first I found that offered the full text free online. This is a continual dilemma for journalists. Not every important study is available without a subscription to the journal in which it's published. Some journals charge more than $30 to access a single study. The abstract is always free, but I hate to reference studies I haven't read. The most telling details are often in the graphs and charts. I end up paying for some; others come to me from friends, colleagues, and occasionally the researchers themselves. But most of the studies I use are either from the *Journal of Strength and Conditioning Research*, to which I subscribe, or free online.

Small spinal fractures: Soler and Calderon, "The prevalence of spondylolysis in the Spanish elite athlete," *American Journal of Sports Medicine* 2000; 28 (1): 57–62. I heard about this study in a lecture by Eric Cressey at the 2011 Perform Better Functional Training Summit in Providence, Rhode Island.

Injuries that become problems years later: I found a specific case-study description on page 53 of *Low Back Disorders* (Human Kinetics, 2002), by Stuart McGill, Ph.D., professor of spine biomechanics at the University of Waterloo in Ontario. I also refer often to Dr. McGill's other book, *Ultimate Back Fitness and Performance* (Wabuno Publishers, 2004). You can find both at backfitpro.com.

Jonathan Fass, DPT: Jon is currently the private physical therapist and sports manager for His Royal Highness Prince Alwaleed bin Talal. He's based in Riyadh, Saudi Arabia. You can find more info at jonathanfass.com and hear him on thefitcast .com.

Back pain statistics: I got these from the second edition of *Rehabilitation of the Spine: A Practitioner's Manual* (Lippincott Williams & Wilkins, 2007), edited by Craig Liebenson, D.C. Most of the stats are on pages 52 and 53. Others are on pages 4 and 34. The information about the risk of sitting is on page 300.

But I'd be selling the textbook short if I pretended this is the only information I used. Along with Dr. McGill's books, *Rehabilitation of the Spine* was on my desk throughout the writing process, thoroughly highlighted and bookmarked.

Twins: Nyman et al., "High heritability for concurrent low back and neck-shoulder pain: a study of twins," *Spine* 2010 (epub ahead of print).

Muscle imbalance and knee injury: The New Rules of Lifting for Women (Avery, 2007), p. 121.

Chapter 4

"Break the Work Out/Pig Out Cycle": This is from prevention.com. I found it by Googling "work out pig out," and was surprised to see it was written by my friend Martica Heaner, Ph.D. (for the record, one of the smartest and most compassionate people I know in the industry). By pure coincidence, Martica supplied me with some of the weight-loss studies I used in this book. If you decide to find and read the article, make sure you check out the comments at the end. Last time I looked all the comments were from spammers who claimed to have lost weight by (1) wearing magic shoes; (2) taking magic supplements; (3) watching a magic TV show (*The Biggest Loser*); and (4) driving a Cadillac without brakes. If we ever get to a point when spambots write better comedy than actual comedy writers, civilization will officially have ended.

Twelve-week exercise program: King et al., "Dual-process action of exercise on appetite control: increase in orexigenic drive but improvement in meal-induced satiety," *American Journal of Clinical Nutrition* 2009; 90: 921–927.

Problems using fat for energy: Hopkins et al., "The relationship between substrate metabolism, exercise, and appetite control: does glycogen availability influence the motivation to eat, energy intake, or food choice?" *Sports Medicine* 2011; 41 (6): 507–521. I referred to this review study for the entire section.

Metabolic effects of strength training: Although a lot of the information in the second half of Chapter 4 falls under the category of "stuff everyone in the fitness industry acknowledges to be true," I used information from this research review: Strasser and Schobersberger, "Evidence for resistance training as a treatment therapy for obesity," *Journal of Obesity* 2011, Article ID 482564.

Increased efficiency and slower metabolism following weight loss: Rosenbaum et al., "Energy intake in weight-reduced humans," *Brain Research* 2010; 1350: 95–102.

Chapter 6

Skepticism about value of core training: There's certainly an opposing view to our approach to core training. In an earlier draft of *NROL for Life*, I described some of the pushback, using these sources: "To Crunch or Not to Crunch: An Evidence-Based Examination of Spinal Flexion Exercises, Their Potential Risks, and Their Applicability to Program Design," by Bret Contreras and Brad Schoenfeld, *Strength and Conditioning Journal*, August 2011. Okada et al., "Relationship between core stability, functional movement, and performance," *Journal of Strength and Conditioning Research* 2011; 25 (1): 252–261. See also "Are Crunches Worth the Effort?" by Gretchen Reynolds, *New York Times*, August 17, 2011.

Chapter 7

Definitions of strength and power: Essentials of Strength Training and Conditioning, Second Edition (Human Kinetics, 2000), p. 35.

Chapter 8

Importance of squatting: This comes from *Athletic Body in Balance*, by Gray Cook (Human Kinetics, 2003), p. 46.

Self-limiting exercises: This is another Gray Cook concept, found in *Movement* (On Target, 2010), pp. 231–233.

Vulnerable shoulder position: Kolber et al., "Shoulder injuries attributed to resistance training: a brief review," *Journal of Strength and Conditioning Research* 2010; 24 (6): 1696–1704. This paper, which rounded up all the available research on the subject, found a handful of exercises consistently linked to shoulder pain and injury: barbell bench press, behind-the-neck lat pulldown and shoulder press, parallel-bar dip, barbell back squat, and chest flies. I discuss the study at length in Chapter 12, which covers pushing exercises. I mention it here because the back squat forces your shoulders into a vulnerable position, where your arms support a load that often exceeds your body weight.

Chapter 9

Bad back/strong back: This is from *Advances in Functional Training*, by Mike Boyle (On Target, 2010), p. 115.

Cook hip lift: Also from *Advances in Functional Training*, pp. 106–107. The exercise is called the Cook hip lift, after physical therapist Gray Cook, whose work is cited for Chapter 8.

Chapter 10

In-line lunge: Yet another test from Gray Cook. This one is from *Athletic Body in Balance*, pp. 52–53.
Origins of knee pain: Boyle, *Advances in Functional Training*, p. 66.

Chapter 12

Shoulder injuries: Kolber et al., "Shoulder injuries attributed to resistance training."
Barbell bench press descriptions: It's been so long since I did this exercise that I wasn't sure if I was up to speed on current recommended form. So I relied heavily on *Maximum Strength*, by Eric Cressey and Matt Fitzgerald (Da Capo, 2008).

Chapter 13

Disparaging dumbbell one-arm row: The New Rules of Lifting (Avery, 2006), pp. 147–148.

Chapter 16

Lance Armstrong/New York City Marathon: "Armstrong Finishes NYC Marathon in Under Three Hours," Associated Press, November 5, 2006. "How Fast Could Lance Armstrong Run a Marathon?" by Amby Burfoot, *Runner's World*, published online September 29, 2006.

Chapter 18

Alan Aragon/The Fitness Summit: Alan writes the outrageously informative *Alan Aragon Research Review* each month; check it out at alanaragon.com. I met Alan in 2008, when he presented at The Fitness Summit for the first time. He's been back every year since, where he joins an annual lineup of speakers that includes some of the most interesting and forward-thinking fitness and nutrition professionals in the United States (including Alwyn in 2007). It's held in May each year; find out more at thefitnesssummit.com.

Leucine importance: Kim et al., "Dietary implications on mechanisms of sarcopenia: roles of protein, amino acids, and antioxidants," *Journal of Nutritional Biochemistry* 2010; 21 (1): 1–13.

Chapter 19

Weight of average Americans: "Poor Choices, Not Aging, Pack on Pounds," by Nancy Helmich, *USA Today*, June 23, 2011. The data in the article came from the National Center for Health Statistics. I clipped the article when I was in Las Vegas to speak at the International Society of Sports Nutrition annual conference, and was so intrigued by the data that I went to the NCHS website to find the rest of the data that I put in the chart.

We move less: The New Rules of Lifting for Abs (Avery, 2011), pp. 193–194.

Wired to store fat: Rethinking Thin: The New Science of Weight Loss and the Myths and Realities of Dieting, by Gina Kolata (Farrar Straus Giroux, 2007).

Capitalism: The End of Overeating: Taking Control of the Insatiable American Appetite, by David A. Kessler, M.D. (Rodale, 2009).

Corn: Fat Land: How Americans Became the Fattest People in the World, by Greg Critser (Houghton Mifflin, 2003), and *The Omnivore's Dilemma: A Natural History of Four Meals,* by Michael Pollan (Penguin, 2006).

Your friends make you fat: A good explanation can be found in "Beating Obesity," by Mark Ambider, in the May 2010 issue of *The Atlantic*. A good refutation can be found in "Catching Obesity from Friends May Not Be So Easy," by Gina Kolata, in the *New York Times*, August 8, 2011.

Bad choices/messy lifestyles: Mozaffarian et al., "Changes in diet and lifestyle and long-term weight gain in women and men," *New England Journal of Medicine* 2011; 364 (25): 2392–2404.

Nineteenth-century gluttony: At Home: A Short History of Private Life, by Bill Bryson (Doubleday, 2010), pp. 81–82.

Size of U.S. presidents: I'm a sucker for anything that combines health and fitness with history. I got the presidential proportions from a variety of sources; my favorite is "Medical History of U.S. Presidents" at doctorzebra.com.

Volume of food needed to gain weight: Katan and Ludwig, "Extra calories cause weight gain, but how much?" *Journal of the American Medical Association* 2010; 303 (1): 65–66; Barry Levin, "Why some of us get fat, and what we can do about it," *Journal of Physiology* 2007; 583.2: 425–430; Hall et al., "Quantification of the effect of energy imbalance on body weight," *The Lancet* 2011; 378: 826–837. At the time I wrote the manuscript, the groundbreaking research by Dr. Kevin Hall's team hadn't gotten any mainstream media coverage that I knew of. But right around the deadline, Jane Brody wrote a series of articles in the *New York Times* focused on the obesity epidemic. "Why Even Resolute Dieters Often Fail," published September 19, 2011, focused on Dr. Hall's studies.

Food alone explains weight surge: Swinburn et al., "Increased food energy supply is more than sufficient to explain the U.S. epidemic of obesity," *American Journal of Clinical Nutrition* 2009; 90 (6): 1453–1456.

Movement to counteract weight gain: Lee et al., "Physical activity and weight gain prevention," *Journal of the American Medical Association* 2010; 303 (12): 1173–1179.

Food palatability and weight gain: This is from the Barry Levin study cited immediately above.

Denis Leary quote: It's from *No Cure for Cancer,* his 1993 comedy album. I edited the quote, leaving out an obscenity that doesn't change the basic idea.

Don't gain weight in the first place: Also from the Levin study.

"Know your Kryptonite": This advice comes from Nate Miyaki, a personal trainer and bodybuilder, whom I interviewed for a feature called "Smash Your Records" in the September 2011 issue of *Men's Health.*

Brian Wansink: Dr. Wansink's research is catnip for journalists. There's always something interesting and counterintuitive. The Cohen and Farley study cited below for Chapter 20 mentions several of his studies. Three others that I looked at but didn't use in Chapter 19: Wansink and van Ittersum, "Shape of glass and amount of alcohol poured: Comparative study of effect of practice and concentration," *British Medical Journal* 2005; 331: 1512–1514; Werle et al., "Just thinking about exercise makes me serve more food: physical activity and calorie compensation," *Appetite* 2011; 56 (2): 332–335; Wansink et al., "The sweet tooth hypothesis: how fruit consumption relates to snack consumption," *Appetite* 2006; 47 (1): 107–110.

Chapter 20

Automatic behavior: Cohen and Farley, "Eating as an automatic behavior," *Preventing Chronic Disease* 2008; 5 (1): A23.

Self-control: de Ridder et al., "Taking stock of self-control: a meta-analysis of how trait self-control relates to a wide range of behaviors," *Personality and Social Psychology Review* 2011: epub ahead of print. I also referred to "The Sugary Secret of Self-Control," by Steven Pinker, in the September 4, 2011, issue of *The New York Times Book Review*. Dr. Pinker reviewed *Willpower: Rediscovering the Greatest Human Strength* (Penguin, 2011), by Roy Baumeister and John Tierney. Dr. Baumeister is one of the coauthors of the de Ridder et al. study.

Adaptive thermogenesis: Tremblay et al., "Role of adaptive thermogenesis in unsuccessful weight loss intervention: a historical perspective and definition," *Future Lipidology* 2007; 2 (6): 651–658.

Metabolism decline: Goldsmith et al., "Effects of experimental weight perturbation on skeletal muscle work efficiency, fuel utilization, and biochemistry in human subjects," *American Journal of Physiology: Regulatory, Integrative, and Comparative Physiology* 2010: 298 (1): R79–88.

Six-month rule: The tips come from our friend Mike Roussell, Ph.D. Mike wrote the sidebar to "Stay Lean for Life," an article I wrote for the May 2011 issue of *Men's Health*. He also alerted me to the research on weight maintenance, cited below. You can read more of his thoughts and tips at mikeroussell.com.

Easier for some to cut calories and increase exercise simultaneously: Annesi and Marti, "Path analysis of exercise treatment-induced changes in psychological factors leading to weight loss," *Psychology and Health* 2011; 26 (8): 1081–1098; Annesi, "Behaviorally supported exercise predicts weight loss in obese adults through improvements in mood, self-efficacy, and self-regulation, rather than by caloric expenditure," *The Permanente Journal* 2011; 15 (1): 23–27.

Weight maintenance: Stuckey et al., "Using positive deviance for determining successful weight-control practices," *Qualitative Health Research* 2010; 21 (4): 563–579. This study came from a research team at Penn State Hershey Medical Center led by Chris Sciamanna, M.D., whom I interviewed for the *Men's Health* article mentioned above.

Chapter 21

Becoming Human: I TiVo'd this from PBS during a rebroadcast in 2011. At the time it was also available for free viewing at pbs.org. If it's no longer available, you can rent the DVD from Netflix or buy it at any online retailer.

Lessons from cave-dwelling forebears: Some readers will notice that I describe the currently trending "paleo diet" without using that term. I have two reasons. First, I don't think the advice to eat foods close to their natural state is any different from what we advocated in the original *NROL*, when we talked about "clean eating" in Chapter 22. Second, I'm uncomfortable with the term "paleo" because it implies there was a single diet all early humans followed. The archaeological record suggests they ate anything and everything, including the brains and bone marrow of animals they hunted or scavenged. Some in warmer climates may have subsisted on near-vegetarian diets at different times, while those farther north may have eaten more like their carnivorous cousins, the Neanderthals. Furthermore, with industrial-scale food production I'm not sure it's possible to replicate any version of a true paleo diet. The air, soil, and water would've been so different from ours that the plants and animals that fed on them would've had different nutritional profiles.

John Berardi, Ph.D.: Alwyn and I have known John for many years. John first got attention as a prolific writer for T-nation.com, and then coauthored *Scrawny to Brawny* (Rodale, 2005) with another mutual friend, Mike Mejia. Since then he's done terrific work on- and offline. You can check out his articles and programs at precisionnutrition.com.

Billy Beck III: I heard Billy speak at the 2011 ISSN conference in Las Vegas, where I was impressed by both his energy and the creative ways he approaches all-too-common problems with training and nutrition. Although I used his basic idea of fire, fuel, and free meals, I scaled back the application for this book's readers. For Billy's take on his own system, check out http://www.billybeck.com/blog/effective-eating/nutrition-cycling-the-ultimate-body-transformation-diet/.

Galina Ivanova Denzel: Galya was a successful author and health-club owner in her native Bulgaria who now counsels clients in the United States. We know each other through the JP Fitness forums (forums.jpfitness.com), where she also met my friend Roland Denzel; they got married in 2011. Her website is eatloveandtrain.com.

Chapter 22

Creatine articles: In "The All-Star Diet" (*Men's Health*, October 2010) I included creatine in a roundup of the latest information on sports nutrition. "Powder to the People" (*Men's Health*, November 2001) focused on creatine exclusively.

Creatine research: Waters et al., "Advantages of dietary, exercise-related, and therapeutic interventions to prevent and treat sarcopenia in adult patients: an update," *Clinical Interventions in Aging* 2010; 5: 259–270.

Index

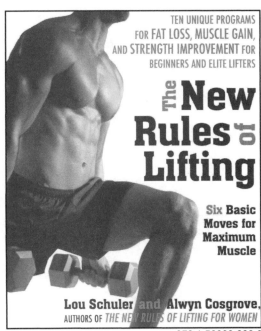
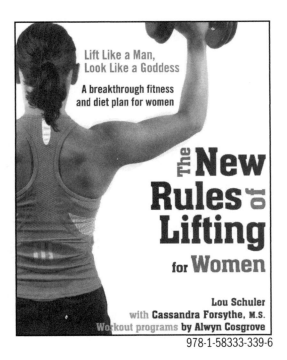
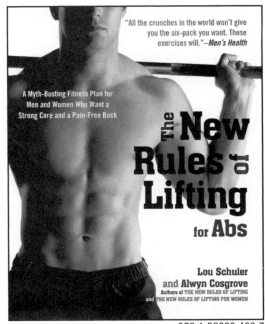

KALEIDOSCOPES & QUILTS

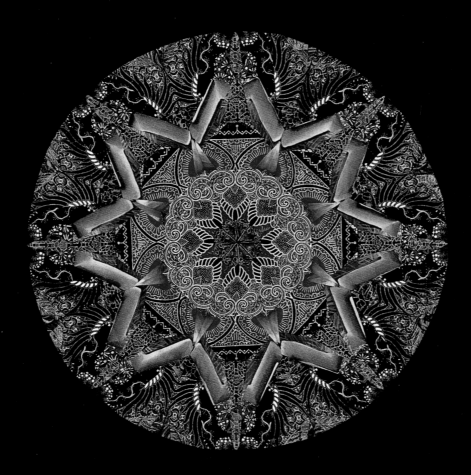

PAULA NADELSTERN

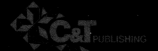
C&T PUBLISHING

Editor: Lee Jonsson
Technical Editor: Joyce Engels Lytle
Copy Editor: Judith M. Moretz
Illustrator: Kandy Petersen
Book Design: Irene Morris, Morris Design
Cover Design: Jill Berry, Artista Artworks
Quilt photography: Karen Bell, New York City, NY, unless otherwise noted.
Illustration photography: John Woodin, Philadelphia, PA, unless otherwise noted.

Attention Teachers:
C&T Publishing, Inc. encourages you to use this book as a text for teaching. Contact us at 800-284-1114 or www.ctpub.com for more information about the C&T Teachers Program.

We take great care to ensure that the information included in this book is accurate and presented in good faith, but no warranty is provided nor result guaranteed. Since we have no control over the choice of materials or procedures used, neither the author nor C&T Publishing, Inc. shall have any liability to any person or entity with respect to any loss or damage caused directly or indirectly by the information contained in this book.

Ruler designs Copyright 1986, 1995, OMNIGRID®, Inc. All rights reserved.
U.S. Patent. 4,779,346; Ca. Pat. 1,297,286
8/8 Cross Section is a product of Canson-Talens, Inc.
Liberty is a registered trademark of Liberty of London Prints Limited.
Omnigrid is a registered trademark of Omnigrid Inc.
Pilot SCA-UF is a registered trademark of the Pilot Pen Corporation of America.
Sesame Street is a trademark of Children's Television Workshop.
Singer Featherweight is a registered trademark of Singer Corporation.
Template-Graph is a product of Quilter's Rule, International.
Ultrasuede is a registered trademark of Springs Industries, Inc.

Library of Congress Cataloging-in-Publication Data

Nadelstern, Paula.
      Kaleidoscopes & quilts / Paula Nadelstern.
               p.   cm.
      Includes index.
      ISBN 1-57120-018-5 (paper trade)
      1. Patchwork—Patterns. 2. Kaleidoscope in art. I. Title.

TT835.N33   1996
746.46'041—dc20   96-17491

Published by C&T Publishing, Inc.
P.O. Box 1456
Lafayette, CA 94549
http://www.ctpub.com

Printed in China
10   9   8   7   6   5

TABLE OF CONTENTS

ACKNOWLEDGMENTS

I would like to give my heartfelt thanks to the following people:

My friends The Manhattan Quilters: Teresa Barkley, Karen Felicity Berkenfeld, Jeanne Lyons Butler, Vikki Berman Chenette, Judy Doenias, Susan B. Faeder, Yvonne K. C. Forman, Iris Gowen, Marilyn Henrion, Katherine Knauer, Leslie Levison, Emiko Toda Loeb, Diana Goulston Robinson, Carmel Roth, Diane Rode Schneck, Robin Schwalb, Judy Speezak, John Swiatek, and Margaret Pohlman Zipkin, who give me the benefit of their enthusiasm, humor, snacks, and joint genius.

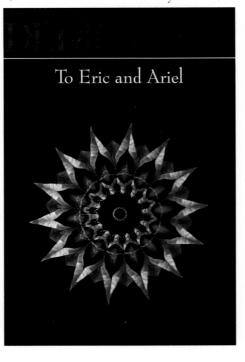

To Eric and Ariel

Todd Hensley and all the creative people at C&T Publishing, for the respect they gave to my ideas. I especially want to thank my new friends Lee Jonsson and Joyce Lytle, whose cross-country, good-humored support and technical expertise arrived in the nick of time. Special thanks to Irene Morris and Diane Pedersen, who worked very hard to capture my design sensibility in the book's design. I also want to remember Louise Townsend, whose encouraging words and wonderful smile in the midst of a frenetic Quilt Market aisle caused me to finally launch this project.

Karen Bell and John Woodin, photographers par excellence, for their keen focus.

Selim Benardete, Esther Zielinski, Lisa Hamm, Kirsten Vogel, and David Lochner (Benartex, Inc.), Fiona McKelvie (Liberty of London Prints Limited), Irwin Bear and Jennifer Sampou (P & B Textiles), Nancy Crow (John Kaldor Fabricmaker), Sandy Muckenthaler (Hoffman California Fabrics), Mickey Lawler (Skydyes), Tina Ruytil (Textil), Dorothy Brown (International Fabric Collection), Lois Griffin (Sparklers) and Peggy Schaefer (Omnigrid Inc.) for donating gorgeous goods and valuable products.

Cozy Baker, for sharing her kaleidoscope collections and connections along with invaluable personal and professional support. Research for "The Kaleidoscope Renaissance" was derived solely from books by Cozy Baker.

Kaleidoscope makers Charles Karadimos, Randy and Shelly Knapp, Peggy Burnside and Steve Kittelson, Adam Peiperl, Kay Winkler, and Sue Rioux who willingly shared their expertise and their slides.

My friends in The Brewster Society, for their enthusiastic acceptance of my attempts to fabricate kaleidoscopes, especially Mary Lou Donarski, a kaleidoscope and quilt enthusiast, who telephoned me on March 12, 1990, after she saw my quilts in *Quilter's® Newsletter Magazine*, and gave me Cozy Baker's phone number.

Quiltmakers Bonnie McCaffery, Sue Spigel, Margaret Zipkin, Diana Goulston Robinson, Margit Echols, Akiko Osugi, Noriko Ikegami, and Noriko Noseki, for their generosity, and to Emiko Toda Loeb, for connecting me to her students, reinforcing my notion that I can always rely on the kindness of quilters.

To friends and colleagues in the quilt world: Mary Leman Austin and Karen O'Dowd (QNM), Victoria Faoro and Mary Lou Schwinn (AQS), Paul Pilgrim, Gerald Roy, Doreen Speckmann, and Marty Bowne, for their active interest and encouragement.

Shelley Zegart and Velma Vaughan, for their generous contribution of photography of antique kaleidoscope quilts, and for understanding the dilemma of a deadline.

Cathy Rasmussen, for her courage, encouragement, and research skills.

The staff at Quilter's Passion in Manhattan, NY, Sew Brooklyn in Brooklyn, NY, and The Country Quilter in Somers, NY, for their friendship and support.

The New York Foundation for the Arts, who, by awarding me an Artist's Fellowship in 1995, did more to encourage my faith in my art than I can express.

My family, Ralph and Clara Lyman, Mark Lyman and Ginnie Salman, Sara and Harold Taubin, Amy Orr and John Woodin, Eva and Mark Nadelstern, Ruth and Neil Pariser, and family friend Rosie Steinberg, whose support of my unusual choice of profession has always been appreciated.

And special thanks to the quiltmakers I met in my classes who encouraged me to write this book. We who have been touched by the camaraderie of quiltmaking are the lucky ones.

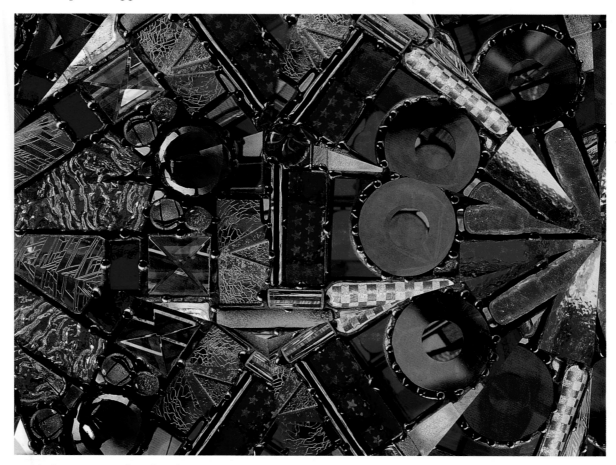

▲ Kaleidoscope interior by Bob and Sue Rioux
◄ Kaleidoscope interior by Adam Peiperl

I make my quilts on the same block in the Bronx where I grew up. The view from our ninth-floor window is one of the most northern exposures in New York City, showcasing acres of tree-filled park and empty sky. My daughter Ariel is the third generation of my family to live in this neighborhood that prides itself on a sense of community and cooperative spirit. She grew up with the expectation that she might bump into either set of grandparents when she walked down the street.

In spite of these images evoking small-town America, I am a New Yorker wrapped up in the fabric of city life. I settled into full-time quiltmaking by way of the playground park bench. That's where city moms on a hiatus from previous lives hang out and share ideas—like organizing quilt novices into making a raffle quilt for the local cooperative nursery school. One good quilt led to another and another. By the time I gave up my place on that bench to a new generation of moms, I had the expertise and repertoire for a comprehensive book on group quilts, and was stitching my way toward a new career.

In 1987 my co-author and I (we met on a park bench) turned in the manuscript for *QUILTING TOGETHER: How to Organize, Design, and Make Group Quilts,* and in the celebratory moment of accomplishment, I resolved to stop smoking. Within a few days my head felt as if it were stuffed with a very fat batt. I couldn't think or write, plan dinner or make a quilt, but—trooper that I was—I could still go shopping. And that's when it happened: I was struck by a bolt of fabric.

At 36 inches wide and $16 per yard, buying a quarter yard of Liberty™ of London fabric seemed sinful. I literally circled it for over an hour. "Anywhichway'll be OK" surfaced through the haze obscuring my thoughts. I think I knew the bilateral symmetry of the beautiful print had the potential to reconnect into graceful kaleidoscopic designs. The results were fascinating, prompting lots of those "what if" kinds of ideas that propel you along a creative path (see *KALEIDOSCOPIC I,* page 12). I was encouraged to make more kaleidoscope quilts (over fifteen at this writing, teeming with an eclectic assortment of scopes) to buy more Liberty™ of London fabric and to explore the world of actual kaleidoscopes for further inspiration.

Another factor played strongly in the development of my personal approach to design and technique. Historians have suggested that the block-style method of quiltmaking evolved in response to the cramped quarters of early American life. My family's living arrangement in an urban environment creates similar considerations that, unwittingly, I resolved in much the same way.

My workspace in our two-bedroom apartment is the forty-two-inch round kitchen table. My fastidious husband shares the living room with the ironing board, and dinner shares the kitchen table with a forty-five-year-old Singer Featherweight™. Fabrics find shelter everywhere: novelty fabrics sleep under the bed; luxury imports reside in the living room wall unit; Ultrasuede® scraps hide in an elaborate Indian treasure chest on the window sill. A foolishly narrow closet next to the bed hoards a hodge-podge of see-through boxes jumbled with fabric sorted by color, along with an arsenal of beads and threads. There's a file cabinet full of paperwork behind the door to Ariel's room, and art supplies are camouflaged in the linen closet.

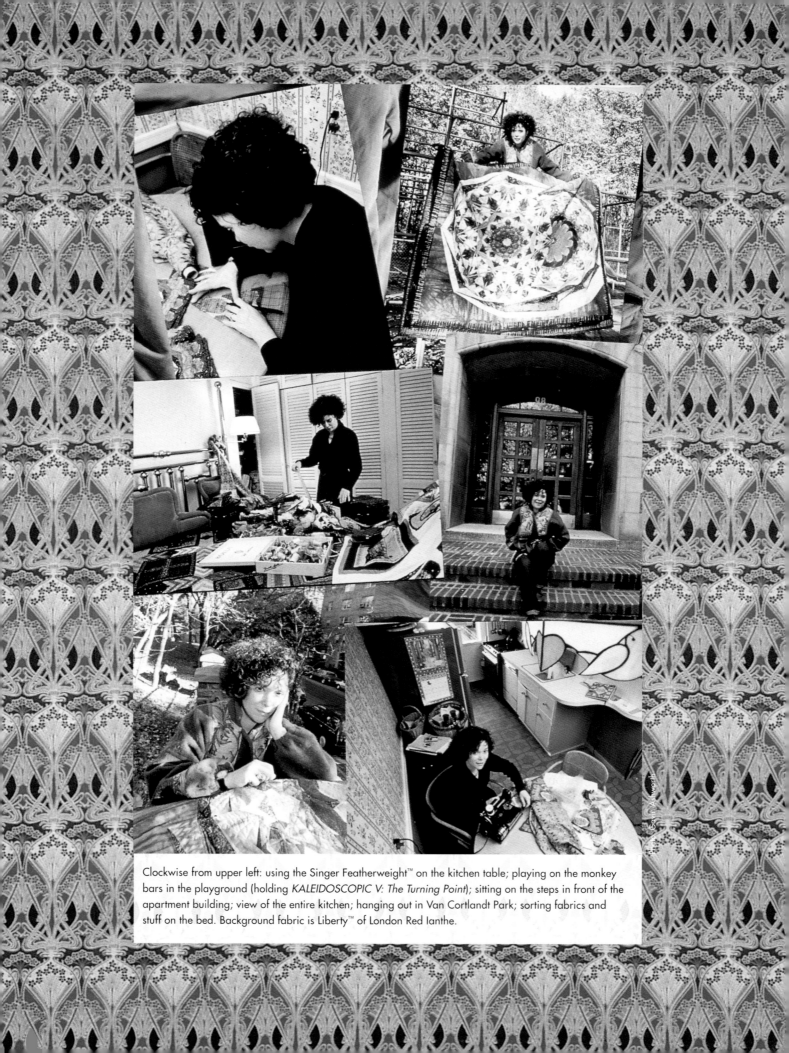

Clockwise from upper left: using the Singer Featherweight™ on the kitchen table; playing on the monkey bars in the playground (holding *KALEIDOSCOPIC V: The Turning Point*); sitting on the steps in front of the apartment building; view of the entire kitchen; hanging out in Van Cortlandt Park; sorting fabrics and stuff on the bed. Background fabric is Liberty™ of London Red Ianthe.

At the beginning of a sewing frenzy I pour this reservoir of goodies onto the bed, sorting and sifting and following tangents until I uncover my palette. I haul my finds around the bend and into the kitchen, where they collect in an unruly pile. I believe in the artistic contribution of a tangled mishmash of cloth. The chance combinations that catch my eye result in unconventional but intriguing relationships between textiles I might not have discovered on my own.

I think the reality of limited space merged with my personality and passion for fabric in shaping the direction of my kaleidoscopic piecework, causing me to rely on intricate detail and inherent symmetry, and to invent a shape that makes the most of limited space. My block-style method is based on a pie-slice sector. Throughout the design stage of a fabric kaleidoscope I focus on a single, full-size triangle drawn on a long sheet of graph paper with an eight-to-the-inch grid. Since there isn't any long-distance viewing space, there are times when I don't see the full impact of my quilt until it is hanging on the photographer's wall.

My ambition is to integrate harmoniously the idea of a kaleidoscope with the techniques and materials of quiltmaking. Making kaleidoscopes is like making magic with fabric. There is an element of abracadabra as the very last seam is stitched, because what you see in one single pieced triangular segment is not what you get in the multiplied sum. The whole is greater than the sum of its parts.

This is probably a good time to mention that, although a quilt may end up seamed from many thousands of pieces, I don't think there is inherent value in teensy slivers of fabric and perfect points. However, while I don't embrace technical achievement as a personal goal, I also don't want technical boo-boos to detract from the visual impact. The truth is, I don't really sew very well.

When quiltmaking first piqued my fancy, no matter how hard I tried, my points never matched, a crucial fabric inevitably lacked a critical amount, and one edge of every quilt wiggled past its significant other. In spite of these indignities, I couldn't wait to start another quilt. There is something optimistic about a palette of portable, colorful, tactile fabric that represses any unpleasant memories left over from a previous project.

So, perhaps you can understand why I thought I was cheating when, over a period of time, a sequence of uncommon techniques evolved which worked for me. Obviously, I was doing it this way because I couldn't do it the right way—compensating, not innovating. When asked, I hesitated to show my method to anyone because I didn't want to defend my cheating ways. The image of the quilt police who point their collective, thimble-encrusted fingers at those of us who sometimes color outside the lines can be demoralizing.

Has the quilt world, and its burgeoning industry, changed so much, or have I? Here I am, eight years and at least one hundred kaleidoscopes beyond that first encounter with a kind fabric, flaunting my *innovations*. I alternate between feeling sorry for the individual who cannot see the quilt for the technique, and being offended by her short-sighted view.

In this book I offer my insights, not techniques that are faster, or better, or foolproof. Making a kaleidoscope block can be tedious unless you enjoy the process. I love it because it allows me to merge control and spontaneity to spark something unexpected. My points appear to match, although oftentimes they don't, and when it comes to fabric, just as I always suspected, more is more!

Remember, I've been making this up as I go along. Now it's your turn. Take what you want. Leave the rest. Until I met quilts I thought I was creative, but not talented. To find something you love to do is a gift. To achieve recognition for it is a miracle. When I am overwhelmed by a longing for functional space complete with a door I can close, I try to remember this.

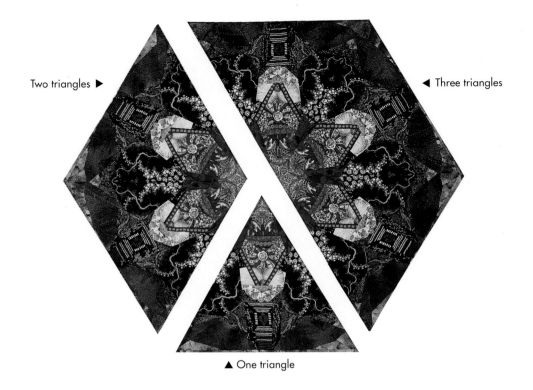

Two triangles ▶

◀ Three triangles

▲ One triangle

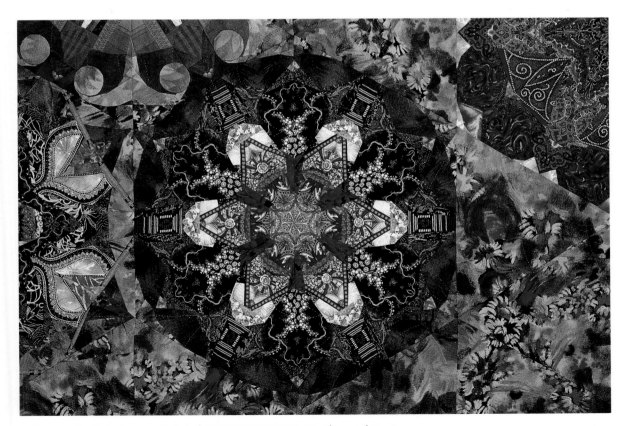

▲ The complete kaleidoscope. Detail of *KALEIDOSCOPIC XII: Up Close and Far Away.*

HOW TO USE THIS BOOK

Writing a book about my personal approach to quiltmaking reminds me of the cartoon where an obviously self-absorbed woman says to her companion: "Enough about me. Let's talk about you. Tell me, what do you think about me?"

At the same time I offer my insights, I am aware of the egocentric nature of this one-sided view. This book is about my interest in the structure of fabricated kaleidoscopes. It focuses on the mechanics involved in the intricate piecework as well as the challenge of finding relationships between fabrics. The underlying assumption of the format is that you are not making your first, or even your fourth, quilt. I don't provide general quiltmaking instructions. Only techniques that are unique to kaleidoscope quiltmaking are covered. The step-by-step directions explain how I do things—by machine piecing, hand quilting, and making lots of templates. If you are a paper piecing person, a rotary cutting connoisseur, or adept at any of the many things I am not, please adapt my strategies to your personal way of doing things.

I've taught this approach to over a thousand people in workshops all over the country. I know where it gets inevitably tedious, where lengthy explanations pay off, where a picture is worth the proverbial thousand words. At this point, more than one hundred kaleidoscopes beyond that first twinkling of a good idea, design and technique are entwined in so integral a manner that separating them neatly for the sake of a how-to discussion laced with clarity seems almost impossible—and definitely artificial. You can't have one without the other. But, in spite of my misgivings, I intend to do exactly that: to isolate these symbiotic companions into first the prerequisite how-to skills, and then the artistic element needed to create something aesthetically satisfying. I'll do this for you, the reader, if you promise to look at both sections before you begin.

In the late 1980's the question put to quilt artists by the media searching for an angle was: "Why quilts?" Within a few years, in response to the flourishing quilt world, the question changed to: "Why are so many people making quilts?" I've always thought the relevant question was: "Why are so many people making so many quilts?"

My goal here is not to answer the question, but to celebrate its implications. We're a phenomenon! An awful lot of us have chosen quiltmaking. There is something in its materials and methods for everyone. Together we create an array of unique personal responses, and a group response that includes both common threads and diverse notions. The state of our art thrives on the lively quality of variety.

I hope that within these pages my quilt persona speaks to yours. Browse through the color photos for inspiration or for amusement. And remember, we came here in the first place to have a good time.

KALEIDOSCOPE

THE GALLERY

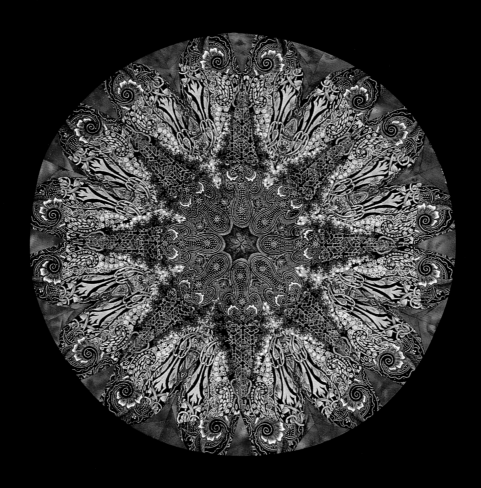

THE GALLERY

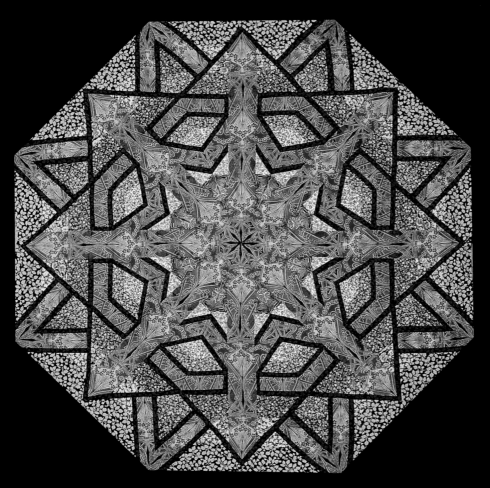

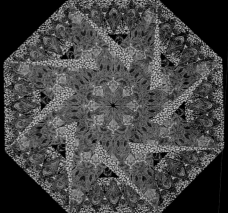

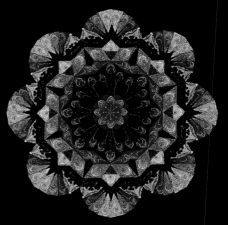

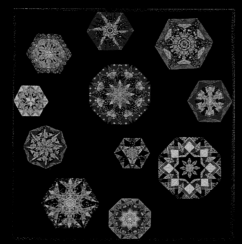

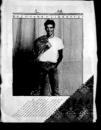

After I finished my first kaleidoscopic quilt inspired by Liberty of London's Red Ianthe cotton, my mother showed me this ad in *The New Yorker.*

An inquiry accompanied by a slide of *KALEIDOSCOPIC* I led to a commission to make sixteen twenty-four inch pillows that were sold in the Rockefeller Center store.

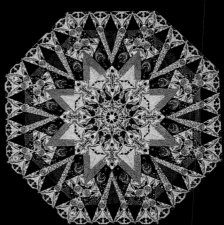

▲ KALEIDOSCOPIC I , 1987, 40" x 40".

▲ The Liberty of London Pillow Commission, 1988, 24" x 24". Machine pieced. Liberty of London Tana Lawns, commercial cottons.

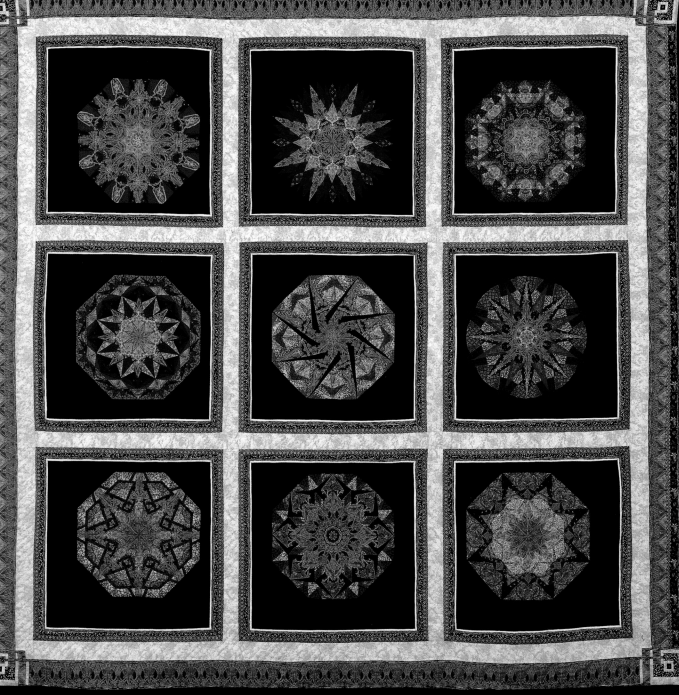

▲ KALEIDOSCOPIC III: Stained Glass Anthology, 1989, 72" x 72", Machine pieced, hand quilted. Cottons, cotton blends.

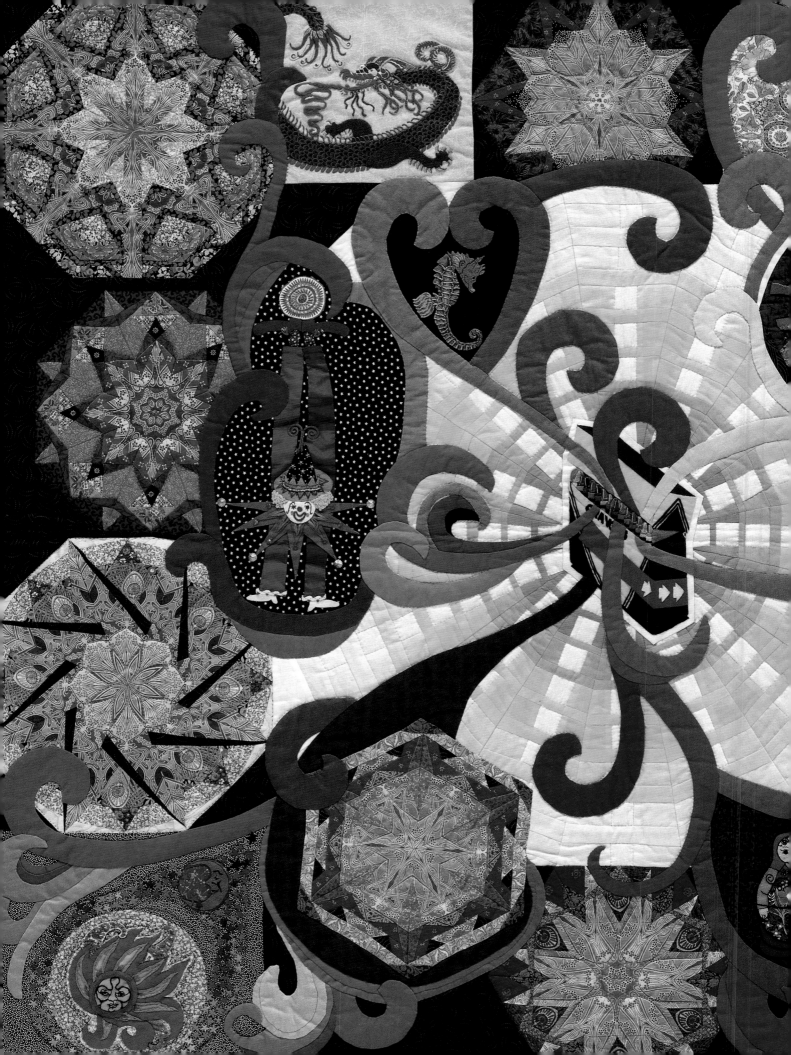

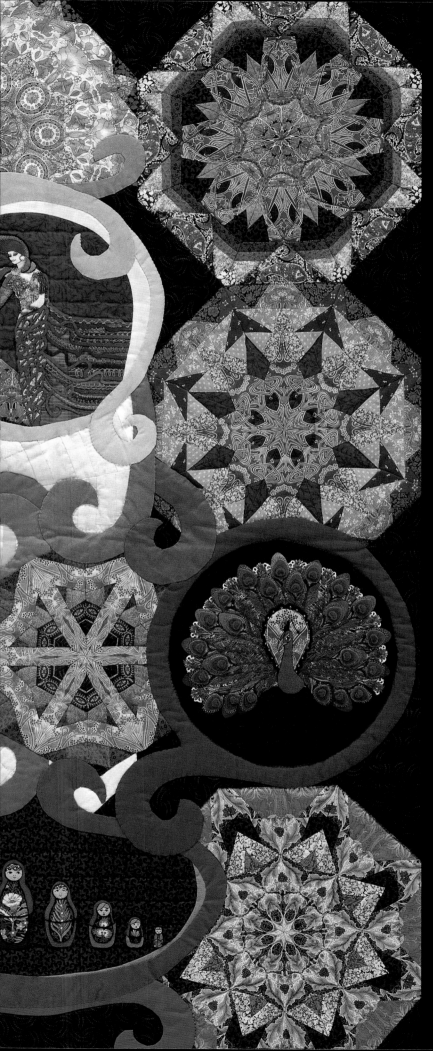

◄ KALEIDOSCOPIC II:
Once Upon a Box of Crayons,
1988, 45" x 54".
Machine pieced, hand appliquéd, embroidered
and quilted. Cottons, cotton blends, Ultrasuede,
found objects.

This crib-sized quilt reflects the endless possibilities
in both childhood and a brand new box of crayons.
As the escaping colors swirl and tumble, they combine
to form kaleidoscopes and magical imagery.
The kaleidoscope piecing and embellished motifs
represent a variety of childhood fascinations
and themes.

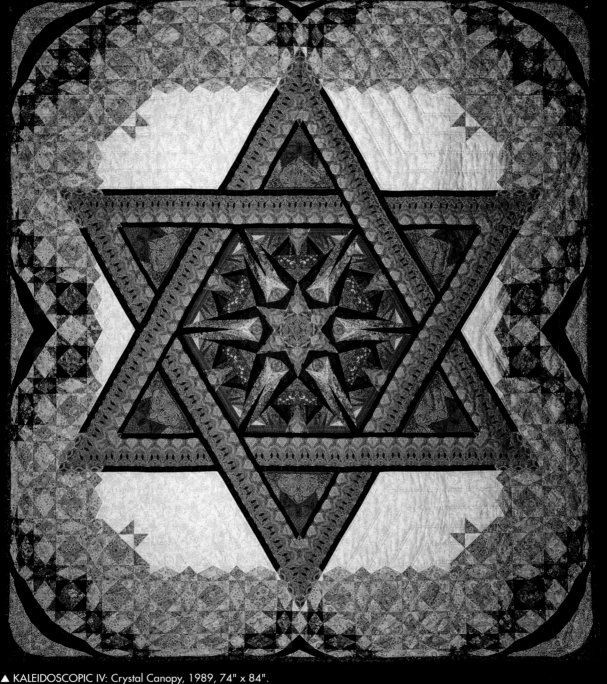

Photo: Bobby Hansson

▲ KALEIDOSCOPIC IV: Crystal Canopy, 1989, 74" x 84".
Designed and machine pieced by Paula Nadelstern; hand quilted by Lynn Della Posta. Cottons and cotton blends.

A Jewish wedding ceremony takes place under a canopy called a *huppah.* Traditionally the wedding ceremony took place outdoors as an omen that the marriage should be blessed with as many children as "the stars of heaven." To separate the ceremony from the marketplace surrounding it, the rabbis sanctioned the use of a huppah. The only laws governing the size, shape, or construction of a huppah is that it must be a temporary structure and open-sided.

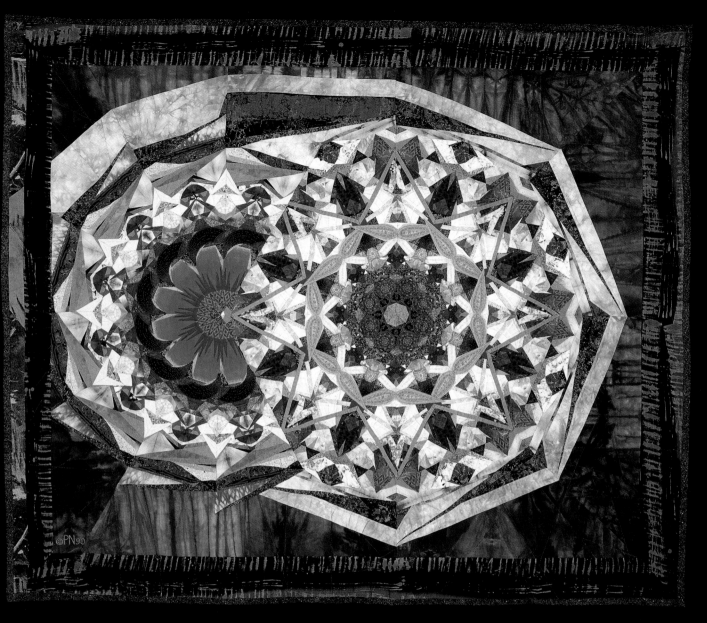

▲ KALEIDOSCOPIC V: The Turning Point,
1990, 74.5" x 62.5".
Machine pieced, hand appliquéd and quilted.
Cottons, cotton-blends, rayon.

The title refers specifically and metaphorically to the
experience of viewing a kaleidoscope. I wanted to
create the illusion of a multifaceted, multi-fractured
surface illuminated by back lighting.

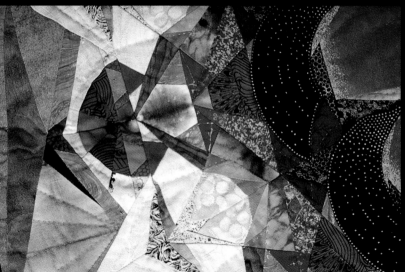

Photo: Bobby Hansson

▲ Detail of KALEIDOSCOPIC V: The Turning Point

17

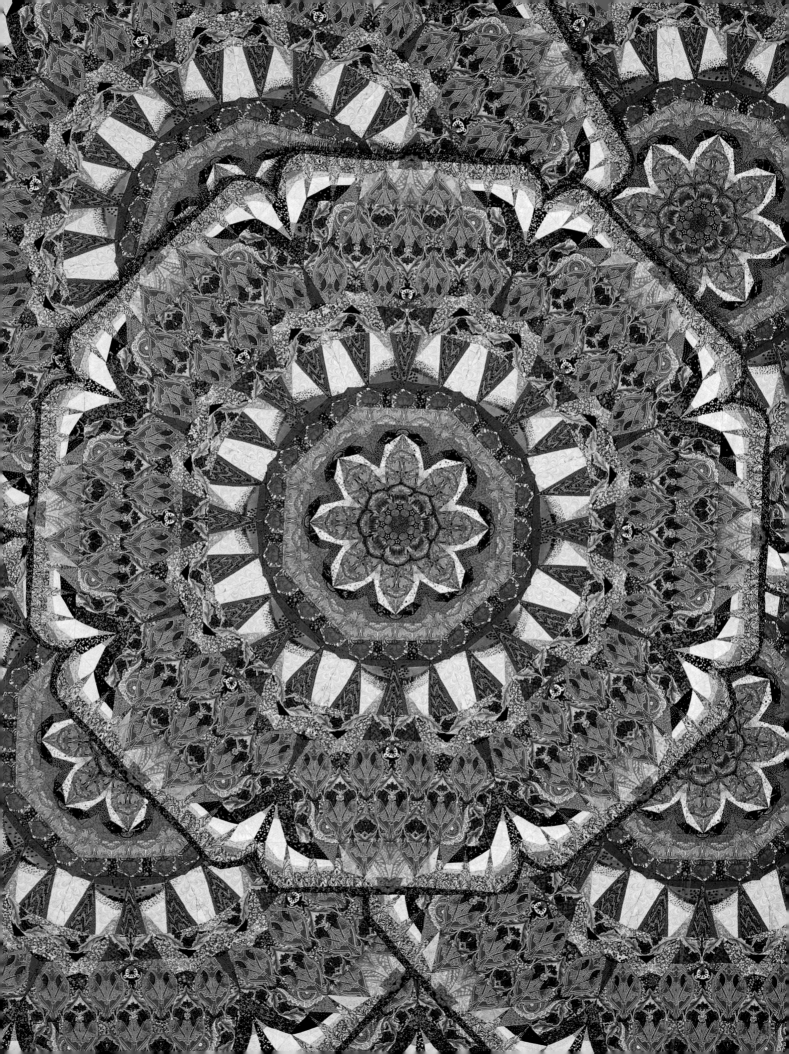

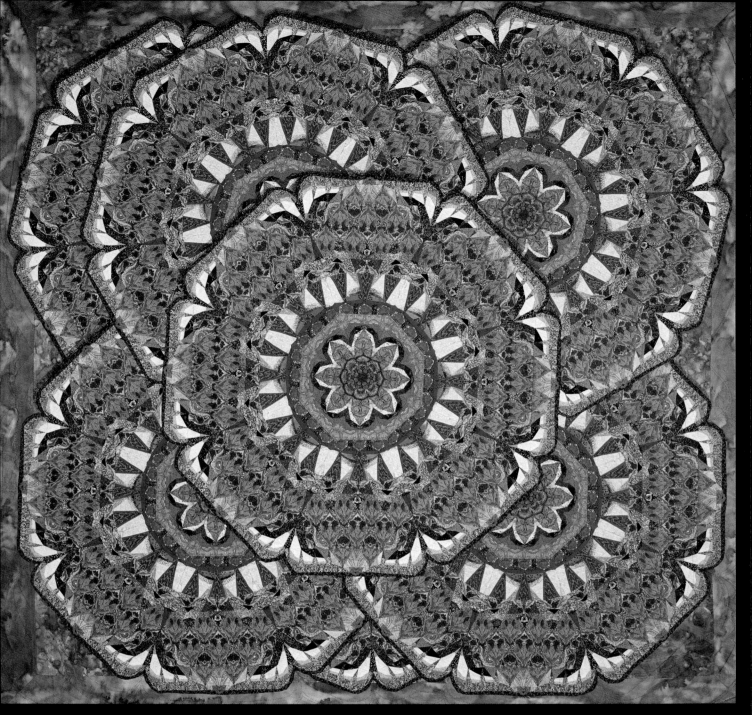

▲ KALEIDOSCOPIC VII: The Natural Order of Chaos, 1991, 85" x 82".
Machine pieced, hand appliquéd, embroidered, beaded and quilted.
Cottons, cotton-blends.

The study of chaos has provided a seemingly paradoxical insight: rich kinds of
order arise spontaneously from the unplanned interaction of many simple things.
I find myself mesmerized by the irregular order that emerges in a haphazard
pile of fabric.

◄ Detail of KALEIDOSCOPIC VII:
The Natural Order of Chaos

Quilt on pages 20 and 21: ▶
KALEIDOSCOPIC VIII: The Sun, the Moon. . .and the Stars, 1991, 88" x 60".
Machine pieced, hand quilted and beaded. Cottons, cotton blends, silk.

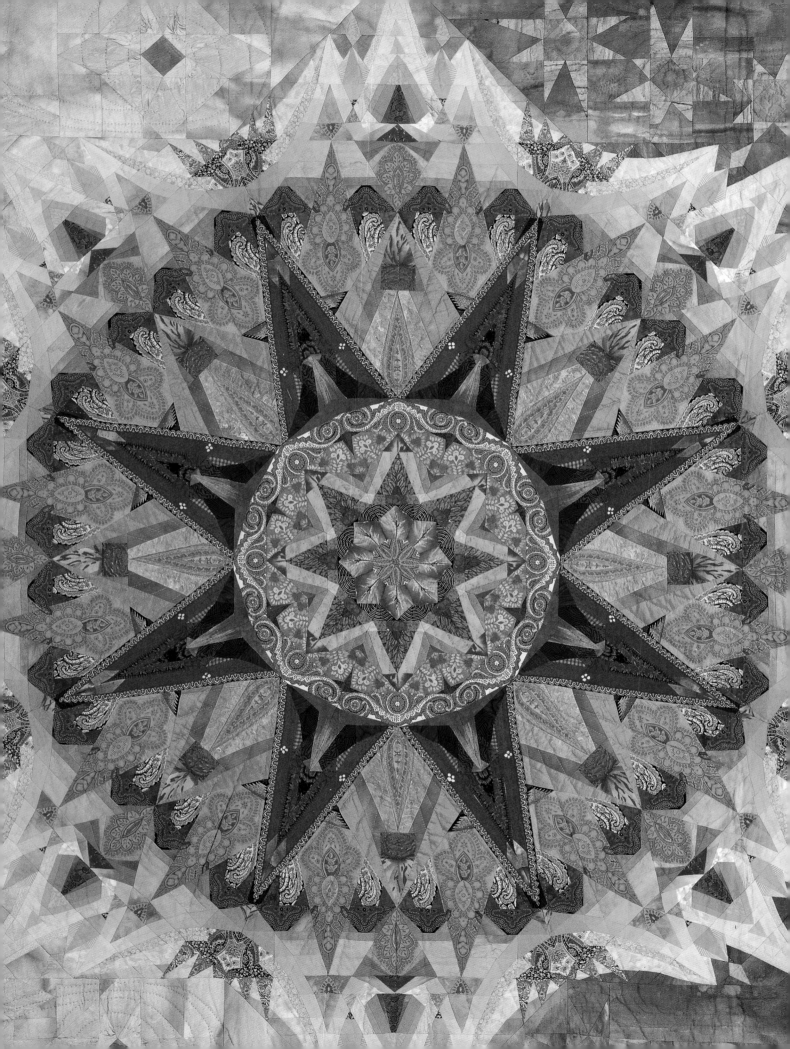

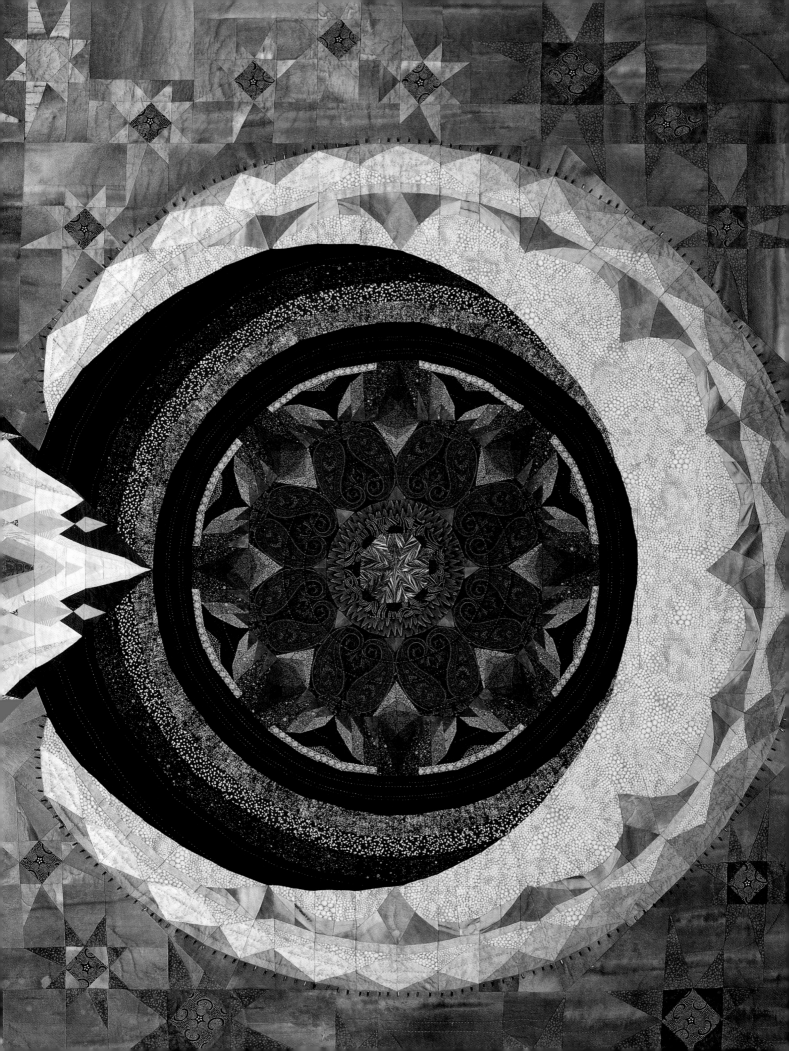

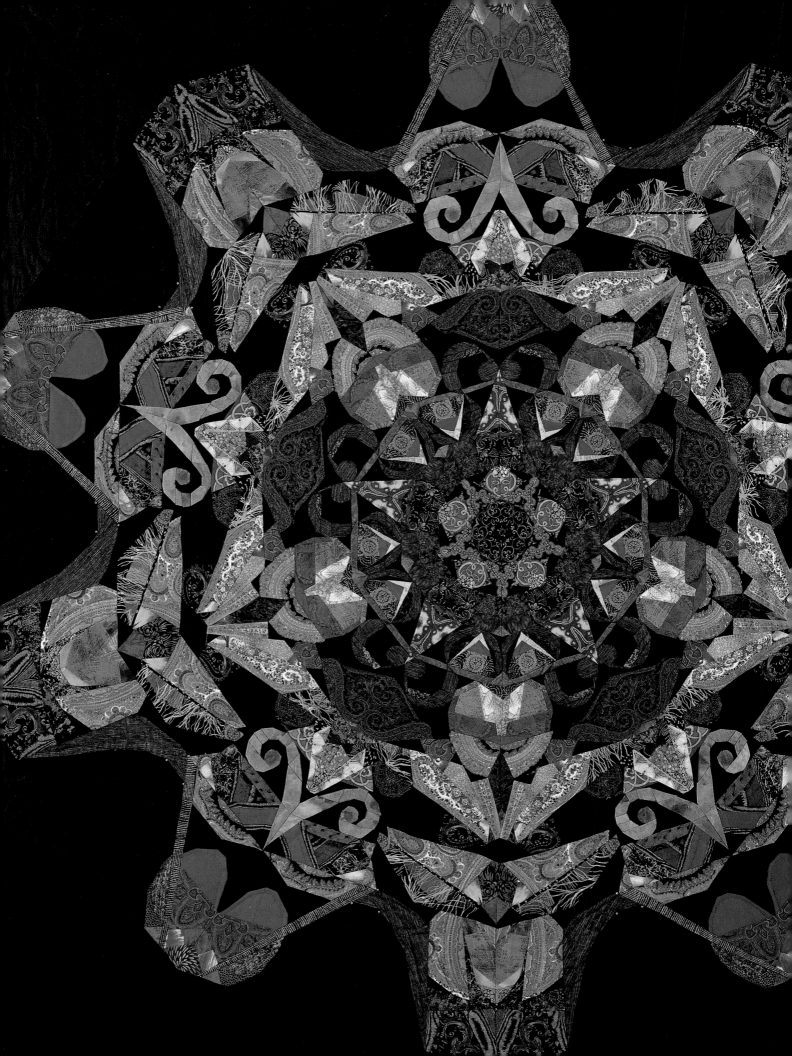

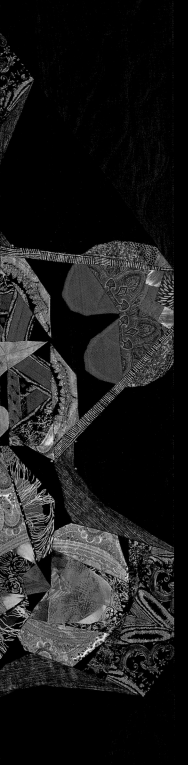

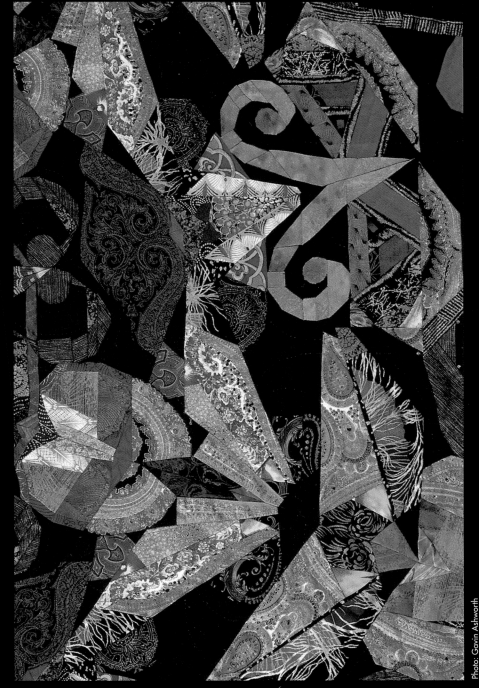

▲ Detail of KALEIDOSCOPIC X: Water from the Moon

◄ KALEIDOSCOPIC X: Water from the Moon, 1993, 52" x 53".
Machine pieced, hand quilted. Cottons, cotton-blends, silk.

This quilt was inspired by a dramatic five-sided scope entitled *Twilight* by Randy and Shelley
Knapp of Ontario, Oregon. This system features a unique side-lighted, fluid-filled object case that
highlights the flame-sculpted dichroic glass against a black backdrop.

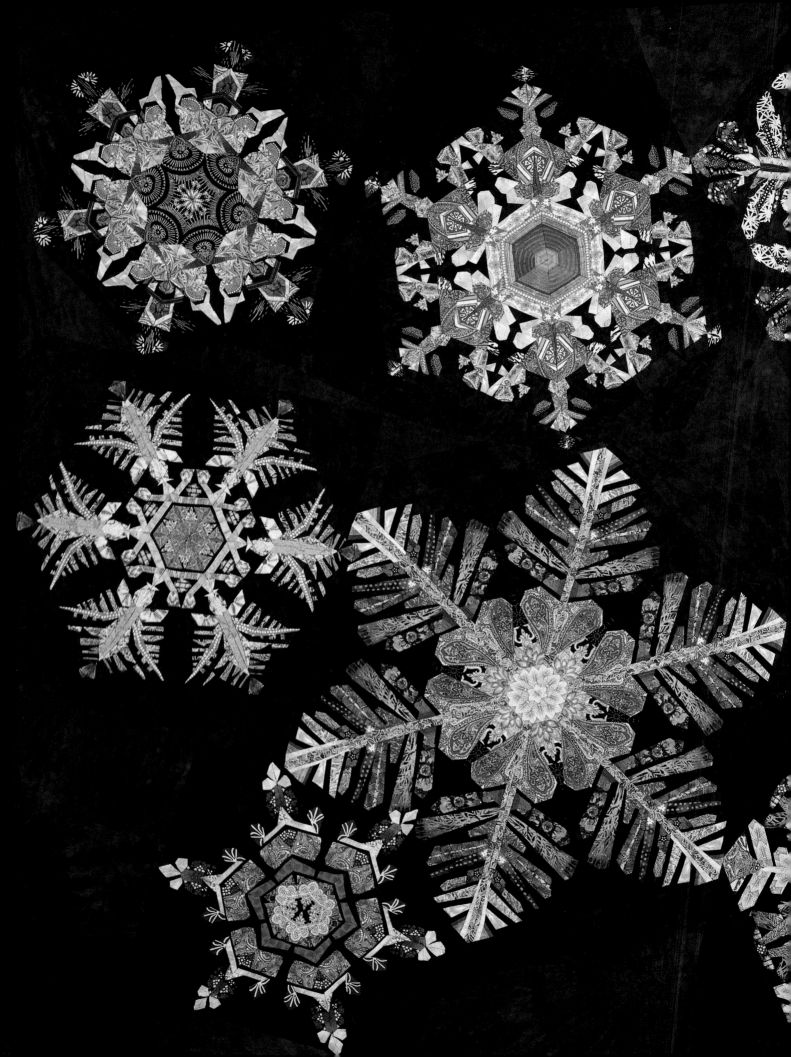

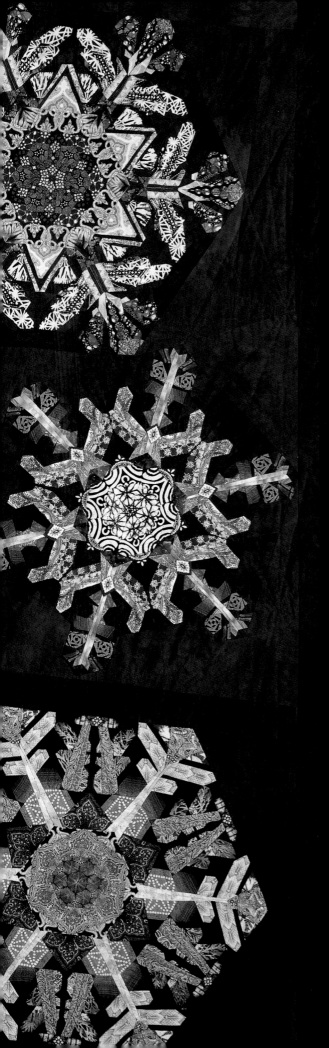

◄ KALEIDOSCOPIC XI: Snowfall,
1993, 63.5" x 60".
Machine pieced, hand quilted. Cottons, cotton-blends, si

Every snow crystal that gently floats to earth is equally
compelling. The pieced snowflakes in this quilt are an
attempt to translate in fabric a few of the over 2,000
photomicrographs made by W. A. Bentley of Jericho,
Vermont, originally published by the American
Meteorological Society in 1931.

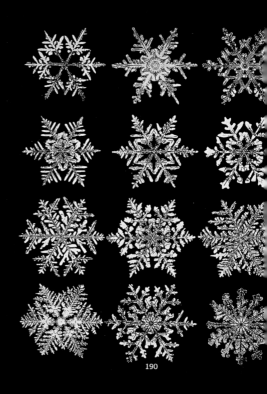

190

▲ Page 190 of *Snow Crystals*, a reprinted edition of Ber
photomicrographs published by Dover Publications.

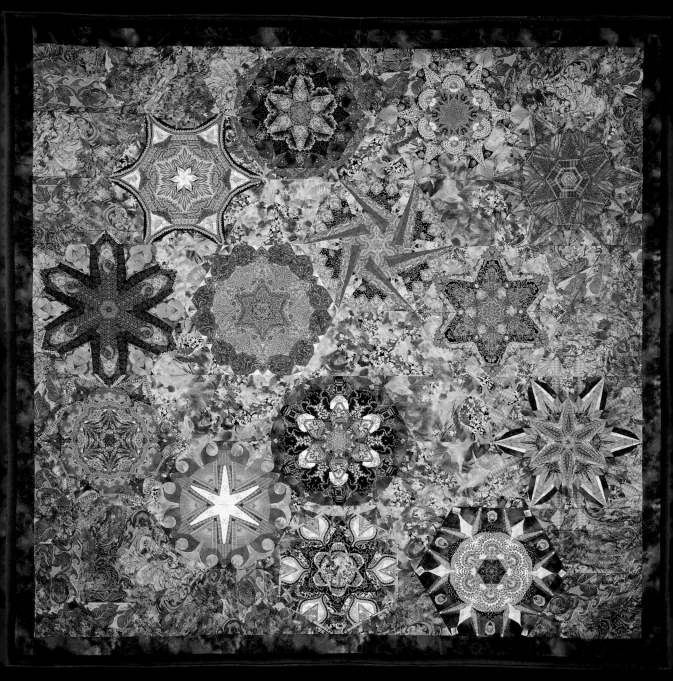

KALEIDOSCOPIC XII: Up Close and Far Away, 1994, 80" X 82".
Machine pieced, hand quilted. Cottons, cotton blends, silk.

James Gleick points out that "nature paints its scenes without regard for conventional order."
I perceive a scene of nature as simultaneously fuzzy and detailed, structured and unpredictable.
This quilt embodies a giant leap along my creative path. Instead of positioning images against
a neutral ground, the background becomes an important element of design.

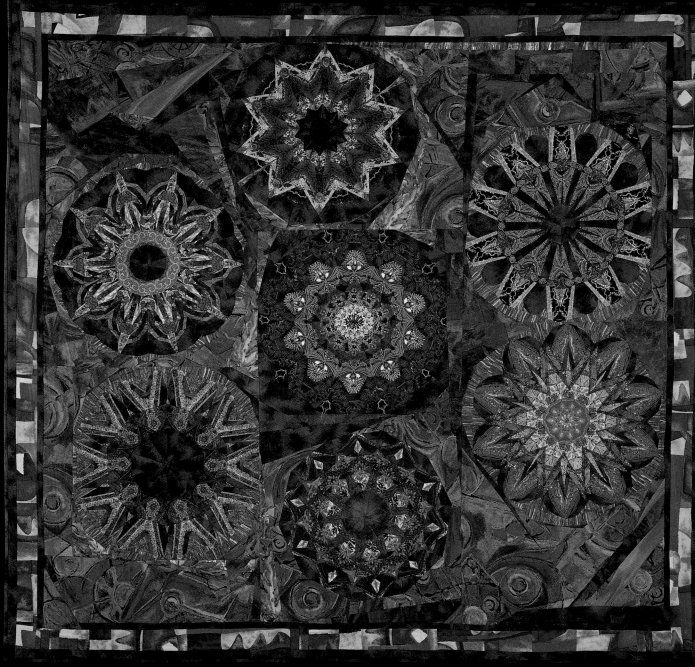

▲ KALEIDOSCOPIC XIII: Random Acts of Color, 1994, 59.5" X 56".
Machine pieced, hand quilted. Cottons, cotton-blends.

The notion that there is no absolute, correct, best selection—that my fabric choices today will be different from ones made tomorrow—is very liberating. Real kaleidoscopes have taught me to rethink my own rules. In these scopes I played with an empty space at the center of some designs.

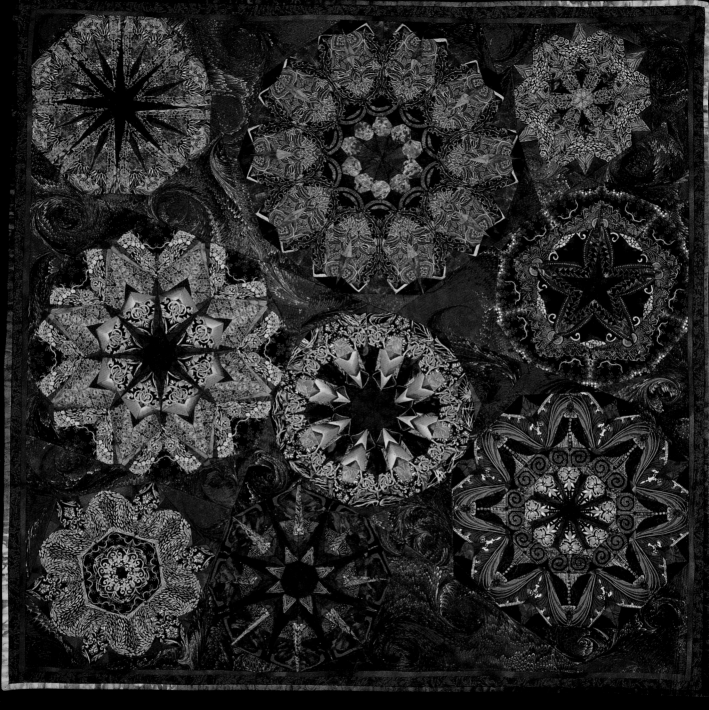

▲ KALEIDOSCOPIC XIV: Myst, 1995, 36" x 36"
Machine pieced, hand quilted. Cottons, cotton blends, hand-marbled silk.

Season: Autumn
Random colors swirl
into prisms of surprise
wrapped in royal silk

This quilt was made for the Manhattan Quilters traveling exhibit entitled "Broadway Haiku" using the theme and 36" x 36" dimensions. The palette was inspired by a hand-marbled piece of silk.

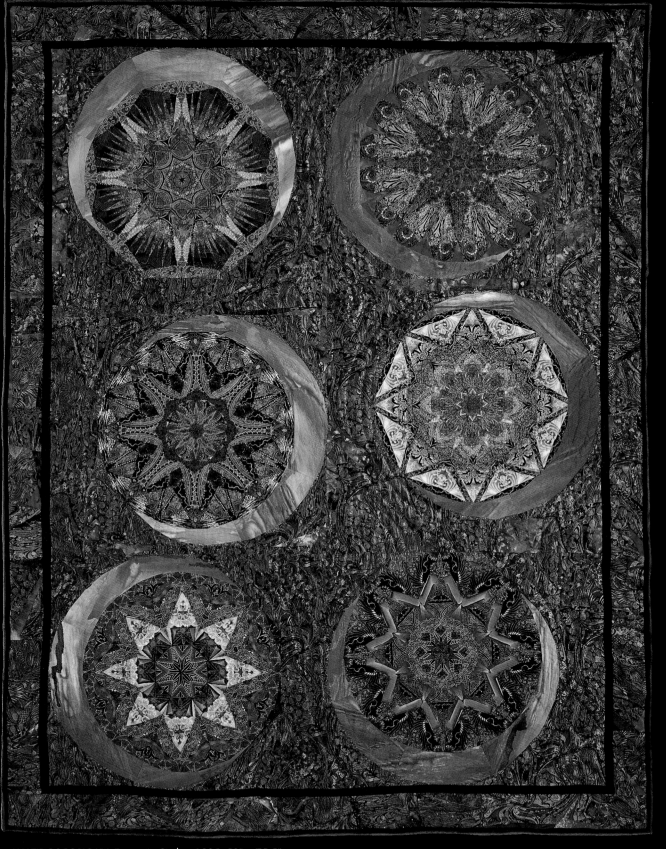

▲ KALEIDOSCOPIC XV: Eccentric Circles, 1995, 59" x 75.5".
Machine pieced, hand quilted. Cottons, silk.

In the body of the quilt, I maintained the nap of the French tapestry-like silk in one direction.
In the fractured border I cut it randomly, hoping to catch the light in different ways.

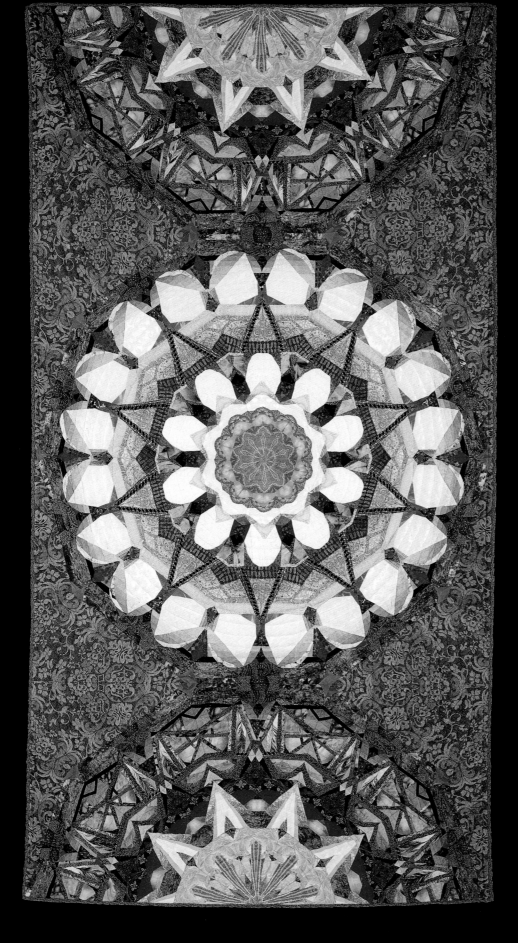

◄ KALEIDOSCOPIC IX:
Public Radio Daze,
1992, 44" x 84".
Machine pieced, hand quilted.
Cottons, cotton-blends, silk.

As I work, I listen
to public radio and
become saturated
with gray-colored
stories of subtle
intricacy, detailed
with touches of
brilliant humor and
flashes of bright hope.

TOOLS OF THE TRADE

Here's a tip for those of us who seem to be wading in the shallow end of the compulsive gene pool. A painless way to bestow a quilt with an air of competence and technical savvy is to use the same tools consistently, from the beginning of a project to the end. It is important that the measuring devices used agree with each other. Otherwise, carefully measured pieces still might not fit together. I've learned to rely on the following implements. They have become the tools of my trade.

1. **Graph paper** with an eight-to-the-inch grid and a bold inch line (hereafter, ⅛" graph paper). Make sure the lines are printed precisely on both sides of the page and measurements are consistent with your other tools. I buy pads of both 11" x 17" and 17" x 22".

2. Sheets of see-through **plastic template material** with an ⅛" grid and bold inch lines. Usually these come in packages with four 8½" x 10¾" sheets.

3. **A thin ruler** made of clear plastic with an accurate ⅛" grid and bold inch lines. I keep a 12" x 2" and an 18" x 2" ruler close by.

■ TECHNIQUE TIP   On some rulers the ⅛" along one edge is narrower—by the barest of smidgens—than the ⅛" on the parallel edge. These rulers are designed to compensate for the width of a pencil line along that edge. Check both sides of your ruler by aligning the ⅛" line along the edge to the grid of the graph paper. Mark along the ruler's edge with a pencil and see if this line falls exactly on the graph paper line or a little above it. Repeat along the ruler's other edge. If one of the ⅛" delineations is wider than the other, make a mark on the ruler's narrow side as a reminder to use this edge consistently.

For drafting I like to use a thin ruler. Thicker ones made to be used with rotary cutters cast shadows and don't allow my pen or pencil to get really close to the ruler's edge.

4. **Well-sharpened pencils** with ample erasers. Lines have not only length, but also width. When you outline a shape, you increase its size by the width of your marking. Regarding erasers, there is at least one virtue to the old-fashioned, attached kind—when you've found your pencil, you know the eraser is not far behind.

5. **A protractor with notations for both whole and half degrees.** The bigger the protractor, the better—since the numbers and marks are easier to read. It's important to be able to decipher and mark the half degrees easily. If possible, collect two or even three protractors of different sizes.

6. **Fabric scissors.**

7. **Template/paper scissors.**

8. **Set-up for rotary cutting**, including a rotary cutter, ruler, and mat.

9. **An extra-fine-point permanent marker.** A marker should glide smoothly without stretching the fabric. I like the PILOT® *Extra Fine Point* Permanent Marker, SCA-UF, because it leaves a thin but visible line. I don't want to waste time searching for a line once it's drawn or increase the size of a patch by the width of a plump line.

Smearing is inevitable with any pen that is brand new and dragged along a ruler. Rulers intended for drafting often compensate for smudging with an elevated bottom surface that doesn't extend completely to the edges of the ruler. These rulers aren't the see-through variety. If smudging bothers you, glue something (like pennies or thick sandpaper) to the bottom of the ruler. Or, sometimes it helps if you wait a beat after marking a line before removing the ruler.

10. **Sewing machine** with a well-defined ¼" seam allowance guide. On some machines the edge of the presser foot is exactly ¼" from the needle. Others, like my aging yet ever-faithful Singer Featherweight™, have a ¼" mark etched on the throat plate. Still others come with a magnetic or screw-on accessory to indicate sewing lines.

If your machine has no markings at all, make your own with a piece of masking tape on the throat plate. Measure from the needle using the same ruler or graph-paper grid you'll be using to draft the design. Check it a few hundred times. This is important. Compulsiveness now will result in well-behaved patches later.

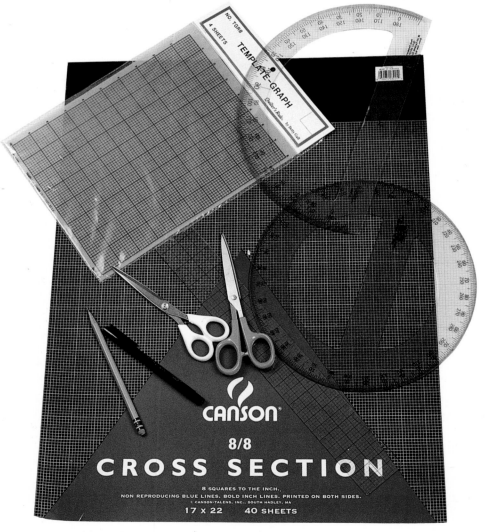

▲ Tools of the trade

KALEIDOSCOPE

TECHNICAL SENSE

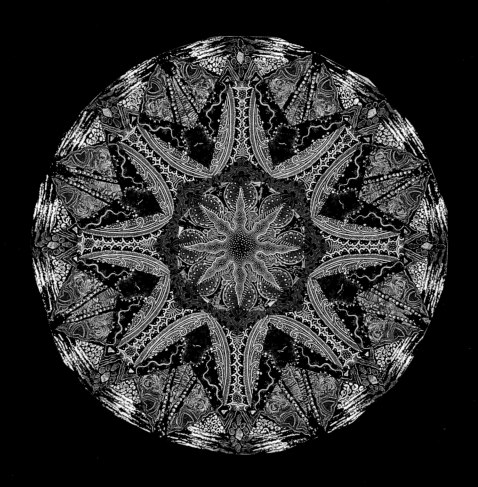

TECHNICAL SENSE

CONSIDERING ALL THE ANGLES

A kaleidoscope-shaped design functions like a circle. In Diagram 1, triangular shaped wedges radiate from the centers of each circle. When fitted together, the sections—no matter how many there are—form a circle.

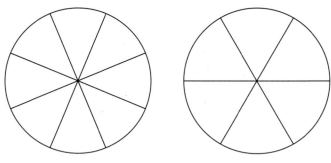

▲ 1   Triangular-shaped wedges radiate from the centers of two circles.

A circle always consists of 360 degrees. This geometric tidbit is the key ingredient in the recipe for piecing well-behaved eight-pointed stars and hexagonal designs. Think of the circle as a *pie,* and the sections as *pieces-of-the-pie.* This means that when any circle is divided into sections, the number of degrees in the angles that meet in the middle must equal 360.

Now that we've established this universally accepted axiom, we can decide how many sections to divide our 360 degrees into. This decision is partially up to your designing druthers and is addressed from that point of view on page 107. Since our quiltmaking legacy includes many evenly divided six-sided hexagonal and eight-sided octagonal designs, that's probably a good place to start.

For a design with eight equal sections, divide 360° by eight. The answer, 45°, is the angle that must be at the apex, or tip-top, of each and every triangle (2A). In other words, the kaleidoscope is created from eight 45° triangles that meet in the middle of the block (2B). Another design alternative is to divide the kaleidoscope into six equal triangles. In this case, divide 360° by six. The answer, 60°, tells us that in order to make a six-sided hexagonal design, each of the triangles must be exactly 60° (3A, 3B).

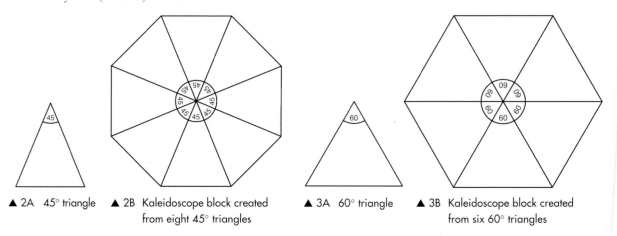

▲ 2A   45° triangle   ▲ 2B   Kaleidoscope block created from eight 45° triangles   ▲ 3A   60° triangle   ▲ 3B   Kaleidoscope block created from six 60° triangles

What happens if your attention is diverted from the drafting task by ringing phones, wafting smells, or unrelenting family members? After all, life makes its demands, and we all make mistakes. You might end up with a triangle that turns out to be, let's say, 61°. Considering I am usually not very persnickety, why should one itty-bitty degree be viewed as such an enormous troublemaker? When a 60° triangle is next to one with 61°, it is hard to see the difference. Is this a case of rampant fastidiousness usurping the design process?

The point is, we're not creating just one triangle. In a hexagonal kaleidoscope, the design calls for six identical triangles. The error is compounded six times by the inherent symmetrical structure of a kaleidoscopic shape. One extra degree attaches to each of the six triangles. In the case of a 61° triangle, 6 x 61 = (uh-oh) 366. When the six triangles meet in the middle, there will be six extra degrees vying for a place in the pie. Count off six degrees on a protractor and you'll have concrete evidence of the extra bulk that's just biding its time, waiting to combine into a dreaded bulge. That seemingly innocuous single degree turns out to be an apocalyptic warning of impending patchwork doom!

Take the time, acquire the tools, and learn the skills for drafting a trustworthy angle. It will become the blueprint you rely on during the entire design process, which, in my case, can be a couple of days or a couple of months. Once I've drafted an angle, I place my confidence in its accuracy, inhibit the voice of that fussbudget within who demands, "If you don't have time to do it right the first time, *blah, blah, blah,*" and release the spirit that yearns to search through beckoning heaps of fabric shouting: Free at last! More *IS MORE!*

HOW TO DRAFT AN ANGLE

The following discussion focuses on drafting the 45° angle needed for an eight-sided kaleidoscope. The technique is the same for drafting an angle of any size.

Diagram 4 shows a sheet of ⅛" graph paper with a right angle in the upper left hand, formed by tracing two perpendicular bold inch lines. In Diagram 5, a line drawn through dots marked at the intersections of the bold inch lines divides the right angle down the center into two equal parts. A right angle always consists of 90 degrees. Therefore, with very little fuss, I drafted a 45° triangle. Well, actually, two of them.

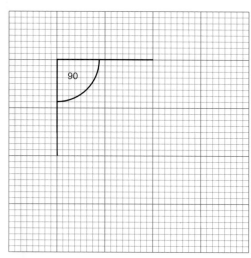

▲ 4 Right-angle corner

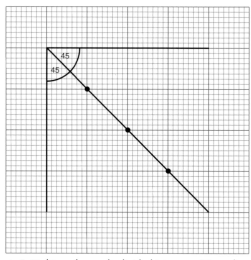

▲ 5 Right angle evenly divided into two 45° angles

Take a look at the shape. What appears as a 45° triangle is really useless for my purposes because it is awkward to work in such an askew format. I may make quilts on the kitchen table, but that doesn't mean I don't have standards.

I want my 45° triangle to be the epitome of a picture book triangle, the kind they invite onto "Sesame Street™." I want it smack in the middle of the graph paper, lined up to the grid with an obvious top, bottom, left, and right, easy to reach and easy to read (6). Pretty soon I intend to be up to my elbows in scintillating fabric. At a glance, I want to know where I am in my design, and where the design is in its space.

To this end, I use the grid of the graph paper to orient me. Mark the words top, left, and right on the graph paper along its corresponding edges (7). Establish which of the bold vertical lines seems to be the center of the graph paper. This line will be the center axis of your design. In geometric terms it is designated the axis of reflection or the axis of symmetry. In Diagram 7 the center axis is marked for you to refer to in the following discussion. ***Do not mark the center axis on your graph paper!*** Every line inside the triangular shape represents a sewing line. By marking this line, you risk interpreting the center axis as a seam later on.

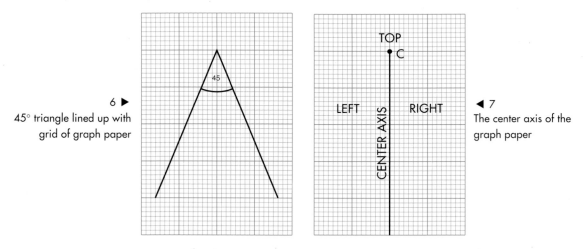

6 ▶

45° triangle lined up with grid of graph paper

◀ 7

The center axis of the graph paper

Toward the top of the page, locate a point where a bold inch line intersects the center axis (7, Point C). This will be the center reference point for lining up the protractor. It will also become the apex of the triangle.

A protractor has three reference marks that must line up accurately with the graph paper (8).

A. The 0s (zeros) on each side of the protractor.

B. The center reference mark along the middle of the straight edge of the protractor.

C. The 90° mark at the center of the semi-circle.

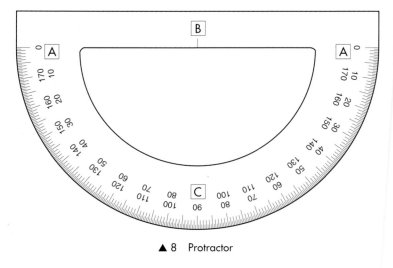

▲ 8   Protractor

Place the protractor so the zeros are aligned with a bold inch line of graph paper. The center reference point and 90° mark line up with the center axis (9). Use as many cues as possible to ensure precision.

Here's the plan. Instead of counting off the entire angle at once, divide those important 45° in half (22½°), and measure half of the 45° to the left of the center axis and the other half to the right. Find Point A in Diagram 9. This is the point where the center axis meets the 90° mark along the circular edge of the protractor. Count off 22½° to the left of Point A and make a visible, but exquisitely delicate, pencil point right there (Point L). Next, go back to Point A, count off 22½° to the right, and mark it with an equally dainty dot (Point R). With a heavy dot, it's hard to be precise when you aim for its center. (For a 60° angle, count 30° to the left and 30° to the right.)

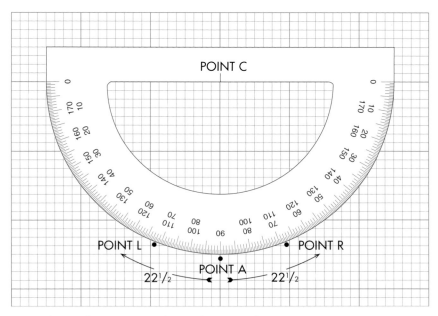

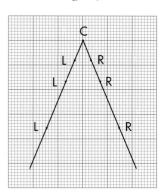

▲ 10 The resulting dots from multiple protractors

▲ 9 Aligning the protractor to the graph paper grid

The next logical step is to remove the protractor and, with a very sharp pencil and straight edge, make a line connecting Point C and Point L and a second line connecting Point C and Point R. Before you do this, I'd like you to consider something.

A line is really a series of points. The more points that connect to make a line, the more accurate the line. In this case, there are two points to connect. If you are making a fairly short line, maybe three or five inches, I'm sure it will be accurate. But what if you base a very *long* line on the strength of those two puny points? The line gets off to an auspicious start by zipping straight through only two points. Pretty soon, there's nothing for the line to aim toward. Even the best intentioned ruler can inadvertently go astray under these circumstances.

After lots of trial and error, with the emphasis on error, I figured out one alternative was to make as many points as possible. In order to achieve an abundance of dots, I use many protractors of different sizes in a single project, lining each one up as illustrated in Diagram 9. Use each protractor to mark 22½° to the left and 22½° to the right of the center axis. Voila! Lots of dots! Because the protractors are different sizes, the resulting dots vary in distance from Point C even though they measure the identical angle (10). Please note that these dots will not necessarily coincide with the paper's grid lines.

A PIECEFUL STRATEGY

During the time it takes to design and piece the kaleidoscope, I'm only going to see a single full-size triangle drawn on a long sheet of ⅛" graph paper. Unless a quilt needs to be a certain size, I won't decide in advance how big the completed triangle will be. I'll let serendipity and my palette of fabric guide the evolving design.

The size of the completed kaleidoscope block is twice the size of a single piece-of-pie. For example, if the piece-of-pie measures 5½", the block will be twice that size, or 11". The final shape of an eight-sided kaleidoscope is a square (11A). Four 45°-45°-90° triangles pieced to every other triangle turn the octagon into a square. A six-sided kaleidoscope block is a rectangle. The four triangles needed to create right angles in the corners measure 30°-60°-90° (11B).

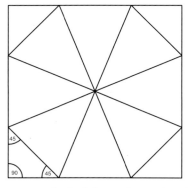

▲ 11A The final shape of an eight-sided kaleidoscope is a square.

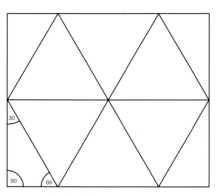

▲ 11B The final shape of a six-sided kaleidoscope is a rectangle.

As simplistic as it sounds, high up on my list of objectives is the desire to create a design that sews together successfully. I rely on a developmental approach, allowing the patches to evolve gradually into sections, combining sections together into bigger and bigger divisions until it all fits together like a puzzle. . .a puzzle defined by two limitations: conforming to the shape set by the designated angle and confining the design to only straight lines. These lines do not have to follow the grid of the graph paper (12).

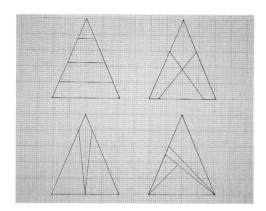

▲ 12 A single wedge divided by straight lines

These criteria are based on my preference to never, ever have to piece my way out of a *corner*, aptly defined by Webster's as "an awkward position from which escape is difficult." As the design progresses into an increasingly more complex map of sewing lines, I continually stay focused on how to divide the wedge into sections that can be sewn together using only straight seams.

There are infinite variations in applying these principles. Kaleidoscope blocks vary in complexity and take various forms. It isn't as if I stare at the empty graph paper diagram and arbitrarily split it into subdivisions. Organizing the wedge into segments keeps pace with the design process, which dominates the decisions and is guided by fabric choices. In fact, the design sequence may not be the same as the piecing sequence (13). Often I design a section and then realize it can't be pieced until later, after an adjacent section is finished. I usually wait until all the sections are complete before I piece them together into the piece-of-pie.

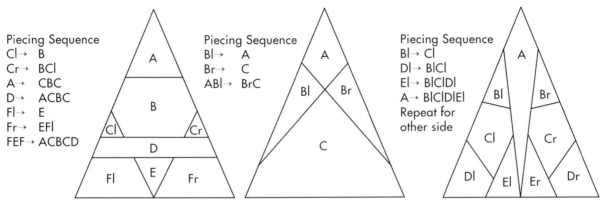

Piecing Sequence
Cl→ B
Cr→ BCl
A→ CBC
D→ ACBC
Fl→ E
Fr→ EFl
FEF→ ACBCD

Piecing Sequence
Bl→ A
Br→ C
ABl→ BrC

Piecing Sequence
Bl→ Cl
Dl→ BlCl
El→ BlClDl
A→ BlClDlEl
Repeat for
other side

▲ 13 Organize the wedge into segments. The design sequence is often different from the piecing sequence.

I prefer not to do a fabric mockup. My standard, glib explanation is that if I knew what it was going to look like, I wouldn't want to do it. Remember, making kaleidoscopic designs satisfies my urge to be the one who makes the magic and the one who feels the surprise. You should do what works best for you. I tend to get absorbed in the act of designing until I'm just about to lose track of the proverbial thread binding my decisions together. That's when I stop to catch my breath, visit the fridge, and transfer every decision to the graph paper diagram.

Starting the design at the top of the triangle, I begin to invent a piecing sequence that fills the body of the triangle. The only rule defining this task is to *stay inside the lines formed by the angle at the top of the triangle.* This governing principle will be interpreted through my palette of fabric. Here's where I balance my confidence in the angle's accuracy with my respect for the fabric and my childish desire to have it all. . .now! An animated back-and-forth exchange develops between the fabric and the graph paper blueprint. The mediator facilitating this collaborative effort—both the peacemaker and the piecemaker—is the template technique.

HOW TO MAKE A TEMPLATE

Along with ensuring an accurate angle, the full-size "piece-of-the-pie" on J" graph paper serves as a blueprint for making clear plastic templates. No matter how complex a shape is, the technique for making a template is always the same. To demonstrate how to make a template, let's say the first patch will be 3G". (This is just an arbitrary measurement to get us started. Usually the patch is shaped by a fabric's motif.)

Mark every decision on the graph paper diagram in pencil so it can be erased when you get an even better idea—or make a mistake. Every pencil line represents a sewing line. That is why I did not want to mark the bold vertical line that functions as the center axis illustrated in Diagram 7 (page 36). I didn't want to risk interpreting it as a sewing line.

Starting at the top of the triangle, count down three bold inch lines and two ⅛" lines. Use a ruler to draw a pencil line across the grid at this point (14A). Use the grid to measure whenever possible; it is quicker than lining up a ruler. One of the most satisfying features of the ⅛" grid is that ¼" and ⅛" dimensions are easily measured. This allows us to be precise and quick when generating a design brimming with intricacy.

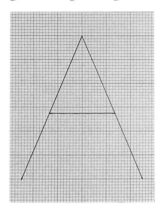

▲ 14A Using a ruler and pencil, draw a line across the triangle 3¹/₄" from the top of the triangle.

▲ 14B Place a sheet of transparent template material over the patch marked on the graph paper, aligning a bold inch line on the template material with the center axis.

▲ 14C Trace the triangle precisely onto the template material with the permanent marker, marking as thin a line as possible.

The plan is to trace the shape of the patch onto the template material using a see-through ruler and permanent marker. Place a sheet of transparent template material over the 3¼" patch marked on the graph paper, aligning a bold inch line on the template material with the center axis (14B). Keeping in mind the guiding principle for placement—*Thou shalt not waste template material*—make sure there's enough space on all three sides to add ¼" for seam allowance.

Trace the triangle precisely onto the template material, marking as thin a line as possible (14C). Remember, every line has width and length. You don't want to increase the width of the template with a corpulent outline. This template will be used to cut eight identical patches for the kaleidoscope. If you inadvertently fatten it up now, the block will be burdened with the extra baggage times eight.

Next, immediately add ¼" seam allowance on all three sides using the see-through ruler. Align the ¼" ruler delineation with the edge of the template line and zip a line along the ruler (15). In other words, on a ruler with an ⅛" grid, two lines will equal ¼". Place the ruler so most of it lies on the template and ¼" extends past the edge.

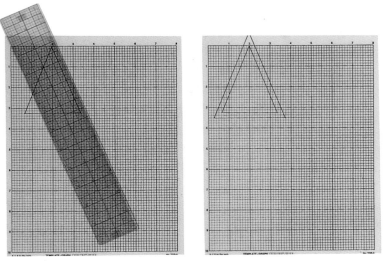

▲ 15 Align the ¹/₄" ruler delineation with the edge of the template line and mark a line along the ruler.

Notice how the seam allowance at the top of the template extends into a point way beyond a true ¼" (16A). Imagine the bulky impact when eight of these oversized angles meet in the middle. Be merciless. Nip that bulk before it gets a chance to bud. Use a ruler to cut it down to ¼" (16B).

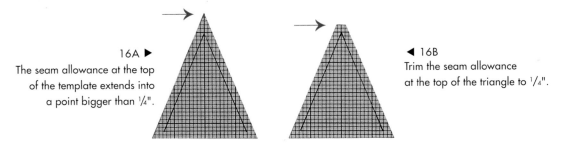

16A ▶
The seam allowance at the top of the template extends into a point bigger than ¼".

◀ 16B
Trim the seam allowance at the top of the triangle to ¹/₄".

■ TECHNIQUE TIP   For patches that are centered along the axis, it is important to make a template that matches the bold lines of the template grid to the corresponding grid of the graph paper. This simple stratagem encourages an accurate mirror-imaged, left/right orientation. For patches that are not positioned along the center axis, matching the template grid to the grid of the graph is not necessary.

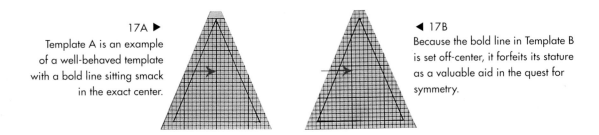

17A ▶
Template A is an example of a well-behaved template with a bold line sitting smack in the exact center.

◀ 17B
Because the bold line in Template B is set off-center, it forfeits its stature as a valuable aid in the quest for symmetry.

HOW TO MARK A TEMPLATE

Using transparent material and marking the seam allowance lines creates a template that functions like a window. It allows you to identify the area that will be visible in the patch and, particularly relevant to this configuration, you can check out what part of the fabric bumps into the seamline. Herein lies the essence of a pieced kaleidoscope. The portion of fabric that winds up along the seamlines connects to its mirror image. Seamlines will disappear, intricacy will reign, and we will get credit for the magic that happens when the whole becomes greater than the sum of its parts.

The top of the triangle, or apex, will eventually take its position in the design's important center. In a radial design, such as a kaleidoscope block, the eye is drawn first into the middle. Therefore, the fabric chosen for the first patch assumes a major role, seducing the viewer into the visually exciting focal point, enticing her to stay for a second look, setting the mood for the scope to come.

To ensure the illusion of graceful continuity in the center, look for a cotton-like border print with perfect bilateral symmetry (see "Our Fabrics, Our Palettes" on page 95). In other words, find a motif printed on the fabric that can be divided into identical halves by a line passing through the center. Give a fabric printed with the capacity to reflect itself in a perfect mirror image the chance to strut its stuff. There will be lots of chances to play with asymmetrical fabric later in the scope.

To decide whether a fabric is design-worthy for this pivotal position, check for two important criteria. First, it must have a sufficient number of repeats to cut an identical patch for each piece-of-the-pie. Second, to promote stability when all the triangles meet in the middle, this first triangle must be cut on a straight grain of fabric. In other words, the center axis of the triangle must line up with either the lengthwise or the crosswise grain of the goods (18). If you fall in love with an exquisite paisley that loops along the diagonal, set it aside for now.

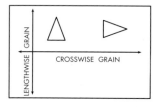

◀ 18
To promote stability when all the triangles meet in the middle, the first triangle must be cut on a straight grain of fabric.

Place the window-like template on the front of the fabric, aligning the center line of the template with the implied center of a motif. Move it up, move it down, turn it upside down. Varying the template's placement even slightly alters the final kaleidoscopic effect (see "The Nitty Gritty of the Very First Patch" on page 110).

When you've decided where to position the template, hold it in place and trace a few lines of the selected motif onto the template with the permanent marker. Trace some of these "clues" or "hints" within the body of the template, making sure several clues spill across the seamlines into the seam allowance. This will facilitate accuracy at the seams (19A).

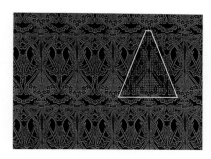

◀ 19A
Trace a few lines of the selected motif from the fabric onto the template with the permanent marker.

Use these clues to superimpose the template identically over corresponding motifs when they occur again on the fabric. Once the template is appropriately placed, trace it on the front of the fabric with the permanent marker. Repeat this process as many times as necessary (19B). Cut accurately, aiming down the center of the marked line. Panel 20 reveals the "holey" quality of much of my stash.

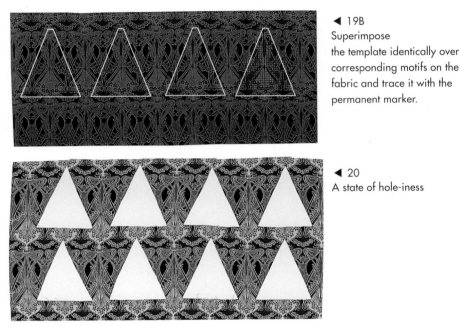

◀ 19B
Superimpose the template identically over corresponding motifs on the fabric and trace it with the permanent marker.

◀ 20
A state of hole-iness

The purists among us are probably asking: "Why on the front?" My answer is: "Why not?" After all, I want to be able to see the fabric clearly in order to recognize identical segments. Also, I'm using a permanent marker that won't bleed to mark a cutting line that will be cut off.

The only time I don't mark on the front is when I can't see what I'm doing. For example, if the fabric is printed with lines that are indistinguishable from ones made by my marker, I'll check to see if the print is recognizable from its wrong side. (In this case, if I am marking a nonreversible template on the wrong side of the fabric, I have to flip the template over; two wrongs make a right). My first choice is always to use the thin, permanent line of the marker. Sometimes on a dark fabric I use a chalk pencil that fits in an electric pencil sharpener.

TEMPLATES FOR SPECIAL EFFECTS

Although the apex of the first patch is predestined by the 45° angle, the contour of its bottom boundary is a design choice. It does not have to be a horizontal line molding the shape into a triangle. Diagram 21 illustrates a few options. Let the fabric shape its own destiny.

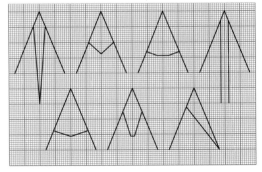

◀ 21
Options for the shape of the first patch

For example, look at the triangle of fabric and its corresponding template (A) in Panel 22. Perhaps lopping off the extraneous stuff in the triangle's corners will highlight the teardrop shape of the fabric's motif. Exactly where to trim the triangle is a decision easily tailored to the fabric. Place the template on the patch (B). Looking through the transparent template, focus on what portion of the design to keep versus what is immaterial. Let the grid lines on the template guide the placement of a cutting line. It will be easier to read and use as an effective measuring tool if lines begin and end at the intersection of grid lines rather than between them.

Note where your choice coincides with a point on the template grid. Next, line up a straight edge with this point and use it to extend an imaginary line toward a second potential grid point. This gives you a chance to experiment visually and survey alternatives for outlining the patch of fabric. In this case, I decided to make the line close to the turquoise contour, eliminating as much of the dark blue circle as possible. Mark the two points on the template and draw a line from point to point (C). Add ¼" seam allowance and cut (D). Use the revised template to reshape the patch of fabric (E).

The next imperative step is to transfer this line onto the graph paper blueprint. Use the template's grid to measure the position of the points. Starting from the top of the triangle, one point is 2⅝" down, on the border line of the triangle. Mark this spot on the graph paper diagram. The second dot coincides with the intersection of the central axis and the bottom edge. Draw a line from point to point (F).

Because the pattern on one side of the center axis is the mirror image of the pattern on the other side, this center line is also called an axis of reflection or symmetry. The pattern can be superimposed on itself by flipping it over. This insight allows me to draw lines only in one half of the graph paper triangle and know that these lines will be identical on the other side (F). The pieces-of-the-pie will replicate more accurately if only one set of lines is used for each adjustment. Flipping the template over, instead of creating a second template, will ensure the line stays fixed.

■ TECHNIQUE TIP   I know it isn't easy for quilters who aren't used to drafting patterns on graph paper to adopt this strategy. But it is exactly the step of marking every sewing line on the diagram that results in a design plan that explains the parts and their relationships. If you give it a chance, you will learn to appreciate the diagram.

I mark sewing lines on the left side of the diagram (probably because I am a lefty). By being consistent, I can assume every template is correctly aligned to a left-sided patch and must be flipped over and used wrong side up to create a mirror-imaged patch on the right side. You should do what feels comfortable for you.

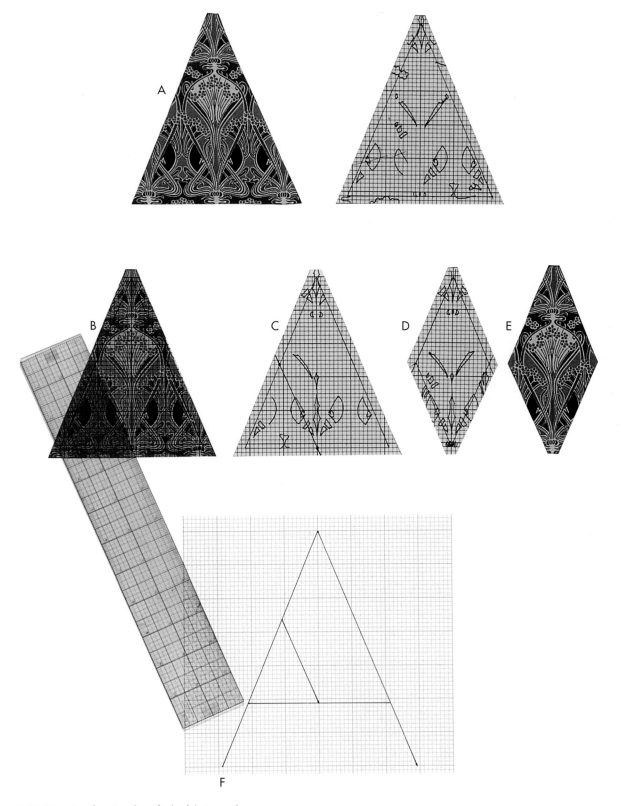

▲ 22 Trimming the triangle to fit the fabric motif

A. A triangle of fabric and its corresponding template.

B. Place the template on the patch. Align a straight edge with the selected point and extend it toward a second potential grid point.

C. Draw a line connecting the points on the template which correspond to your choices for the patch's outline.

D. Add ¹/₄" seam allowance and cut the re-defined template.

E. Use the revised template to reshape the patch of fabric.

F. Transfer this line onto the graph paper blueprint.

VISUAL PROBLEMS, CREATIVE SOLUTIONS

Let the first patch inspire the second. My tendency is to camouflage seams through fabric manipulation, to encourage an uninterrupted flow of design or color from one patch to the next.

Consider this design scenario: What if I select a portion of the fabric used for Patch 1 (A) and use it again in Patch 2, creating a connection between the two that seems to reflect the tear-shaped motif back on itself? Confused? Don't be! There is a picture worthy of the proverbial thousand words in Panel 23 (I). The next couple of paragraphs explain how to create this special effect.

Let the grid of the template plastic serve as a ruler. Place the template on its patch-mate (B). Looking through the transparent plastic, select the portion of the motif you want to include in Patch 2. Orient yourself to the details. Do you want to include all of the purple motif, just a fragment, or none of it? Do you want to end at 2" or 2½" or somewhere in between? As soon as you make a decision, transfer it to the graph paper diagram. Remember, the best way to define a patch is by choosing points along grid line intersections.

I decided to end the patch in a tip at Point Y, capturing the turquoise contour only. I figured out the coordinates of this point by counting grid lines along the center axis, starting at Point X, the intersection of the seamline and the center axis. The result, two bold inch lines and four eighth lines, or 2½", was transferred to the graph paper diagram (C).

Next, I focused on how to shape the patch along the horizontal connecting seamline. Since the goal was to mirror image the turquoise pear shape, it seemed logical to pinpoint Point Z at the little periwinkle flower. Counting from Point X, this point measured 1⅛" to the left of the center axis. After marking the appropriate point on the diagram, I used a ruler to draw lines connecting Points Y and Points Z (D).

Once Patch 2 was outlined on the diagram, I made a template for it by tracing the shape onto template material, aligning grid to grid. Next, I added ¼" seam allowance to every side by the method described in Panel 15, and cut (E).

The goal is for the pattern in Patch 1 to match the motif in Patch 2 exactly. This is remarkably easy to arrange. Line up Template 2 with Template 1, right sides together matching sewing lines and center axes (F). Trace hints from Template 1 onto Template 2, using the permanent marker (G).

Use the cues on Template 2 to find the corresponding motif on the fabric (H). Once the template is appropriately placed, trace it as many times as necessary on the front of the fabric with the permanent marker. This method ensures the two fabrics are accurately aligned when machine-pieced together, because the all-important seam allowance is built into the construction technique (I).

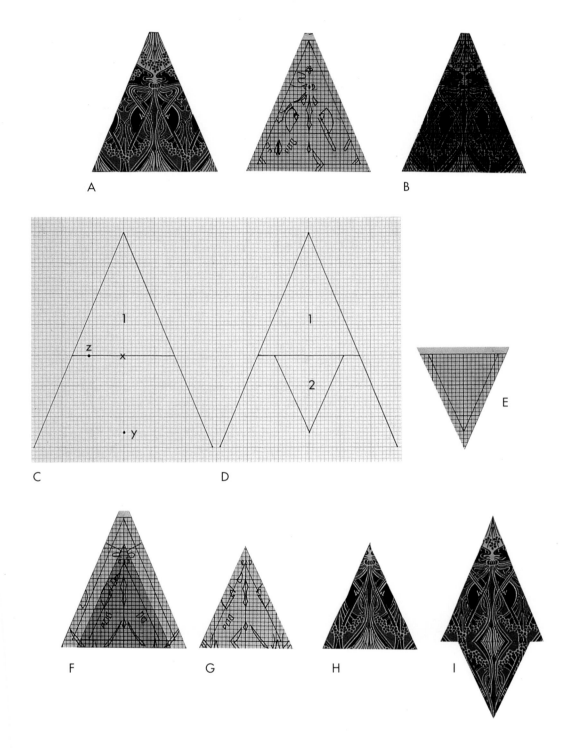

▲ 23 Filling Template 2 with the mirror image of Patch 1

A. The patch and its corresponding template

B. Place the template on its patch-mate.

C. Transfer design decisions to the graph paper diagram.

D. Use a straight edge to draw a line connecting the chosen points.

E. Once Patch 2 is outlined on the diagram, make a template for it by tracing the shape onto template material, aligning grid to grid. Add ¹/₄" seam allowance to every side

F. Place the two templates right sides together, as if sewing them together, matching the bold center axes and sewing lines.

G. Trace hints from Template 1 onto Template 2, using the permanent marker.

H. Use the cues on Template 2 to find the corresponding motif on the fabric.

I. The result: an accurately aligned connection between two patches that appears to reflect the tear-shaped motif.

THE SAME BEGINNING, A DIFFERENT ENDING

What if, instead of filling Template 2 with the mirror image of Patch 1, I want to create the illusion that the two patches aren't interrupted by a seam, as if the design spills across the seamline and resumes the natural flow of the pattern (A)? This idea is explored in Panel 24.

Let's use the shape created in the previous discussion to work out the construction strategy for this alternate design (B). The key to success is provided by the following unusual way to line up Template 2 to Template 1: overlap the bottom seam allowance of Template 1 onto the top seam allowance of Template 2 (C). Match up the bold center axes and the sewing lines. Trace hints marked in the seam allowance of Template 1 where they land on 2 (D). If there aren't enough cues to ensure accuracy, place Template 1 back on its fabric counterpart and add some more hints in the seam allowance.

Place Template 2 on the fabric and find its corresponding position. The easiest way to conduct this search is to first find the spot for Template 1. Keep it there. Line up Template 2 to 1 (E). Trace clues from the fabric onto 2 (F). Copy enough hints to make identifying repeats a cinch (G).

Again, two fabrics are assured accurate alignment when stitched together using a sewing machine because the template technique includes the all-important seam allowance.

THE PACE OF PIECING

Design a little, piece a little, design a little more. Sew identical units at the same time, using an assembly line approach. Whatever I do for one piece-of-the-pie, I do simultaneously to all of its mates. By the time the end is in sight, the six or eight triangles are at identical stages of completion.

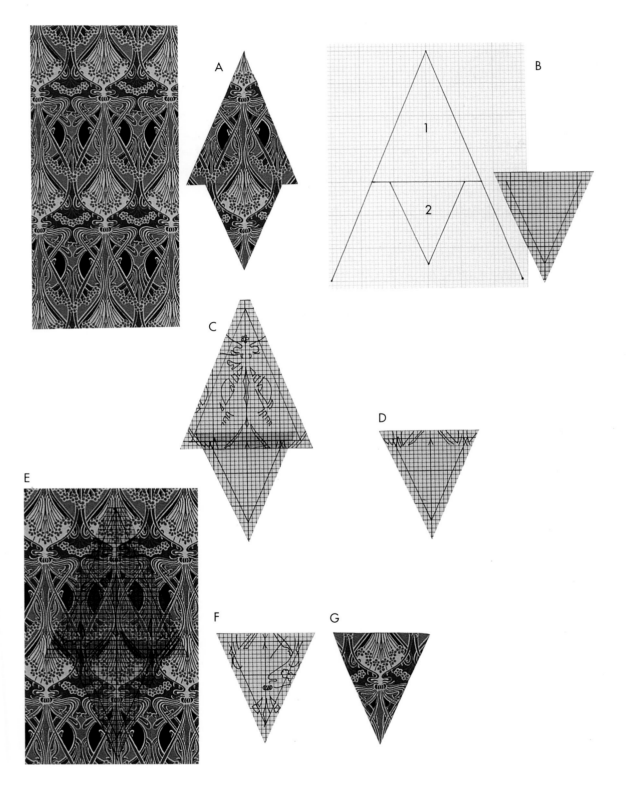

▲ 24 Creating the illusion that the two patches aren't interrupted by a seam

A. The final version.

B. The shape and its corresponding template.

C. Overlap the bottom seam allowance of Template 1 onto the top seam allowance of Template 2, matching the bold center axes and the stitching lines.

D. Trace hints marked in the seam allowance of Template 1 where they land on 2.

E. Place Template 2 on the fabric and find its correlating position.

F. Trace clues from the fabric onto Template 2.

G. The result.

HOW TO PIECE ITSY-BITSY, TEENY-WEENY PIECES

Designing a kaleidoscope block is basically visual invention. There is no "correct" way to continue the piece-in-progress. This time, brainstorming led to surrounding Patch 2 with a reddish-purple outline. I guessed that this would show off the elegant tear-shaped motif and create a chain linking the purple "vees" from a single wedge into a star. The color purple influenced similar colors in the design to dance forward and be highlighted. A sharp demarcation between the background colors of Patches 2 and 3 accentuated the impression of an outline*. An all-over print that read like a solid was my fabric of choice. That was in keeping with my modus operandi: slip a forgiving textile next to a fussy one whenever possible.

(*Although I'm supposed to be demonstrating technique, I can't resist pursuing the design tangent left dangling in the previous paragraph. Try to imagine the alternate effect of a subtle shift in color. Fabrics that evoke a sense of shading translate the translucent nature of a scope's interior on a quilt's flat surface. For example, a fabric flavored with a moody version of Patch 2 will cast a shadow around the silhouette, conveying qualities of depth and dimension (25).)

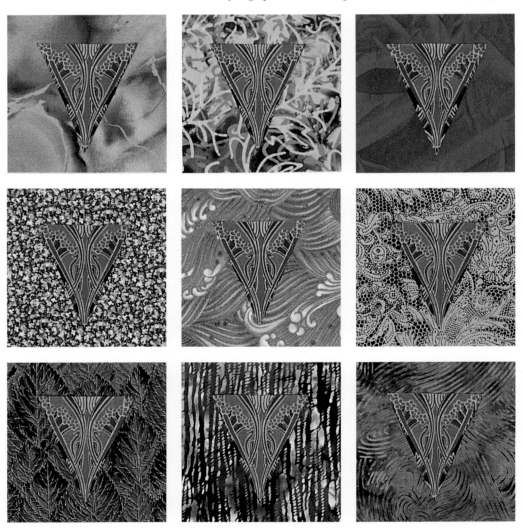

▲ 25 The effect of a subtle shift in color between Patch 2 and the fabric used to create its outline

The first step is to draft the shape of an outline on the graph paper diagram. Our legacy of quilting traditions hands down the notion that an outline must be uniformly even. But a peek into a real kaleidoscope reveals lines capable of infinite variety. Irregular ones suggest spontaneity, randomness, and transience.

I used existing points to begin and end an outline that narrows as it moves from top to bottom. There is a small but significant difference between Diagram 26A and 26B. In 26A the new line comes to the same point as the bottom tip of Template 2. In 26B it ends ⅛" to the left (and the right) of that point, along the same horizontal graph line. Both diagrams create the effect of an outline. But in Diagram 26A at least three patches and their seam allowances converge in the same spot.

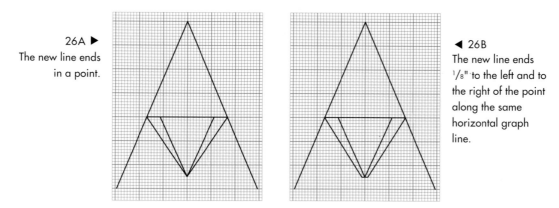

26A ▶
The new line ends
in a point.

◀ 26B
The new line ends
¹/₈" to the left and to
the right of the point
along the same
horizontal graph
line.

This construction scenario is a tad bulky for my taste. I try to avoid a multitude of seams. Whenever I see three or more fabrics about to crash into the same destination, I reroute the drafting lines to avoid a collision. Of course, there are times when this kind of detour isn't possible or desirable. There are also times when rethinking the design because of these considerations makes it even better.

By choosing the outline that ends ⅛" to each side of the point, I've narrowed the options for the final piecing sequence. The only practical conclusion for the version in Diagram 26B is a horizontal line 6½" from the top of the piece-of-pie (27B). On the other hand, the pointy design illustrated in Diagram 26A is open to more than one sewing strategy. The same horizontal line is one possibility. Extending the margins of the outline is another (27A).

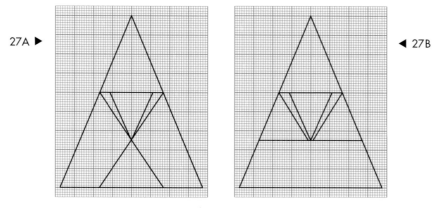

27A ▶

◀ 27B

Options for the final piecing sequence

DO NOT make a separate template for Patch 3. Instead, follow these steps (28).

STEP 1: Make a template that includes Patch 2 and Patch 3. Add ¼" seam allowance and cut. Extend lines that represent sewing lines all the way to the outside edge of the seam allowance. Place this new Template (2+3) on top of Template 2, aligning the bold center lines. Trace hints from 2 in the analogous position on Template (2+3).

STEP 2: Use a rotary cutter to slice a long strip of the reddish-purple outline fabric. How to estimate the required width of the strip is discussed in the next section.

STEP 3: Machine piece one side of each Patch 2 to the reddish-purple strip. Press.

STEP 4: Place Template (2+3) on the strip-pieced unit. First, match the hints drawn on the template with corresponding motifs in Patch 2. Next, adjust the sewing line drawn on the template so it fits directly on the seam between the two fabrics. Holding the template firmly in place, mark around it with a visible, precise line. Cut accurately, aiming the scissors down the middle of the marked line.

STEP 5: Repeat Steps 2 through 4 on the other side.

Voila! An accurately pieced unit, complete with seam allowance and ready for a new assignment. Treat the result as a unit of fabric that was born that way. Doesn't it look as if tiny patches were meticulously cut and perfectly pieced together?

■ TECHNIQUE TIP   In the above scenario, consider Patch 2 the "driver," since being in the driver's seat connotes the position of control. When placing the template on the fabric, the most important areas of alignment are the fussy fabrics that must appear to be meticulously identical. I call these temperamental prints the "prima donna" fabrics. If you have to fudge a bit when aligning templates to fabric—and you probably will at some point—make amends via altruistic, laid-back, all-over prints.

PRESSING ISSUES

Balance the usual rules guiding pressing patchwork with a pinch of logic and an eye toward future quilting. Eliminate as many layers of fabric that congregate at one point as you can. Press seams closed to one side. Whenever possible, press the seam toward the darker fabric, *unless* you are dealing with really tiny pieces. In this case, press toward the bigger patch. (If the ¼" seam allowance is bigger than some portion of its patch, you're looking at trouble come piecing time. This bulk will bump into the sewing machine's seam guide, causing it to slide off its straight-forward path.)

■ TECHNIQUE TIP   When I take the time to press after every sewing step, the inevitable multitude of seams behaves compatibly, adjusting unsightly bulges into a smooth, even surface. If an iron is inaccessible, there is always finger pressing.

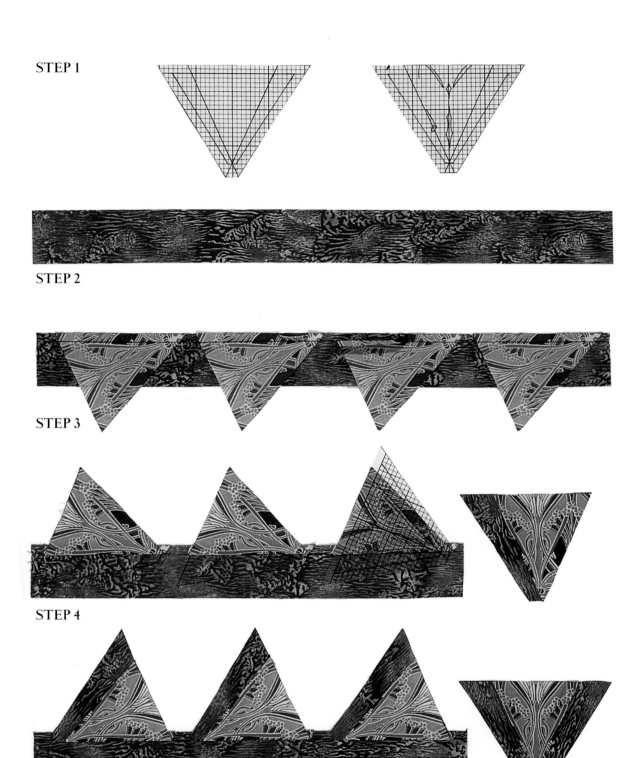

STEP 1

STEP 2

STEP 3

STEP 4

STEP 5

▲ 28　Piecing itsy-bitsy, teeny-weeny pieces

TRIMMING SEAMS

No matter how teeny-weeny a patch may be, it is always surrounded by an entourage of full-sized seam allowances. Adding on patches via strip-piecing can create an excessive bundle of bulk. Use common sense. Trim away just enough to tidy up. This makes it easier to piece the patch to adjacent ones. But don't get carried away—a skimpy amount of material sets the stage for a fate worse than bulk.

HOW TO CALCULATE THE WIDTH OF A STRIP

Use the template to calculate how wide to rotary cut a strip. Place a transparent ruler on the template, aligning the ¼" demarcation (²/₈" in from the ruler's edge) with the sewing line. In other words, ¼" of the ruler is on one side of the sewing line (representing the addition of this amount for seam allowance), and the rest of the ruler lies on the portion of template that represents the piece to be added on.

Read the ruler to see what measurement coincides with the widest point of the template. In this case, a tiny bit more than one inch of template material lies under the ruler. Cut the strip 1¼" to be on the safe side (29).

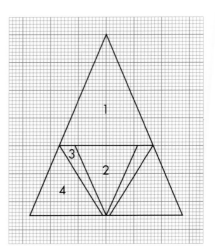

29 ▶
How to calculate the required
width of a strip

HOW TO MATCH TEMPLATES

Diagram 30 depicts the current stage of the design. Find Patch 4. This space can be filled with a single fabric or fractured into two, or three, or many fabrics. The two following principles apply regardless of the number of pieces you choose to make up Patch 4:

1. No matter how many lines divide it, the final patch must be the same exact size as Patch 4, plus seam allowance.
2. The sewing line of Patch 4 must match the sewing line of Patch (2+3).

Here's the predicament: when you align the cut edges of two differently angled shapes, the finished product will be distorted. This is because the sewing lines, ¼" from the cut edge, don't match. Once templates are cut into patches of fabric, there is no guideline to judge how to position the shapes perfectly. The sharper the angles to be pieced, the more difficult it is to eyeball the correct alignment.

▲ 30 The current stage of the design.

54

Here's the solution, made possible through the generous support of the see-through templates (32A). The following discussion refers to the points labeled in Diagram 31.

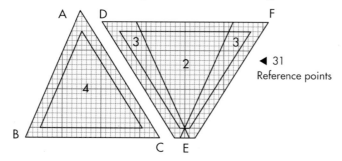

◄ 31
Reference points

STEP 1: Make a template for Patch 4, including the seam allowance.

STEP 2: Line up Template 4 to Template (2+3) right sides together, as if you were going to sew them together, matching sewing lines. Keeping the templates precisely aligned, look at the correlation between Points C and E at the bottom. See how extra plastic from Template 4 peeks out, extending beyond the other template.

STEP 3: Using the rigid edge of Template (2+3) as a guide, mark and trim off the excess at Point C.

STEP 4: This touch of grooming creates neat and tidy templates with evenly matched edges for accurate piecing alignment. (You will find the corner angles of neighboring templates are rarely identical.)

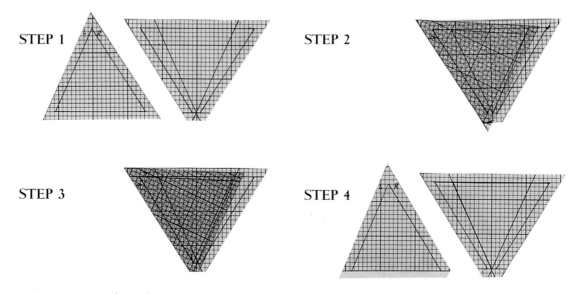

▲ 32A How to match templates

Whenever possible, make this step an essential part of your template habit *before* you cut into the fabric. Align every template to its adjoining templates, right sides together, *sewing line to sewing line*, and trim away any plastic peeping past its partner. There's even an added benefit: you'll simultaneously eliminate excess seam allowance and waste less fabric.

Back to the drawing board. Now consider the relationship between the two templates at the other end of the sewing line, between Points A and D. It is hard to see in the photograph that the templates don't *quite* match. This statement reminds me of an adage about pregnancy. When it comes to templates, there's no such thing as a little bit matched. Templates either match or they don't.

In Diagram 33 you can see how Point A on Template 4 is a sliver bigger than Template (2 + 3). In cases like this, when the angles are similar but not identical, the quiltmaker, in her infinite wisdom, can reshape the existing angle into a more serviceable one. This operation requires two steps:

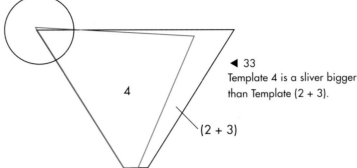

◄ 33
Template 4 is a sliver bigger than Template (2 + 3).

1. Invent a new, blunt angle on one of the templates, preserving approximately ¼" seam allowance. Mark and cut.

2. Transfer the new angle to the corresponding corner of the other template by aligning the templates right sides together, matching sewing lines. Use the edge of the just-cut angle to copy the identical shape onto the second template. Cut.

When this metamorphosis is complete, two previously dissimilar corners emerge as identical twins. Each predicament requires its own unique solution.

Here's how I resolved this case (34). Refer to points labeled in Diagram 31 on page 55.

STEP 1: Begin by trimming the left corner of Template (2+3) at Point D. Prune it any way that seems logical to you. Its seam allowance is more than the requisite ¼" anyway. Trim one side of the template only. At this time there is no accurate way to duplicate an identical angle at Point F.

STEP 2: Align Template (2+3) and Template 4 right sides together, relying on the cropped edges that now match neatly at Points C and E and the sewing lines. At Points A-D, the corner of Template 4 extends past the new edge of Point D.

STEP 3: Mark off the excess and cut.

STEP 4: Now you can use revised Point A to fashion an identical Point F on the right side of Template (2+3). Flip Template 4 over and use it wrong side up. Right sides together, align Template 4 to the right side of Template (2+3). Using Point A as a guide, trim the excess plastic at Point F.

■ TECHNIQUE TIP   Patch 4 is the first shape in this piecing sequence that isn't positioned squarely on the center axis. Therefore, when making Template 4, it is not important to match a bold line of the template grid to the grid of the graph paper. That step ensured the design stayed visually centered.

Another of Patch 4's quirks is that it is an asymmetrical shape. It is nonreversible: the back and the front of the shape are mirror images of each other. For instant orientation, mark asymmetrical shapes with direction cues: T(top), L(left) and/or R(right).

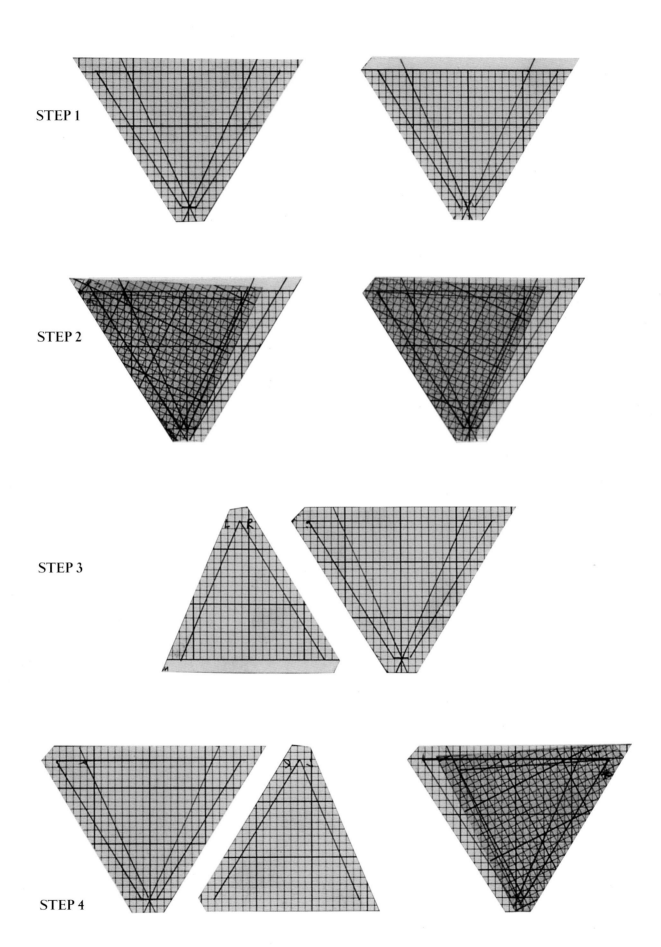

STEP 1

STEP 2

STEP 3

STEP 4

▲ 34   Revise angles of adjacent templates that are similar but not identical.

57

FRACTURED PATCHES

In the previous section I mentioned that Patch 4 could be filled with a single fabric or fractured into many pieces. Let's brainstorm through both options, focusing primarily on elements of construction rather than design.

The design spotlight is no longer aimed along the center axis. Now that we've moved beyond the prominent first patch, the laws of fabric grain are irrelevant. Isn't that a hoot! Lopsided is lovely, as long as the fabric is printed with a wiggle to the left *and* an identical wiggle to the right. Go ahead; catch a falling paisley! Hook a spiraling curlicue!

Patch 4 bumps into its mirror image in the adjacent triangle. This position along the seam inherits certain idiosyncrasies. For example, twice as much of the fabric filling the space in a single piece-of-pie will be seen in the finished product. Keep this in mind. Too much of even a good thing can be boring. On the other hand, a single spark sets off a visually exciting chain reaction, encircling the finished block by punctuating each triangular segment identically.

In the following eight examples, Patch 4 advances through a series of progressively more complex adventures in piecework. Please note, the template-making instructions for these samples are written for the left side. Whenever you need to create a pair—the one-way shape and its mirror image—first mark the template on the fabric right side up, then flip the template over and use it wrong side up. Also, from this point on, please assume that every template automatically includes seam allowance.

EXAMPLE A

Complexity, of course, is not always the preferred route. The first sample is gorgeous and created from a single patch. Positioning an intact Template 4 on an intricate, symmetrical fabric generated a slew of possible solutions (35). A template adorned with clues makes replicating sixteen identical patches feasible. Before cutting into the fabric, align this template to neighboring Template (2+3) and trim away extending points.

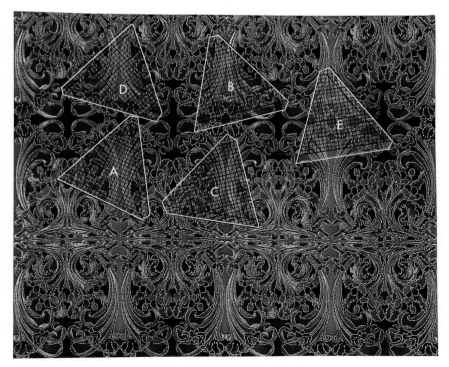

▲ 35   Template 4 positioned on an intricately printed symmetrical design five different ways

By revealing the effect of each option side by side, the five in-progress samples emphasize the visual force of symmetry (36). In each radiating design patterns of inferred lines and visual rhythms begin to emerge. Along the side seams motifs connect to their mirror images and act as if reflected, multiplying into new, never-before-seen patterns. Here's a chance to play the usual guessing game with twice as many clues. Try to predict the effect of these eyecatching elements when their circular journey is finished. Which one is your favorite? Which would you like to revise? How about a twinkle of something unexpected in the corner? How about intercepting the inevitable self-encounter along the seam?

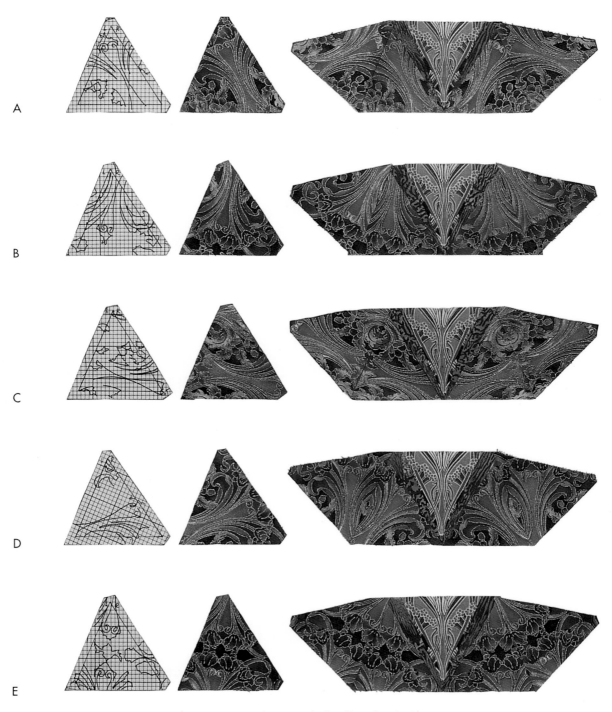

▲ 36 Example A: One prima donna patch; the effect of each alternative placement

EXAMPLE B

A single piece of all-over fabric adds a casual touch to the second example. An unaltered Template 4 can be used to form the necessary patches. Or make Template (2+3+4), as shown in Panel 37, and strip-piece. I like the juxtaposition of elegant, organized Patch 2 surrounded by random doodles scribbled on a murky ground (37).

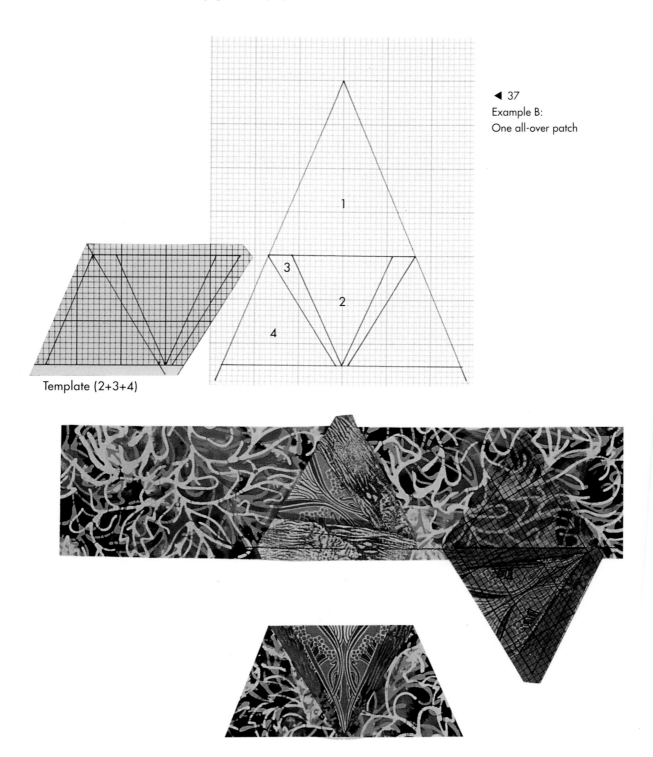

◀ 37
Example B:
One all-over patch

Template (2+3+4)

EXAMPLE C

Paying attention to the prima donnas in your palette is often the best way to start the ball rolling. Once their needs are addressed, they quiet down and do their best to be team players. (Please forgive my tendency to anthropomorphize fabric.) This sample divides Patch 4 in two, combining a prima donna with a deep blue all-over print (38). My idea was to extend the line of Patch 2's purple details into Patch 4. I used see-through Template (2+3) to locate the position of the purple doodads and transfer this point to the diagram. Using a ruler, I drew a line from this point, aiming for the side of the wedge. The only proviso regarding its landing was that I didn't want to drop anchor in the corner.

After I made a template for this shape (Patch 4), I placed it on the prima donna fabric and fiddled until I liked the patch enclosed by the seamlines. Holding the template in place, I traced hints from the fabric onto the template. A second template linking Patch 4 + Patch 5 was crucial for the next step. This template, of course, is our old friend Template 4 marked with a line that divides it in two. I sewed Patch 4 to a long strip of blue fabric and pressed. After aligning Template (4+5) with both the prima donna patch and the sewing line, I marked and cut the desired patches. *Please note*: this time the finished version is shown without seam allowance.

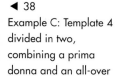

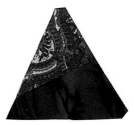

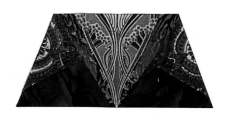

◀ 38
Example C: Template 4 divided in two, combining a prima donna and an all-over

61

EXAMPLE D

I recycled the diagram from Example C to explore an idea coupling two prima donna fabrics (39). Patch 4 stayed the same. I positioned Patch 5 on a fabric printed with gradual shadings from one color to another and used the see-through template to capture a very subtle shift from dark to light (A). My prediction is that this hint of shadow, as innocuous as it seems in a single patch, will intensify into a dramatic ring of translucence when it is multiplied by eight. Because the desired effect required duplicating the identical transition from dark to light, this pseudo-friendly fabric assumed the status of a prima donna and needed a separate template. By coincidence, this patch is cut on grain.

After you make Template 4 and Template 5, complete with seam allowance, remember to match these adjacent templates to each other before translating them into fabric (B). Align the two templates right sides together, sewing line to sewing line, and trim away any plastic peeping out. Again, the finished version is shown without seam allowance (C).

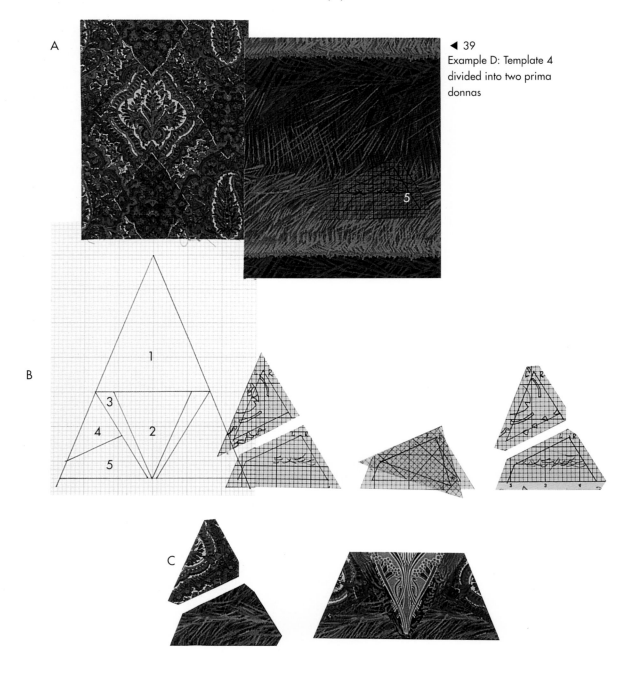

◀ 39
Example D: Template 4
divided into two prima
donnas

EXAMPLE E

It may seem as though the most logical routine is to make all the templates at first. This would allow you to match the edges of neighboring templates to each other before spending time copying them in fabric. Usually all of the patches aren't defined at the beginning of a project. How convenient, this time they are. The diagram for multifaceted Example E is a complete blueprint requiring four templates. Here's a blow-by-blow account of the construction sequence (40).

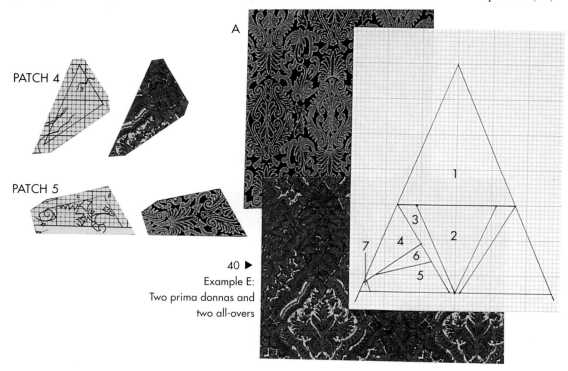

40 ▶
Example E:
Two prima donnas and
two all-overs

STEP 1: Patch 4 and Patch 5 are prima donna fabrics. Each needs its own template. Trace each shape from the diagram onto template plastic, add seam allowance, and cut. Mark T(top), L(left), R(right). Place each template on the appropriate fabric and move it around until it lands on a pleasing motif. Copy hints from the motif onto the template with the permanent marker (A). Mark and cut eight left-sided patches; flip the template and create eight right-sided patches.

STEP 2: Make Template (5+6) by tracing the shape off the graph paper diagram. Immediately add seam allowance. Because Patch 5 is a prima donna fabric, trace hints from Template 5 in the analogous position on Template (5+6) to ensure accurate placement (B).

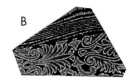

STEP 3: Make Template (5+6+7). Trace a few hints from Patch 5 in the corresponding position on the template (C).

STEP 4: Right sides together, match the sewing line of Template 4 to the sewing line of Template (5+6+7). Trim away extending points. This step ensures templates with evenly matched edges for accurate piecing alignment. Use these revised templates to cut out the fabric (C).

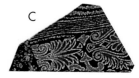

STEP 5: Cut a strip of Fabric 6. Sew the eight left-sided and eight right-sided Patch 5s to this strip (D). Press. Align Template (5+6) to the strip-pieced unit (E). Begin by matching hints on the template with corresponding motifs on Patch 5. Next, adjust the seam connecting Patch 5 and Fabric 6 with the sewing line marked on the template. Mark and cut eight times; flip the template and repeat eight times. Treat this new unit as if it is a single piece of fabric (F).

STEP 6: Cut a strip of Fabric 7. Sew all sixteen Patch (5+6)s to this strip. Press. Align Template (5+6+7) to the strip-pieced units, using fussy Fabric 5 as the "driver," matching seams and sewing line (G). Mark and cut (H).

STEP 7: Sew sixteen Patch 4s to sixteen Patch (5+6+7)s. Press. The resulting shape should be the same as the patch we started with in Example A (I). Sew the eight left-sided units to the left side of Patch (2+3) and the eight right-sided units to Patch (2+3)'s right side (J).

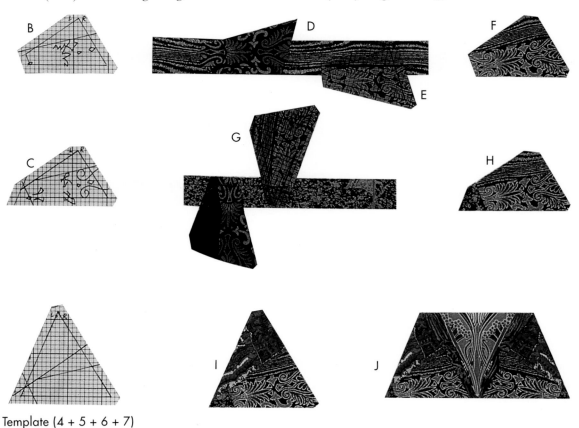

Template (4 + 5 + 6 + 7)

EXAMPLE F

The sixth sample is another version of Example E. Blending a bunch of all-over prints with limited distinction between the fabrics creates a mushy, ambiguous effect. I like it a lot. These subtle but consistent areas of dark and light will combine into flowing, graceful visual rhythms in the completed block (41).

STEP 1: Neither Patch 4 nor Patch 5 needs its own template. Instead, make (A) Template (5+6), (B) Template (5+6+7), and (C) Template (4+5+6+7).

STEP 2: Sew strips of Fabric 5 and Fabric 6 together. Press. Line up Template (5+6) with the seam between the fabrics (D). Mark and cut eight times; reverse the template and repeat eight times. Treat this new unit as if it is a single piece of fabric (E).

STEP 3: Cut a strip of Fabric 7. Piece the eight left-sided and eight right-sided Patch (5+6)s to this strip. Press. Align Template (5+6+7) to the strip-pieced unit, matching seams and sewing lines (F). Mark and cut.

STEP 4: Sew sixteen (eight left and eight right) Patch (5+6+7)s to a strip of Fabric 4. Press. Use Template (4+5+6+7), which is the same shape as the original Patch 4 back in Example A, to mark and cut eight left-sided units and eight right-sided units (G).

STEP 5: Sew these units to Patch (2+3).

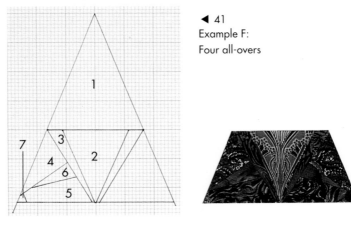

◀ 41
Example F:
Four all-overs

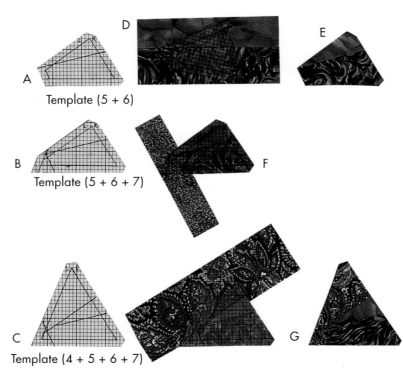

A Template (5 + 6)

B Template (5 + 6 + 7)

C Template (4 + 5 + 6 + 7)

D

E

F

G

65

EXAMPLE G

And now for something completely different. Here's the multiple fractures rendition, for those of us who believe you can never have too many fabrics. Panel 42 illustrates the design sequence on graph paper. Panel 43 explains how to custom make a template for an idiosyncratic fabric.

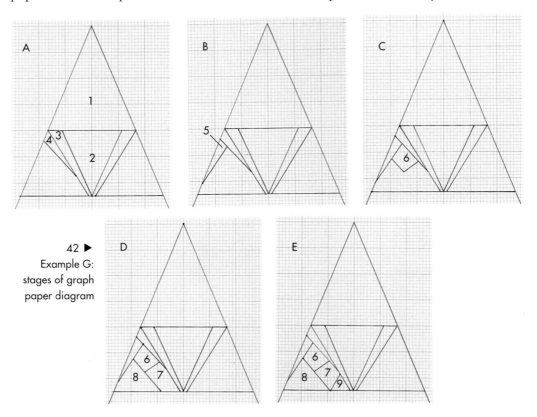

42 ▶
Example G:
stages of graph
paper diagram

I decided to highlight the outline with a thin sliver of new color (Patch 4), predicting that this splinter would multiply into a significant connector (42A). Next, I drafted a shape similar to Patch 4 along the side line, deliberately drawing Patch 5 a bit longer to suggest the irregular unplanned variations that instill a sense of spontaneity (42B). An eye-popping fabric filled with exploding stars seemed perfect for the left-over space. The question was how to fit the fabric into the shape (43A).

By placing a sheet of template material over the diagram (43B) I created a see-through template that represented the final patch (43C). Playing and rearranging the template on the fabric revealed an array of possibilities. I decided to cram a piece of star into the top corner, catching some gold points jutting onto the black background (43D). Tracing the star points onto the template ensured consistency. The criteria for this patch's boundaries were to expose as little of the black background as possible without cutting off the tips of the star. Each of the sixteen patches does not have to duplicate the exact same portion of the star. The irregular, fragmented points of a star suggests constant movement and change.

By counting gridlines on the template, I transferred this patch to the diagram (42C). Wow! This turned out to be a quirky little shape. Before another fabric had a chance to grab my attention, I ensured the final design was composed of straight lines that sewed together. Using a ruler, I extended the left bottom edge of Patch 6 until it hit the wedge's horizontal boundary (42D). Now the shape was divided into three sections, Patches 6, 7, and 8. By using all-over prints around the prima donna star patch the whole shebang can be strip-pieced.

Let's talk colors. At this point in the design, choices aren't arbitrary. They must relate to (not match!) the evolving pattern. Patches 1, 2, 3, and 6 are already established. Look over the diagram and see if it suggests ways to visually connect patches (that aren't necessarily next to each other) via color.

Surrounding the star patch with black-background prints keeps the star popping by camouflaging the seams connecting adjacent patches (44). The positions of Patches 7 and 8 gave me the idea to find two different fabrics with an interesting relationship: dark/light, sharp/fuzzy, positive/negative. I had a yen for erratic black and white polka-dots. I chose small white and gray flecks (Patch 7) merging into puffy white dots (Patch 8). This combination suggested one further addition: little gold blotches on a barely visible black ground (Patch 9), ringing the tip of Patch 2 and complementing the gold contoured star (42E). Imagine the effect as this threesome ebbs and flows around the circle.

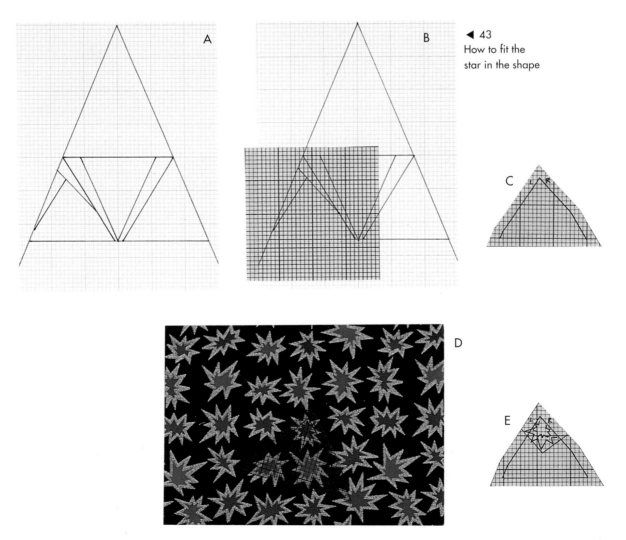

A

B

◀ 43
How to fit the
star in the shape

C

D

E

The column of templates and corresponding patches in Panel 44 explains the sequence of template making. At the bottom of the column is the final pieced version, shown without seam allowance. As is often the case, the design sequence for this example differs from the piecing sequence. Diagram 45A is labeled according to the design sequence. Diagram 45B is marked in the order of the piecing progression.

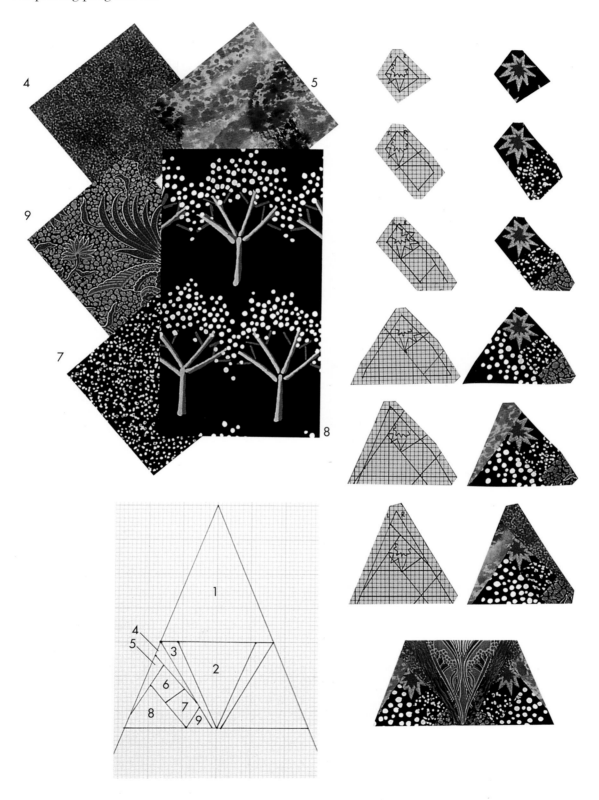

▲ 44   Templates and corresponding patches for Example G

68

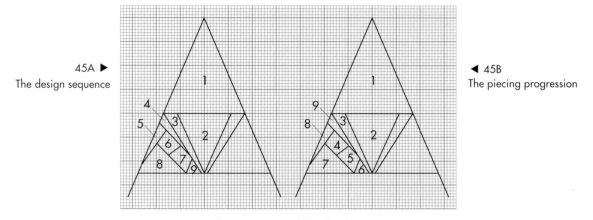

45A ▶
The design sequence

◄ 45B
The piecing progression

In Example G, the design sequence differs from the piecing sequence.

EXAMPLE H

I got carried away with a kiwi (46).

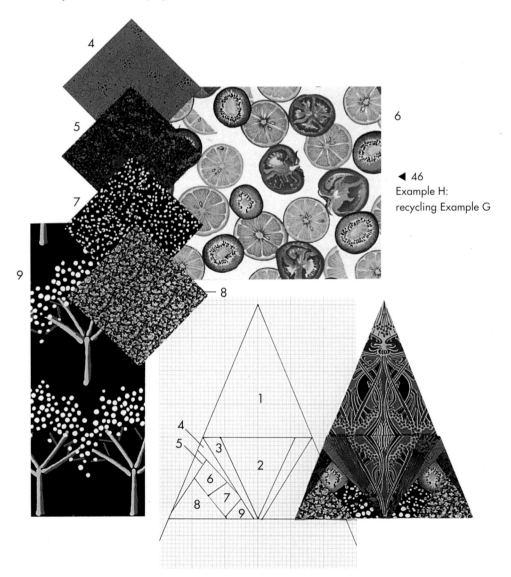

◄ 46
Example H:
recycling Example G

BACK ON GRAIN

In order for the finished kaleidoscope to behave as a block of good breeding should, stability must be provided at the two opposite ends of the piece-of-pie. Fabrics at the apex and the designated bottom edge must follow the grainlines (47A). Otherwise the block might give in to its proclivity to wiggle when you were counting on it being nice and flat.

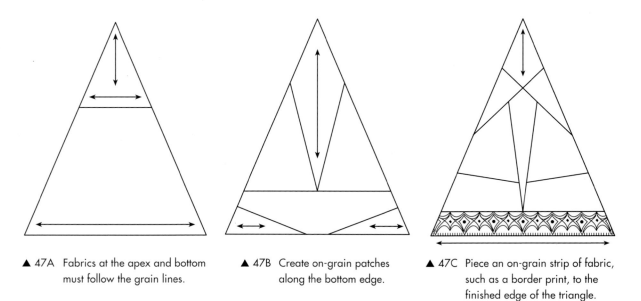

▲ 47A Fabrics at the apex and bottom must follow the grain lines.

▲ 47B Create on-grain patches along the bottom edge.

▲ 47C Piece an on-grain strip of fabric, such as a border print, to the finished edge of the triangle.

The parameters for choosing the first patch which graces the important center is discussed on pages 42 and 110. Remember, to promote stability when a gaggle of wedges meets in the middle, this first shape must be cut on a straight grain of fabric.

The outermost edge of any patch forming the bottom boundary of the triangle should also follow the grainline. Think of the outside border as a girdle, encircling the block, binding it into a shapely silhouette with firm control. Fabrics that surround the block should line up with either the lengthwise or the crosswise grain of the goods.

Keep this in mind when figuring out a piecing strategy for the patches that fall on the block's periphery. Check to see if strip piecing will provide the correct grainline alignment. Often, at this close-to-the-end position in the wedge, a shape needs to be cut directly from its own template to ensure an on-grain patch (47B). Handle it with the care bestowed on a prima donna, even if the fabric is an all-over pattern. If the adjacent fabrics are all-over prints that lend themselves to the strip-piecing method, make the template for this patch first. Then create templates with as many add-ons as needed.

There is another way to ensure that the piece-of-pie ends on-grain. Piece a strip of fabric cut along the grainline to the finished edge of the triangle. Border prints are good candidates for this assignment (47C). Or, for a completely different look, consider using the same fabric that will be used in the corner triangles to square off the design (see "The Sample" on page 128).

TO STRIP OR NOT TO STRIP

Here's the long and short of all the previous stuff, a veritable thimble-full.

A prima donna fabric that demands to be treated "just so" requires its own template—"sharing" is not a word in this textile's vocabulary.

Fabrics falling in the "to-be-strip-pieced" category are all-over prints that can be cut randomly.

Never make a separate template for a patch designated for strip-piecing. The beauty of this technique is that it allows you to add diminutive, uncommonly shaped patches, no matter how small, by strip-piecing.

There is no limit to the number of strips that can be added to a unit.

Match each template to its adjacent templates, as described on pages 54-57, before cutting it into fabric.

When joining two angles that are not the same, remember to align the sewing lines, not the cut edges. Trim away any points that stick out. Or reshape one side into a new angle, and match the partner to the new angle.

If the shape must be cut on-grain in order to provide stability, and strip-piecing will create an off-grain direction, cut the shape from its own individual template.

IS IT A CIRCLE OR ISN'T IT?

One day I was hit on the head by the truth in the following sentence: *a line is a series of points.* After I came to, my perspective was reversed. Instead of connecting points to make a line, I could draw any line and break it up into points. The wizardry in this logic was an eye-opener for an unadventurous seamstress like me. Now I'm a whiz at dissecting a curvaceous contour into a chain of straight lines or smoothing an austere shape into a gently rounded arc.

Usually I begin by drawing the curvy line on the graph-paper diagram with a pencil. Sometimes I draw the curve freehand. Other times I use a compass to draft a true circle. Lots of times I create the effect completely by accident. *KALEIDOSCOPIC VIII: The Sun, the Moon. . .and the Stars* (48), and *KALEIDOSCOPIC XV: Eccentric Circles* (page 29), are extreme cases of illusory curved piecing.

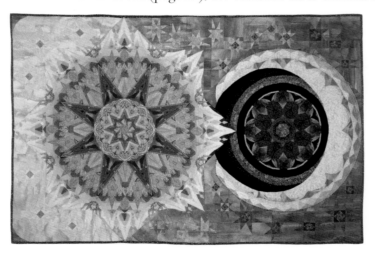

◀ 48
*KALEIDOSCOPIC VIII:
The Sun, The Moon...
and the Stars*

Any curve can be reformed into straight lines. The key is: don't rely on the inaccurate eyeball method to approximate alignment between adjacent patches. Instead, make sure the edges of neighboring templates match each other before copying them in fabric, using the method described on pages 54-57.

With a compass, I drew the circular line defining Patch 2 in Panel 49A. When all eight wedges connect, this line will form a perfect circle. Think of the design possibilities! Imagine Patch 1 erupting out of a dramatic black hole or glowing on a hot yellow sun. Next, I identified the points where this line begins and ends. Remember, it is always easier to distinguish points if the line travels from grid line to grid line rather than between them. Line up a ruler from the starting point to the end of the line. If there isn't much discrepancy between the straight edge of the ruler and the curve, use the ruler to draw a line connecting the dots (49B). Erase the original curvy line.

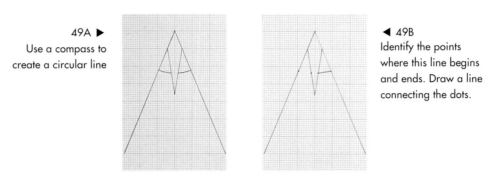

49A ▶
Use a compass to
create a circular line

◀ 49B
Identify the points
where this line begins
and ends. Draw a line
connecting the dots.

A lengthy wide curve probably needs to be separated into more than one straight line. Here are the steps dividing the curve formed by positioning a compass at the X in Panel 50.

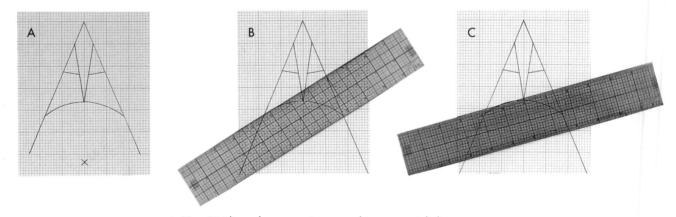

▲ 50   Dividing a long curve into more than one straight line.

STEP 1: Starting at one end, place the straight edge of the ruler along the curve. Note where the straight edge begins to diverge from the curve. Mark this point with a dot (50B).

STEP 2: Reposition the ruler so that it is alongside the dot and once again, try to follow the contour of the curve (50C). If this second maneuver reaches the end of the line, draw a line from the dot to the line's end. Erase the original curve.

STEP 3: If the second dot falls within the curve, repeat Step 2 as many times as necessary. If more than three joints are required, try stretching each link into a slightly longer line in order to need fewer divisions. When they are fused together, the lines will blend into the illusion of a curve, even if it's not a perfect rendition of the original line. Revising the design so it is less complex, but still provides a rounded effect, is a reasonable approach. Translating curves into fabric involves a lot of precise piecing. A long sequence of steps can get tedious.

The construction sequence for this example requires three templates: Template 1, Template (1+2), and Template (3+4) (51A,B). Coincidentally, the cut edge of Template (1+2) already matches the cut edge of Template (3+4).

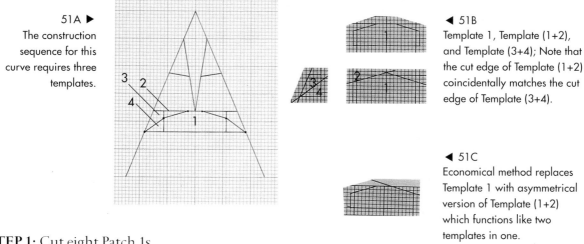

51A ▶
The construction sequence for this curve requires three templates.

◀ 51B
Template 1, Template (1+2), and Template (3+4); Note that the cut edge of Template (1+2) coincidentally matches the cut edge of Template (3+4).

◀ 51C
Economical method replaces Template 1 with asymmetrical version of Template (1+2) which functions like two templates in one.

STEP 1: Cut eight Patch 1s.

STEP 2: Sew a strip of Fabric 2 to the left side of each Patch 1. Press. Use Template (1+2) to cut eight Patch (1+2)s. Repeat on the right side.

STEP 3: Strip-piece Fabric 3 to Fabric 4. Press. Align Template (3+4) to the seam. Mark and cut eight left-sided and eight right-sided patches.

STEP 4: Sew Patch (3+4) to Patch (1+2), eight times on the left and eight times on the right. For accurate alignment, pin at the junction between the seams.

Here's an alternative method that eliminates the need for Template 1. Instead, make Template (1+2) as shown in Panel 51C. This asymmetrical template is ambidextrous! It's two templates in one: the shape of Patch 1 on the left side and the shape of Patch (1+2) on the right side. Use the left side to form one side of Patch 1, then flip the template over and complete the shape. Sew a strip of Fabric 2 to these patches. Use the right side of the template to mark and cut the appropriate number of patches from this strip-pieced unit. Continue from Step 3 (above).

REDEFINING THE POINT SYSTEM

Patchwork etiquette favors distinct, well-matched points. Our quiltmaking legacy is filled with sharply defined triangles. But unconventional shapes are more in line with a kaleidoscope-inspired design, simulating the spontaneity and randomness synonymous with scopes.

It is difficult to match and stitch thin shapes with acute angles accurately. There are two solutions to this predicament. One, reshape severe points into more user-friendly forms. Points don't have to come to points to read as points. The interior of a scope by Charles Karadimos illustrates this well (52).

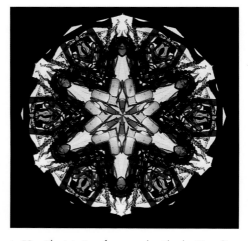

▲ 52   The interior of a scope by Charles Karadimos

73

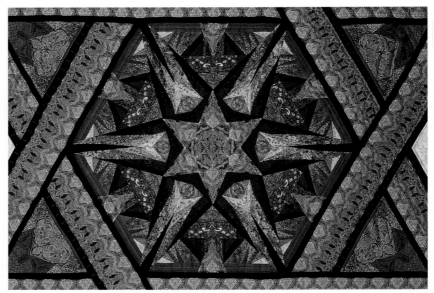

53 ▶
Detail of
KALEIDOSCOPIC IV:
Crystal Canopy

Use the ⅛" graph paper to draft lines that meet one-eighth or one-quarter inch apart instead of assuming that two lines must always meet at the same point.

Two, accept that it is OK for these kinds of points to join together unevenly. Irregular stabs of color might even enhance the design and be perceived as pulsating, momentary vibrations. There is a good example of this effect in *KALEIDOSCOPIC IV: Crystal Canopy*, above. (Imagine my dismay when I stitched the six twenty-inch-long pieces-of-pie together and beheld a pouffy disaster. After drying my tears, I remeasured and found out the 60 degree angle was accurate at the top, but narrowed as it moved through the twenty inches. It was missing one half inch at each bottom corner, which was a lot when multiplied by twelve. I fixed it by adding the long, thin piercing points of dark blue.) Notice how the dark blue fabric outlining the star emerges as a lance-like slice into each of the six corners of the large hexagon? Each of the final tips pierce the quilt's surface at a different place.

Evaluate every fussy point. Does it really have to be a precise barbed tip to enhance the design? Often the answer is yes. But sometimes a fabric's lovely details end up eliminated when an elaborate motif is crammed into a narrow point. Use intricate fabrics to their best advantage by applying the window-like template technique described on page 42. By following the route of the print, you might create a shape that's easier to sew and a design that either reads like a point or is even better (54). Sharp points destined to rendezvous along the side seams are rendered best in simple all-over prints. Then the assembly process does not demand matching both an intricate pattern and seam joints.

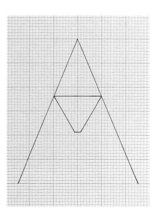

◀ 54
Following the route of the fabric creates a shape that is easy to sew and reads like a point.

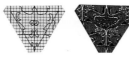

THE FINAL SCRUTINY

This discussion focuses on the need to look over the blueprint critically to see if it is piece-able. Don't wait until the last minute to examine the graph paper diagram for piecing blunders. Probe it as it evolves with an analytic, construction worker point of view. Demand cooperation from both sides of your brain: be a creator and a problem-solver. Before you make templates, do a dry run. Go through the blueprint step by step to check for bloopers that will interrupt the piecing sequence.

Be prudent. Redraft sewing lines to disperse a potential crowd of seams, making the union between them—and adjacent patches—easier (55). Avoid creating excessive bulk at the long seams of a piece-of-pie. You need complex math skills, or basic common sense, to predict the quantity of cloth involved when a party of points rendezvous with their mirror-imaged counterparts escorted by a complete entourage of seam allowances.

Remember, you're the boss. You are never limited to a specific solution. Strike a balance between the textiles' suggestions and the network of pencil lines. If the final version doesn't fit together, or if it is just plain sloppy, it won't matter how drop-dead gorgeous the original vision was.

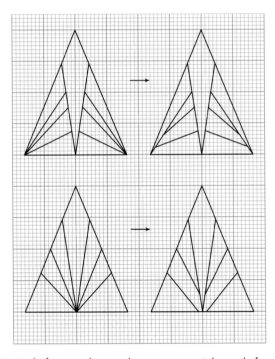

▲ 55   Redraft sewing lines to disperse a potential crowd of seams.

THE FINAL PIECING SEQUENCE

When I decide the number of "pieces of pie," I consider two factors. The more triangles there are, the greater the chance for a bumpy and bulky concussion at the important center. The second factor involves my personal sewing prerogative: I only sew straight seams.

A design divided into an even number of divisions can be constructed much more easily than one with an odd number. In an evenly numbered design, half of the triangles pieced together will form a straight edge.

Here is the piecing sequence for an eight-sided design (56A):

STEP 1: Sew each triangle to another, creating four pairs.

STEP 2: Piece one pair of triangles to another duo. Repeat, creating two sets of four.

STEP 3: Sew the two halves together.

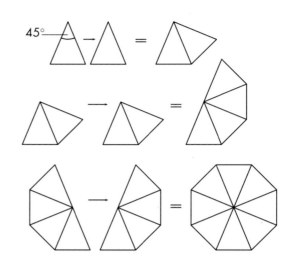

▲ 56A   Piecing sequence for an eight-sided design

The piecing sequence for a six-sided design follows (56B):

STEP 1: Sew one triangle to another. Repeat, creating two pairs.

STEP 2: Stitch one triangle to each of the pairs, creating two units comprised of three triangles.

STEP 3: Sew the two halves together.

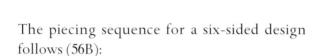

▲ 56B   Piecing sequence for a six-sided design

A ten-sided design is quirky. Three hundred and sixty degrees divided into ten pieces-of-the-pie is a slim thirty-six degrees. When all ten converge at a single point, expect a densely packed crowd. The piecing sequence for a ten-sided design is (56C):

STEP 1: Sew four triangles to four other triangles, creating four pairs.

STEP 2: Piece one pair of triangles to another duo. Repeat, creating two units of four triangles.

STEP 3: Add one triangle to each of the units, creating two units of five triangles.

STEP 4: Sew the two halves together.

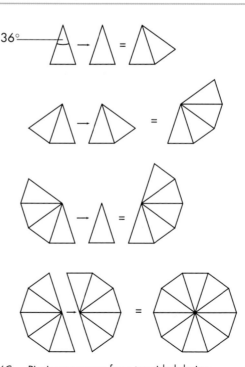

▲ 56C   Piecing sequence for a ten-sided design

JOINING TOGETHER

This next-to-last construction step will benefit from a moment of philosophical reflection. Stop and consider the kaleidoscopic nature of the whole shebang. Repetition from one piece-of-pie to another and another and so on creates visual pathways that camouflage seams. The whole becomes greater than the sum of its parts. My point? A couple of mismatched joints are not going to be noticed in an image filled to the brim with complexity.

In other words, season the usual rules of piecing with a generous dose of common sense. Yes, coherence between triangular segments is fundamental. But this quality is already guaranteed by the symmetry built into a design that unites identical sections radiating from a central point. Success does not mean that every one of the many joints along the sixteen borders of eight segments will make a perfect match. Many will, some won't. Even in a real kaleidoscope, every multifaceted image isn't reflected flawlessly. It depends on the optical quality of the mirrors, the critical angle of the mirror set-up, and the seams where the mirrors connect. Just like its quilted counterpart, the objective is to eliminate as many distractions as possible.

The goal is to prevent joints along the seamline from acting like visual barricades. Deal with the prima donna fabrics first. If these fabrics become victims of piecing interruptus, they will spitefully sabotage the visual flow, shattering the illusion of seamless continuity from one segment to another.

Right sides together, match and pin through corresponding joints. Use thin, sharp-pointed silk pins. I rarely baste; it doesn't seem to make the alignment more accurate, especially when big bulky seams bounce the presser foot off its intended path.

Follow the aforementioned policy: spoil the prima donnas and fudge with the all-overs. Begin by matching Patch 1 at the top to its twin. Next, align the prima donna fabrics. Then ease in the more forgiving all-overs. It is to our advantage that patches along the diagonal edge of the piece-of-pie are often cut on the bias. Here's where we benefit from its natural "give." Be gentle, but forceful; make it give you neatly joined seams.

Sew *slowly*. Begin from the skinny tops of Patch 1 and aim toward the raw edges at the bottoms of the pieces-of-pie. Backstitch at the end. If the presser foot bumps off the ¼" seam, stop. Rip. Remove any leftover threads. Realign. Re-stitch, overlapping a few of the leftover previous stitches with new ones.

Sometimes one or two of the finished pieces-of-pie are definitely crooked. In this case I make a master template of the entire triangle, lining up a sheet of plastic to the graph paper diagram, matching the bold center axis of the diagram to a prominent inch line of template plastic. Copy a few of the longest sewing lines, tracing enough of the original to provide enough cues for aligning the template to the fabric triangle. To conserve template material, make a template of only the left half of the triangle and flip it over to investigate the right side (57). For really *big* triangles, tape pieces of template material together. Although long rolls of ¼" template material are available, I find it difficult to store the lengthy size neatly.

Line up the master template with two key components on the patchwork triangle, the all-important on-grain first patch and the center axis. Don't expect every clue to match a sewing line. I use the master plan to provide a sense of how "off" the pieced triangle is: where the temperamental areas are, where the seam allowance is too narrow, when the sensible plan of action is to stop, rip, and repair. Sometimes identifying one unruly seam is enough to adjust the design.

There is an art to compensating. A triangle that ends up too big can't be automatically "fixed" by chopping off the excess along the two side seams—unless the guilty party is a compliant all-over print whose only crime is being bigger than a ¼ inch. I admit that sometimes I give in to the temptation to prune all-overs on the triangle's edge if this step makes the shape fit the master template. But I never trim those spiteful prima donnas without weighing the consequences. The long vertical side seams are where the actual attention-grabbing matching takes place. If motifs inside the body of the triangle are askew, it won't matter—they will still read as identical when the viewer's eye moves around the scope from wedge to wedge.

Another remedy for healing a warped wedge is to mark the actual sewing line on the long side seams. Otherwise, there is an underlying assumption the edge of the triangle is accurate and can be relied on to align adjacent triangles. Make a full-size template *without* the seam allowance (58). Line it up on the wrong side of the wedge, first to the top patch, then to the center axis. Holding the template carefully in place, trace around the edge of the plastic with a well-sharpened regular or chalk pencil, or trace lightly with the fine-pointed permanent marker. Make a line that is visible, but doesn't go through to the front of the fabric.

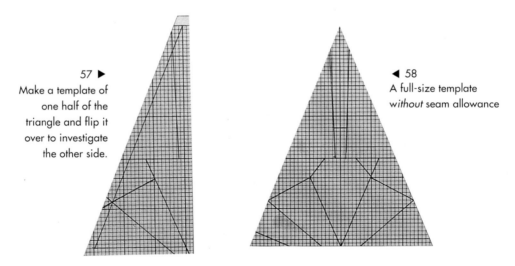

57 ▶
Make a template of
one half of the
triangle and flip it
over to investigate
the other side.

◀ 58
A full-size template
without seam allowance

Now, when the two triangles are aligned right sides together, pin through points where the marked sewing lines coincide at a seam joint. This may create a seam allowance that is not a full ¼-inch seam allowance. If it is very narrow, use a small stitch length and reinforce the seam a few times.

Use the same criteria described above to align, pin, and stitch the two halves together. To ensure a finished product that lies flat, make sure the long edge of each half is straight. If it isn't, the error is probably due to an inaccurate seam between two pieces-of-the-pie. Use the full size template to determine which triangle is the culprit. Then muttering under your breath, *I think I can, I think I can...*, start at one end and sew together toward the other.

SQUARING OFF THE CORNERS

The theory is simple: add a right triangle to the piece-of-pie in each of the four corners to make a square. The problem is calculating the dimensions of the triangle needed to square off the design.

At first, figuring out the measurements of this shape by drawing it full size on graph paper seems the logical route. This allows you to draft a template right from the diagram, remembering to add seam allowances on all sides. Obviously, it is easier to do this when the size of the finished block is more modest than humongous.

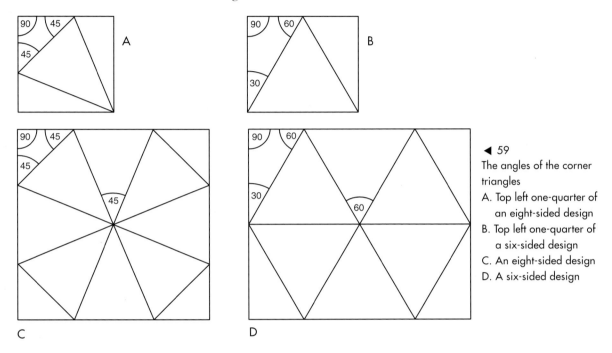

◀ 59
The angles of the corner triangles
A. Top left one-quarter of an eight-sided design
B. Top left one-quarter of a six-sided design
C. An eight-sided design
D. A six-sided design

The geometric explanation of what is going on is based on the following blast from your high school past: the angles of a triangle added together equal 180° (59). An eight-sided design squares off with a 90°-45°-45° triangle (A). The corner of a six-sided pattern requires a 90°-60°-30° triangle (B). If you are handy with a protractor, you can draft the appropriate triangle to the bottom boundary of a piece-of-the-pie by plotting the correct angles (60). Make sure there is enough room on the graph paper to accommodate this shape. If there isn't, tape another piece of graph paper to the original, matching bold inch lines.

60 ▶
Adding a right triangle to the piece-of-pie

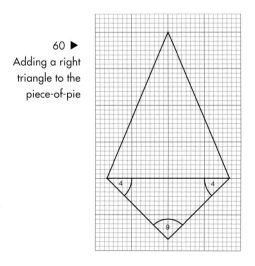

61 ▶

Drafting a corner triangle using a protractor
A. Count off 45°.
B. Draw a line connecting the corner and this point.
C. The two lines intersect along the center axis and
   create a 90° angle.
D. Erase pencil lines that extend past the intersection.

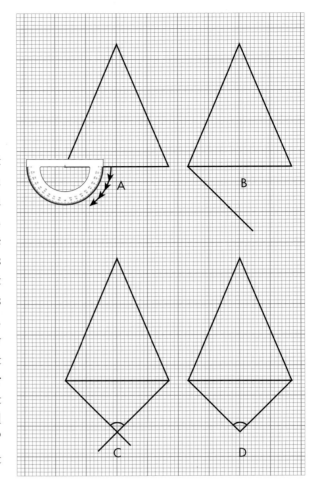

Let's work with the octagon design first. Start by positioning the protractor on the graph paper diagram. Align its center reference mark to the left bottom corner of the piece-of-pie. Make sure the 0s (zeros) on each side of the protractor line up accurately on the pie's bottom horizontal gridline (61A). Beginning at the right zero, measure 45°, counting left towards the 90° mark at the center of the semi-circle (61A). Mark this point. Remove the protractor and draw a line from the left corner through this point (61B). Move the protractor to the right corner and repeat in reverse. Draw a line from the right corner to the second point. The two lines will intersect along the center axis and create a 90° angle (61C). Erase pencil lines that extend past the intersection (61D).

The Omnigrid® 98L-Right Triangle turns out to be a friendly instrument. This product creates right-angle triangles up to 12 inches. Although it wasn't designed for this specific task, I find it adapts with a couple of limitations. The good news is, its markings along the center facilitate accurate alignment with the center axis of the graph paper diagram. The inevitable bad news is that alignment along a horizontal grid line relies on the technically imprecise eyeball method. The Omnigrid triangle is marked with yellow quarter-inch lines and black half-inch lines. Regrettably, the shape we want to create doesn't fall neatly on the lines of the graph grid. Also, the size of the Omnigrid restricts its use to a piece-of-pie under eleven inches. And, obviously, it only works with an eight-sided design.

Once you understand and accept these conditions, it is a functional method. Here's how to use this tool to draft the correct size triangle on graph paper. We're going to add a right angle triangle to the bottom of the finished piece-of-pie, so make sure you have enough room for this appendage. During the following steps, ignore the pre-calculated seam allowance line on the Omnigrid ruler. Pretend it isn't there at all.

Place the Omnigrid triangle so the arrows labeled GRAIN are aligned with the horizontal lines of the graph paper. Orient the long side of the acrylic triangle by lining it up to the very last line of the piece-of-pie. Slowly slide the Omnigrid triangle toward the top of the pie-shaped graph paper wedge. Stop when the edges of the acrylic triangle touch the corners of the piece-of-pie exactly. This is the size and shape of the required corner patch. Holding the acrylic triangle securely in place, use its straight edges to trace this shape on the graph paper. Draft a template, adding seam allowance to every side of the template (62).

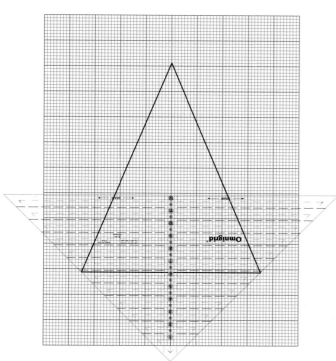

One of the gifts of quiltmaking is the camaraderie of smart, kind folk willing to share their knowledge. Margit Echols, a Manhattan quilter whose exquisite quilts are based on a love and understanding of geometry, suggests the following procedure. You need a compass, a ruler, and the size of the finished piece-of-pie. Double that number. Draft a square on graph paper that size and mark its center. For example, if the pie-shaped wedge measures 6⅜", make a square 12¾" (63). If the dimensions are large, try drafting the square "to scale" instead of full size.

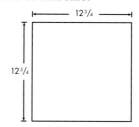

▲ 62   Using the Omnigrid® 98L-Right Triangle to create the corner triangle for an eight-sided kaleidoscope

▲ 63   Draft a square on graph paper twice the size of the finished piece-of-pie.

Place the pointy tip of the compass on a corner. Keeping it in place, open the compass just enough to let the pencil point touch the center of the square (65A). This distance is the keystone, so maintain this length securely. With the pointy tip still on the corner, swing the compass to the left and right. Mark where it intersects the sides of the square (65B). Repeat this maneuver in each of the three remaining corners, creating eight marks in all. Use a ruler to draw a line connecting the two marks on either side of each corner (65C). The result is four faithfully-sized right triangles. Use one to create a template. This protractor-free technique is limited only by the size of your compass. Check out art supply stores for large ones. Omnigrid's Ruler and Compass (1C & C) make circles up to twelve inches.

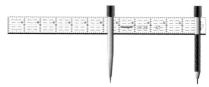

▼ 65   Drafting corner triangles using a compass

▲ Omnigrid's Ruler and Compass (1C & C) makes circles up to twelve inches. When the lead point gets dull, use an emery board or sandpaper pad to sharpen it.

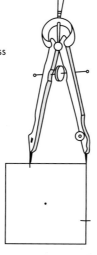

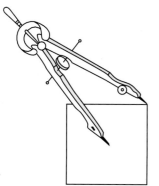

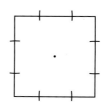

A. Place the pointy tip on a corner and the pencil point on the center.

B. Swing the compass left and right and mark where it intersects the sides.

C. Use a ruler to connect the marks on either side of a corner.

Regarding a hexagon block, it is easier to draft the required 30°-60°-90° corner triangle to one side of the piece-of-pie, instead of adding it to the bottom (66). This scheme aligns the drafting lines with the graph paper grid. In this example I drafted the triangle onto the left side of the triangular wedge. Start at the tip-top of the piece-of-pie. Use the grid lines of the graph paper to extend a line left from this point. This line creates a 60° angle (66A). Move to the bottom left corner of the piece-of-pie. Extend a line up toward the first line. The corner rarely falls on a grid line exactly, so expect to make your own ruled line. The angle created should measure 30°. Because you followed the straight lines of the graph's grid, the intersection is automatically a 90° angle (66B). Use the protractor to check the accuracy of all three angles. It is important to realize that a hexagonal design requires two left sided corner triangles and two right-sided triangles. Use the template twice in one direction, then flip it over and repeat two times.

Extend a line from the
apex.

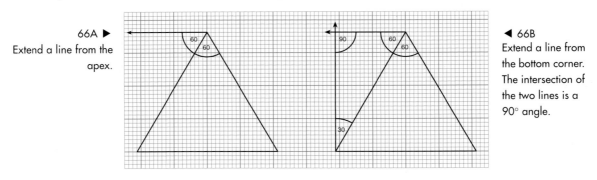

◀ 66B
Extend a line from
the bottom corner.
The intersection of
the two lines is a
90° angle.

Adding a corner triangle to a six-sided design

In *KALEIDOSCOPIC IX: Public Radio Daze* (page 30), I fumbled my way through the geometry of a ten-sided design. The geometric construction of this 36° triangle (360 divided by ten sides) created an unwelcome enigma at the corners of the quilts. I was flabbergasted to find something other than the single, well-behaved, right-angled triangle I had come to rely on (67). After I calmed down, I realized that figuring out the angles and shapes required dredging up geometry stuff from some previous life. I remembered that (1) the angles that form a straight line equal 180° and (2) the angles of a triangle added together equal 180°. I drafted a full-size, forty-inch kaleidoscope, and used these two axioms and a protractor to check the accuracy of the drafting lines.

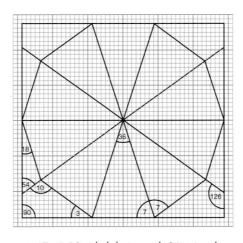

▲ 67   A 10-sided design with 36° triangles

THE QUILT SANDWICH

The Batting

The choice is simple. A patchwork textured with a multitude of seams needs exceedingly thin loft that needles easily (like butter!). It is hard to get tiny even-tempered stitches on a quilt fraught with seams. I hesitate to name a brand. The batting manufacturers are in touch with quiltmakers' needs and expand the market with a steady stream of innovations and improvements.

The Backing

My regard for the quilt backing has evolved from an attitude shaped more by frugality than design, to its current status as an integral part of the design package. This is where I indulge my romantic notion that good things come in beautifully wrapped packages.

Picking the backing fabric deserves more than an afterthought. It is not just another step toward finishing the quilt. The backing collaborates with the quilt top in a relationship that affects the visual impact. It has to seem as though some connection beyond mere chance has brought them together. Compatibility isn't achieved by settling for something bland. I want a fling with a fabulous fabric that commands a presence in its own right. After all, the backing's personality sets the stage for the grand unveiling.

I always choose a print fabric rather than a solid, preferably a striking all-over nondirectional printed with a generous dose of terrific color that looks great from close up and far away. Is that so much to ask? My stitches are better off camouflaged than displayed for the world to see. The mommy in me usually adds her two cents and cautions that maybe it won't show as much dirt.

The choice of a cotton fabric for the quilt backing is comforting. I am experienced enough to know that I don't have to go looking for trouble. My quilts are a field of seams. I fight off the seduction of tightly woven fabrics dyed with rich, vibrant colors. They sabotage my quilting stitch by acting like barricades against the needle.

QUILTING

I quilt by hand with a hoop in my lap, marking the quilt pattern as I go. Chalk lines show up better than penciled ones on a surface crowded with multicolored pieces. When possible, I use masking tape to mark straight lines. I devised a quilting pattern for *KALEIDOSCOPIC XIV: Myst* (page 28) that accommodated straight lines of tape (68). Subjecting the background silk to any other kind of mark seemed risky for the silk and frustrating for me.

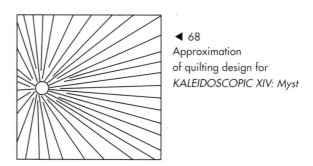

◄ 68
Approximation
of quilting design for
KALEIDOSCOPIC XIV: Myst

Since I don't want my stitches to show, a thread color that blends with both the feel of the quilt top and the backing fabric is my preference. I like the soothing rhythm of hand quilting. I don't know how to machine quilt, but I admire the skill of those who do it well.

The new-fangled batts have pretty much freed us from choosing quilting patterns for their anchoring potential. This leaves rapport between the pieced top and the quilting design as the guiding criterion. Like every other aspect of solving design problems, there is never a single right answer.

I quilted my first kaleidoscopic images by following their interwoven patterns with simple outlines to emphasize the circular flow. A quilted, textured background surrounded the kaleidoscopes. My current approach is to devise an underlying design that unites the whole quilt, preferably a grid with irregular spacing and built-in flexibility. An accommodating pattern that allows the quilting line to adapt to the erratic needs of an uneven surface is ideal. I want to avoid being bogged down in areas dense with seams. A truly enjoyable quilting event lets me zoom across the tightly packed seams in a kaleidoscope's interior, and mosey along at a leisurely pace in the just-as-important ground.

For example, in *KALEIDOSCOPIC XIII: Random Acts of Color* (page 27), nine loopy lines of quilting stitches snake across the width of the quilt from selvage to selvage. They leap across the seams as quickly as possible, and meander in the open spaces of background leaving tangles of curls. The stitches carrying the viewer's eye along their textured, indented paths convey a casual rhythm (69). In *KALEIDOSCOPIC XII: Up Close and Far Away* (page 26), a spider web pattern starts at the top of the quilt, not in the quilt's center. The columns of the web narrow as the rows progress down the length of the quilt (70).

69 ▶
Approximation of
quilting design for
*KALEIDOSCOPIC XIII:
Random Acts of Color*

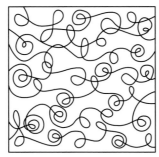

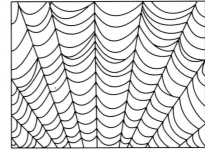

◀ 70
Approximation of
quilting design for
*KALEIDOSCOPIC XII:
Up Close and Far
Away*

The textured repetition of concentric circles sets up a vibrating rhythm and echoes the theme of *KALEIDOSCOPIC XV: Eccentric Circles* (page 29). Note that the circular quilting pattern does not radiate from the center of a kaleidoscope. Instead, the compass was aligned with the midpoint of the larger circle that encompassed the crescent shape. Lucky me! When I showed this quilt-in-progress at a Manhattan Quilters Guild meeting, Teresa Barkley, a consummate quiltmaker, offered the following excellent method for marking and quilting circles accurately. Teresa gave me permission to share her idea in this book.

Mark the concentric circles on a piece of muslin or stiff woven interfacing. Teresa, a patternmaker in the garment district, used a stiff woven interfacing, and recommends the following steps. Cut away the excess material around the outside circle so that the muslin pattern is a circular shape. Position the muslin pattern in the appropriate place on the quilt by aligning the corresponding midpoints. Pin or baste the pattern in place.

The key here is that you are going to quilt from the outside-in, instead of the usual center-out. Stitch along the edge of the outermost circle. When you finish quilting the circle, cut the muslin away up to the line of the next inner circle. Continue this scheme of quilting progressively smaller circles until completed (71).

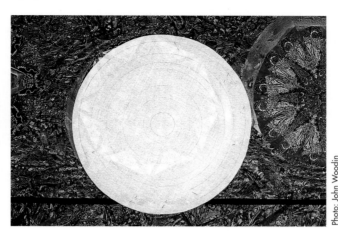

71 ▶
Marking concentric circles for quilting
KALEIDOSCOPIC XV: Eccentric Circles

Photo: John Woodin

Instead of a whole-quilt design scheme, *KALEIDOSCOPIC VIII: The Sun, the Moon. . .and the Stars* (pages 20-21) is quilted in components. Radiating lines beam out from the center of the sun. Tightly packed circles create a crater-like texture on the moon. Spiraling lines entice the eye to cross the darkening sky.

SIGNS AND LABELS

By its very nature, a quilt tells a story about the person who made it. An anonymous quilt is missing a vital piece of the plot. I am sad I didn't know enough to label quilts that were given away years ago. A signature can make such a difference.

Embroidered on the front of my quilts, in the lower right hand corner, is an unobtrusive copyright sign followed by my initials and the year the quilt was finished. A muslin label sewn on the back reports the title of the quilt, the size and date, my name, address, and phone number. Recently, a quilt traveling home from a large national quilt show escaped from its cylindrical packing tube. An attentive delivery service representative was able to call me using the information on the label.

The antidote for my initial bout of autograph deficiency seems to be excess. A third identifying device on each major quilt is an embellished Ultrasuede facsimile of my dominant left hand appliquéd to the quilt back. This unique trademark coordinates with the essence of the quilt. After I draw my name, the year, and a design on the back of the Ultrasuede, I cut it out with a very fine scissors. This gets appliquéd to a fabric chosen because its multicolored print pops out of the cut-out design. Details of beads and glittery threads tie the image together. A second printed fabric mediates a pleasing relationship between the hand and the quilt backing (72, 73, 74).

■ TECHNIQUE TIP   I count Ultrasuede among my blessings. It is my kind of fabric: the edges don't ravel, it is easy to pierce with a sharp needle, and it comes in more flavors than gourmet ice creams. The bad news is, it is very expensive.

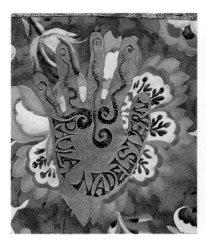 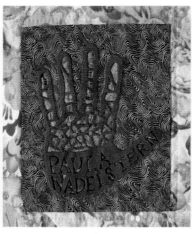 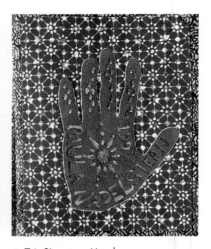

▲ 72 Signature Hand:
KALEIDOSCOPIC XV:
Eccentric Circles

▲ 73 Signature Hand:
KALEIDOSCOPIC XII:
Up Close and Far Away

Photo: Mellisa Karlin Mahoney;
courtesy of *Quilter's Newsletter Magazine*

▲ 74 Signature Hand:
KALEIDOSCOPIC XI: Snowfall

NAME THAT QUILT

As a beginning quiltmaker I thought that titling a quilt was pretentious. My first time out I took a deep breath, picked something colorless and literal, and looked around self-consciously to see if anyone noticed.

Now I like titles. They round off the work and contribute to closure. Choosing a satisfying name is like solving the final piece of a puzzle. You know you've made a perfect match when a title trips off your tongue effortlessly.

Some think a title's function is to set the stage. Others want it to be evocative. And, of course, there are those who believe a title inhibits the viewer's involvement and personal interpretation. In other words, the work should stand on its own. Whether or not you name your quilt, and what kind of title you give it, may be a function of how you perceive quilts: as art, folk art, or craft. Or perhaps you simply need a name to put on the entry form for a quilt show.

A title is helpful in identifying a piece and keeping it in the viewer's mind. A mundane title may not be very interesting, but it is easier than trying to remember something called Landscape No. 17. Some titles are literally what they are, like *KALEIDOSCOPIC VIII: The Sun, the Moon. . .and the Stars.* Others act like shorthand, shifting the perception of the design, adding another dimension, truly enhancing the quilt. When an image is enigmatic, a title offers access to it.

PHOTOGRAPHY

Try to keep a photographic record of the finished product. Any time I've ignored this important stage, I've regretted it.

KALEIDOSCOPE

DESIGN SENSIBILITY

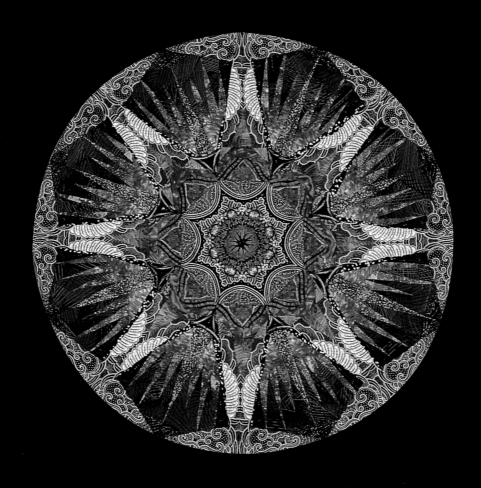

DESIGN SENSIBILITY

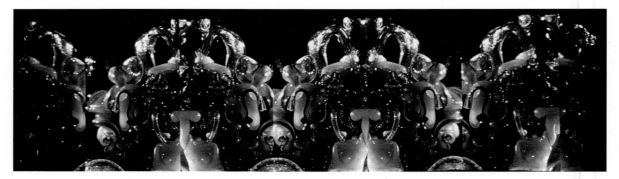

Kaleidoscope—the very word promises surprise and magic, change and chance. Exploding with visual excitement, a kaleidoscopic design organizes an abundance of light and color, form and motion into a complex and coherent image, capturing a moment of infinity.

I can give a few design guidelines here, a little color theory there. But it is the unique qualities synonymous with the kaleidoscope personality that catapults this kind of design way beyond the ordinary. During the design stage I rely heavily on the innate order that arranges the parts into a complete and artistic unit. This confidence, based on over one hundred pieced kaleidoscopes, allows me to be both the one who makes the magic and the one who is surprised. For me, the thrill of creating is in the process.

ELEMENTS OF A KALEIDOSCOPIC DESIGN

Symmetry

Trust in symmetry. Use its force. The symmetrical repetition of a design radiating in multiple repeating segments creates a visual pattern of inferred lines. The patches along the side seams of the pie-slice sector connect to their mirror images and act as if reflected, multiplying into new, unique pathways.

Human beings are symmetrical creatures. Midline orientation is innate. Consequently, symmetry is comforting to us. There are two lessons to gain from this notion. First, too much of a good thing can be bland and boring. This condition is easily remedied in a symmetrical configuration. A pinch of something unexpected, i.e., color, shape, texture, becomes a pulsating punctuation point due to its identical placement from wedge to wedge, reinforcing the visual rhythm.

The second notion is akin to the first. A motif that seems awkward and unrelated in a single wedge will be well accepted in the finished product when it's peppered identically throughout the design.

Intricate Detail

The word "kaleidoscope" conjures up images brimming with elaborate details and interlaced patterns. In an actual kaleidoscope, the complexity of the pattern is determined by the angle of the mirrors. The resulting image doesn't seem cluttered or ambiguous because of the underlying organization and symmetry.

One way to achieve an effect of complex detail and dramatic impact is to use textiles printed with elaborate patterns. A second effective technique is to facet one shape into an unexpected network of pieced-together patches.

Luminosity

Kaleidoscopes rely on the reflection of light rays from the mirrors. When you look into one end, your eye intercepts light that entered the opposite end and is then reflected one or more times from the mirrors. Choosing fabrics that evoke a sense of shading and transparency creates the translucent nature of a scope's interior on a quilt's flat surface.

A Fleeting Instance of Infinity

It is the nature of a kaleidoscope to generate an inexhaustible supply of endlessly changing, mandala-like images. There is no beginning or end. Each inevitable metamorphosis results in a marked or complete change of character. This provides the viewer a rare opportunity to witness the visual expression of infinite images extending beyond measure.

I try to create a visual sense of the spontaneity and transience reminiscent of the chance interlinkings and seemingly endless possibilities synonymous with kaleidoscopes. An unconventional combination of fabrics simulates its random nature.

Becoming a kaleidoscope aficionado has made me more adaptable and creative both artistically and intellectually. The notion that there is no absolute, correct, best selection is very liberating. After all, a breathtaking collision of color in a scope will maneuver into something different, something slightly new, during even the instant it takes me to hand it to you.

The Whole Is Greater than the Sum of Its Parts

It is the nature of a kaleidoscope to reflect and refract the loose bits and pieces in the end case into a symphony of shape and color. The viewer is compelled to synthesize its components into a visual whole rather than analyze the elements separately.

Because of the techniques used to piece a fabric kaleidoscope, it is not hyperbole to suggest the whole is greater than the sum of its parts. There is an air of abracadabra as the very last seam is stitched because what you see in one single triangle is not what you get in the multiplied sum. Often effects more wonderful than I had imagined occur and I am hypnotized by the result.

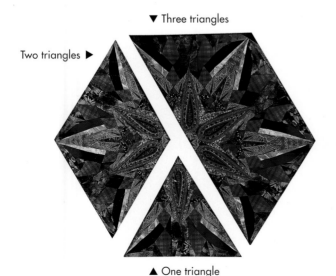

◀ Two triangles ▶

▼ Three triangles

▲ One triangle

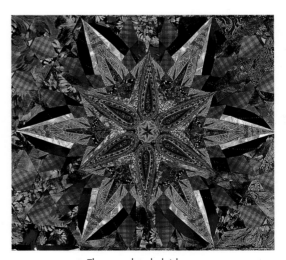

▲ The complete kaleidoscope

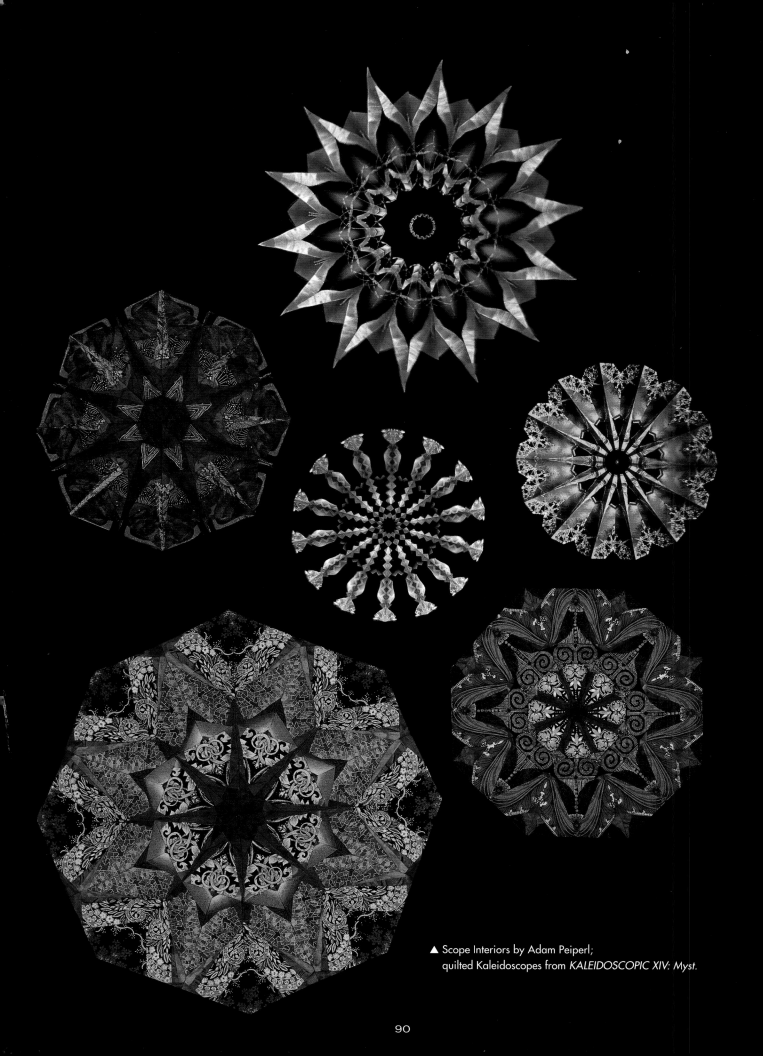

▲ Scope Interiors by Adam Peiperl;
quilted Kaleidoscopes from *KALEIDOSCOPIC XIV: Myst.*

90

ELEMENTS OF ANY GOOD DESIGN

Many of the fundamental principles of design are inseparable characteristics of the kaleidoscope form. Understanding these properties provides us with a common language. We can use the terms to articulate what we think will happen, and to critique the final result. A welcome consequence of acquiring this theoretical knowledge is that mentally trying out principles of design turns out to be a credible method for unblocking creative blocks.

While reviewing the following list, keep in mind the unique qualities of the kaleidoscope. Above all, it is a dynamic entity. The most effective kaleidoscopic designs create the illusion of motion, a suggestion that the image is fleeting and bound to change in another second. Learn to manipulate the following physical properties in order to inject a feeling of motion into an otherwise static image.

Unity

A good design implies visual unity. Visual unity is achieved when the whole pattern is noticed before its parts. The good news is that the viewer instantly searches for a coherent unity because chaos isn't really all that appealing. A pieced kaleidoscope is a complicated structure unified by its repetitive patterns. Its formal organization, characterized by rigid repetition, arranges for each element of the design to be duplicated identically, thereby establishing a relationship between the parts.

However, it is possible to create a pattern so overly unified that the result offers visual boredom rather than satisfaction. My advice, in this case, is to go back and add more. . .fabric, color, a dash of something unexpected. In an effective kaleidoscopic design the ordered quality of unity balances the lively quality of variety.

I rely heavily on the unifying element of repetition. In my first kaleidoscopic experiments, variety in color and fabric is present but in a more subtle way. This is apparent in *KALEIDOSCOPIC III: Stained Glass Anthology* (page 13). Familiarity with my subject has granted me the confidence to stretch this artistic principle wide open. My color and fabric choices are now bolder and more haphazard. But clearly I wouldn't be comfortable taking risks now if I hadn't first experimented with the basics back then.

Focal Point

A radial design directs the viewer's attention into the important center, the primary focal point. The eye travels around the design, making connections between recurrent motifs and searching for secondary focal points and accents. Eventually the central element draws your attention back to the primary focal point.

There can be more than one focal point. In general, a focal point or visual emphasis results where there is contrast between one element and another. Keep this in mind when choosing components such as color, fabric, or shape for the pie-slice sector. When the design is veering too close to the edge of boredom, stimulate some visual diversity by injecting a deliberate accent. Although the viewer has the impression that she doesn't know where to look, it is not actually true; her eye will take her where it wants to go.

In fact, a definite focal point is not required to create a successful design. In *KALEIDOSCOPIC XII: Up Close and Far Away* (page 26), the idea of a focal point is ignored. The large, all-over cotton print used as the background fabric creates an effect which is both interesting and ambiguous. There is a feeling of depth and light, but no one area stands out.

Balance

Balance is innate. In fact, the task of the developing infant in the first eighteen months of life is to integrate normal equilibrium reactions, which provide a stable base of support for more complex activity. Consequently, lack of balance disturbs us. In assessing artistic balance, the viewer unconsciously presumes a center vertical axis and expects to see equal distribution of visual weight on either side—which is precisely the modus operandi of a kaleidoscopic design.

In symmetrical balance identical elements are repeated in the same position on either side of a central vertical axis. One side, in effect, becomes the mirror image of the other. Radial balance tames even a cluttered pie-sliced sector, molding it along with its clones into a unified and coherent visual statement. That's why I advocate audacity in some of the fabric choices, restrained by a sense of patchwork decorum.

Trying to impose a specific type of balance, for example, balancing dark, light, and medium values is not appropriate in a radial design. The final image sorts itself out into areas of dark and light in relation to the whole. Symmetry—not the designer—is responsible for the ultimate balancing act, automatically arranging order from unanticipated combinations.

Rhythm

The idea of visual rhythm refers to the movement of the viewer's eye. As a principle of design it is based on repetition, causing the eye to move from element to repeated element. Repetitive visual patterns compel the eye to keep moving about, encouraging the viewer to experience a dynamic quality.

Visual rhythm is a natural consequence of the kaleidoscope form. Predicting the exact pathway of the viewer's eye around the final image isn't possible, but that doesn't mean we shouldn't try. Influencing the result by introducing accents is part of our job as the designer.

The rhythmic pattern also causes an emotional response in the viewer. Some visual rhythms are flowing and graceful, others are abrupt and dynamic. When I begin a kaleidoscope I am vaguely aware my intention is to establish a rhythm that will seem, for example, graceful or, perhaps, staccato. Initially, I have a general "mood" in mind. The character of the rhythm results partially from the palette of fabric and partially from the shapes and lines of the faceted patches.

Line

In geometry a line is defined as an infinite number of points. Art defines it as a moving dot, reinforcing its inherently dynamic quality, since the viewer's eye must move to follow it. Designing a kaleidoscope block involves two different kinds of lines. One kind is implied lines created by the position of identical elements, so the eye tends to connect them automatically.

Secondly, within the pie-sliced sector lines facet the body of the triangular wedge again and again into a network of adjacent patches. Some of these lines eventually become camouflaged seams, while others are highlighted and command attention.

Line turns out to be a very expressive tool. By understanding the characteristics of directions, you can infuse a quality of motion onto a flat surface with a minimal effort. A horizontal line suggests quiet and repose, perhaps because it is reminiscent of the sleeping position. A vertical line is interpreted as more visually active. But the diagonal line most strongly implies movement, contributing to a dynamic, motion-filled image and evoking the impression that change is imminent.

A line is capable of infinite variety. It is a form that has length and width. Remember that in a kaleidoscopic design there are no rules. The width can vary in thickness. It does not have to stay even, like a lattice or a binding. Irregular variations serve to maintain the viewer's interest.

RANDOM ACTS OF COLOR

There's something about an actual kaleidoscope that makes the viewer gasp out loud with delight. Maybe it's the layer after layer of uninhibited colors tumbling irrepressibly into unpredictable harmony. After all, what can be more satisfying than witnessing order conquering chaos, over and over again, right in the palm of your hand?

Approach color choices playfully and with an open mind. Seek the unexpected—better yet, embrace the unexpected and take credit for it. Browse through life looking for unusual combinations of color, and you'll recognize them when they bump into you. Explore every-day resources filled with an abundance of hues: tropical fish, fine wrapping papers, oriental rugs. When your attention is caught, mentally dissect what grabbed it.

A pieced kaleidoscope is an opportunity to use color intuitively. There is no formula. But since the viewer's perception of the complete scope is based on the relationships between colors, we can deliberately use color's spatial properties to create the illusion of depth. Some of the classic theories employed by artists work in a kaleidoscope design while others are irrelevant. So let's be flexible and tuck a few pertinent guidelines into the sewing basket.

Value and Contrast

Value and contrast define the kaleidoscopic image. Value is the artistic term for light and dark. Value contrast refers to the relationship between areas of dark and light. Often the design choice is not "purple" or "green," but how dark or light a purple or green to use. The visual unity of the whole pattern is based on contrasts and comparisons between light and dark. The relative color values organize the design into areas of sharp and mild contrast. This arrangement happens in spite of you, so don't agonize too much.

Value creates a sense of depth, the perception that some shapes are in front and some shapes are in back of others. In general, light values appear to advance and dark values appear to recede. High-value contrast seems to come forward, to appear actually closer, while areas of lesser contrast retreat, suggesting distance.

The eye is drawn to sharp contrasts. When the contrast between values is minimal, the effect is calm and subtle. Highly contrasting values suggest drama and excitement. Colors "pop" when there is strong dark and light contrast with their backgrounds.

In *KALEIDOSCOPIC IX: Public Radio Daze* (page 30), the color strategy was to keep the values within a limited range in most of the areas, and sprinkle contained groupings with intense, deeply saturated color. The smaller areas of bright color balance the much larger areas of neutral color, keeping a complicated design organized and coherent. The seams between the closely related patches are barely discernible. The high-contrast colors advance and dominate the areas of lesser contrast.

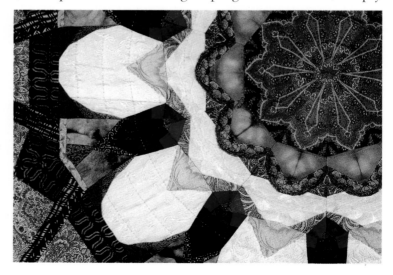

▶

Detail of *KALEIDOSCOPIC IX: Public Radio Daze*

Color Characteristics

There is a direct relationship between color and the visual impression of depth. The cool blues and greens have a tranquil, airy, far-away feel. They tend to recede into the background. As objects recede, any brilliance of color becomes more neutral, finally seeming to be gray-blue. Yellow-green through violet is the cool side of the color wheel. The warm side ranges from yellow through red-violet. The hot reds and oranges provide a stimulating, opaque, earthy effect. These colors catch the eye and advance from the ground.

Colors are never isolated entities. The term *spreading effect* refers to the way colors change depending on what colors and fabrics they are next to. Even the warmth or coolness of a color is relative to its surrounding colors. Some colors are more susceptible to change than others. Pure, vibrant colors are less vulnerable to the influences of adjacent neighbors, while muted colors modify their appearance depending on the context. That's why olives and strange greens turn out to be versatile foils, setting off other colors by contrast.

White has a tendency to expand and overflow its boundaries. The "spreading" of white affects its adjacent colors by creating a slightly washed out or tinted effect. Black achieves the opposite effect. The darkness controls the spreading effect, letting each color display its own true sensation, visually rich and clear in tone.

KALEIDOSCOPIC XI: Snowfall (pages 24-25) is an example of a true blue quilt. The effect is not only harmonious, but generally quiet, restful and very, very cool. It demonstrates how color values are important in creating spatial illusion in spite of the monochromatic color scheme. The snowflakes do not seem flat and one-dimensional. A visual illusion of depth is created where the high-contrast values come forward and the low-contrast areas recede. *KALEIDOSCOPIC XII: Up Close and Far Away* (page 26) is an example of a warm color scheme. *KALEIDOSCOPIC VIII: The Sun, the Moon. . .and the Stars* (pages 20-21) runs hot and cold, true to the literal nature of the quilt's subject matter.

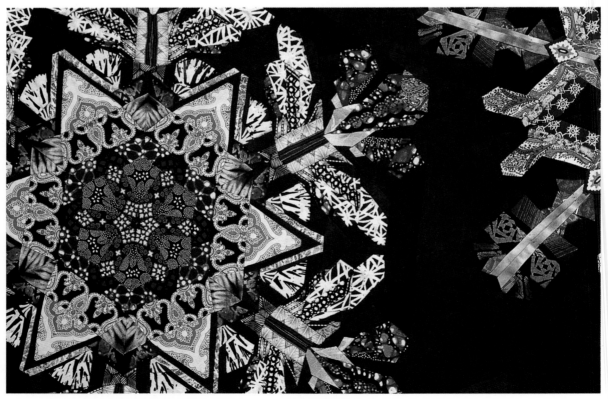

▲ Detail of *KALEIDOSCOPIC XI: Snowfall*

Color Discord

Discord has gotten a bad rap. When we say that colors clash, we mean that they seem to pull away from each other rather than relate harmoniously. This isn't necessarily bad, since the results are exciting, eye-catching, unexpected combinations. A discordant color contributes to the visual surprise. Well, don't we want our kaleidoscope to be full of surprises? It's even OK for colors to compete for attention. Make those eyeballs spin! The radial structure and repetitive nature of the whole shebang will harmonize the final result.

KALEIDOSCOPIC XIII: Random Acts of Color (page 27) is a showcase of mildly discordant eye-catching color combinations.

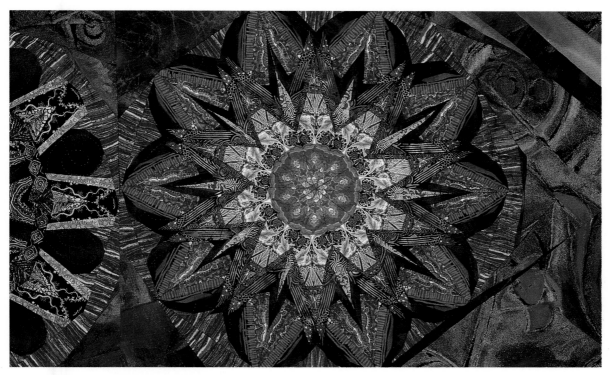

▲ Detail of *KALEIDOSCOPIC XIII: Random Acts of Color*

OUR FABRICS, OUR PALETTES

The more I am exposed to state-of-the-art kaleidoscopes, the more I am enticed by their magic. However, my love for kaleidoscopes does not compel me to make quilts. I make quilts because I love printed textiles.

On the whole, I'd much rather go fabric shopping than write about it. Some quiltmakers clearly have a knack for this material pursuit. The key element separating the master fabric collectors from the wannabees is: *attitude.* Above all, be your own advocate. Cloth is as valid a palette as paint. Never make excuses for the size of your stash. A vast selection promotes in-depth, on-site exploration and increases the odds that the perfect fabric antidote is waiting on your shelf. Remember, just because you buy a lot of fabric doesn't mean you are materialistic.

You've probably figured out by now that I'm not a purist. When it comes to textiles, I'm your basic eclectic out to have a good time. I look for medium-weight, firmly woven fabrics, but I'm willing to consider whatever catches my eye and doesn't leave its mark all over my fingers or all over the floor. That is the only reasonable way to explore the treasures of New York City's garment center.

My quilts are not functional. I don't make them expecting to throw them into the washing machine, but I do make them expecting the unexpected. I choose materials with this in mind and prepare them accordingly.

My hometown paper, *The New York Times*, once quoted me in the following way: "'We don't do calicoes,' said Paula Nadelstern of the Bronx, speaking for those who consider their quilt making an art." (From "Mild-Mannered Quilters Pursue Quarry," by Cara Greenberg, May 2, 1993). This soundbite might be too glib. Calico began not as a print, but as a cotton cloth, and of course I love cottons. The pliable nature of its weave makes it ideal for machine-piecing and hand-quilting. It's the best stuff to rely on when you find yourself cast in a piecing adventure that is threatening to take you places you never wanted to go.

I don't use true cotton solids. I think they are appropriately named. According to the dictionary, a solid tends to keep its form rather than flow or spread out. I read them as visual periods. The image in a pieced kaleidoscope should be tinged with the promise of things to come. Printed fabrics tickle our imaginations. Their versatility lets them adapt to countless moods: playful, enigmatic, charming, sophisticated, or plain and simple. They blend; they fade; they dodge; they dance; they dazzle!

I don't feel the same way about solid-colored silks. Many contemporary kaleidoscope makers are incorporating innovations that include dichroic glass. The unique quality of this substance, invented for the space program, is that it shows different colors depending on the angle of light falling on it. For example, the same piece can be blue, pink, or yellow. The effect is an interior image that glows. Sometimes I interpret this quality with a sprinkling of silks that reflect different colorations depending on the viewing angle.

In the past year I entered brand-new textile territory by exploring the wonderful world of fusibles. It all started when I was seduced by nine feet of hand-marbled magenta/maroon/plum silk swirling with olive and a profusion of other colors. (To create this effect, nonsoluble inks are floated across a liquid base, drawn into a design, and picked up by the fabric.) I know it sounds wicked, but I turned that silk into cotton by using a fusible woven interfacing. Losing the "drape" of the goods was an asset for piecing; it stabilized the cloth, making it easier to cut with a rotary blade and needle (see *KALEIDOSCOPIC XIV: Myst*, page 28).

When I first started exploring kaleidoscopic imagery, I was more timid in my fabric selections. I played by the rules. Eventually I left civilized patchwork for uncharted frontiers and learned to regard the rules as guidelines. Now I try to free myself from a conventional sense of fabric orderliness and commit random acts of fabric. Conveying a quality that suggests the succession

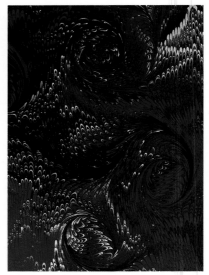

▲ Silk fabric used in
KALEIDOSCOPIC XIV: Myst

of chance interlinkings synonymous with kaleidoscopes is an important design objective. Creating visions of sparkling crystal and jewel-like images is another. Evoking a sense of luminosity is perhaps the easiest of the three to translate into textiles.

Certain kinds of fabric work best in a kaleidoscopic design. Variety in a single block provides visual texture. My inclination is to balance glamour and usefulness. When possible, place a forgiving textile next to a fussy one. Consider the weight and fiber content of adjacent fabrics. It's nice when fabrics play well together.

AND THE CATEGORIES ARE:

I seem to have invented a personal vocabulary for colorful patterned textiles that defines them according to personality and function. There are four categories. Prima donnas are simultaneously temperamental and charismatic. All-overs are reliable and forgiving. Directionals are dynamic. Novelty prints are unexpected contributors of highlights and shadows.

The Prima Donnas

Any motif that needs to be duplicated precisely needs its own template. If it can't be strip-pieced, it is a prima donna. Accordingly, prima donnas need to be lavished with attention. In exchange, these powerful design elements make strong, memorable statements.

I figure out how much to buy by counting off eight or sixteen repeats. Usually my purchase is between one and two yards, depending on the size of the repeat, previous acquisitions, how much I like it, and the state of my cash flow.

MOTIFS SET IN STRIPES WITH BILATERAL SYMMETRY

I search for patterns printed with perfect bilateral symmetry. By definition, a repeating pattern can be superimposed on itself. If a line can be drawn in the pattern so that the pattern on one side of the line is the mirror image of the pattern on the other side of the line, then the pattern can be superimposed on itself by flipping it over so that the line stays fixed. This motion is called reflection, and the mirror line is called an axis of reflection (1,2,3).

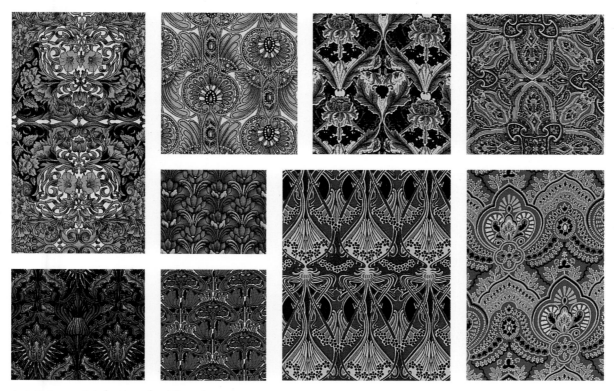

▲ 1 Patterns printed with perfect bilateral symmetry

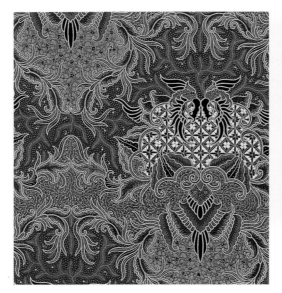

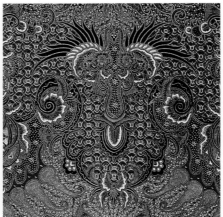

◀ 2
These stunning patterns with bilateral symmetry and oversized motifs require lots of yardage to ensure sufficient repeats.

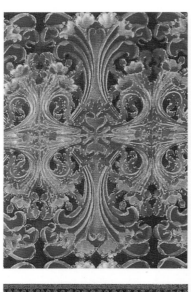

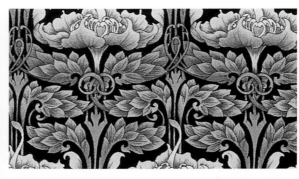

◀ 3
These slightly "off" renditions of symmetrical motifs behave admirably when handled with care, resulting in a looser image that seems less formal.

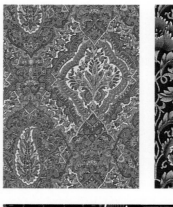

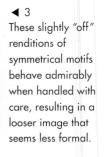

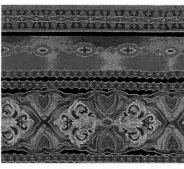

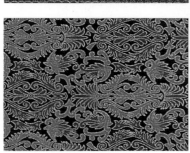

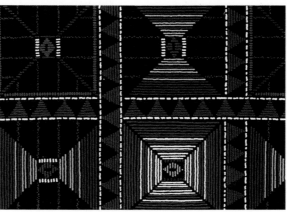

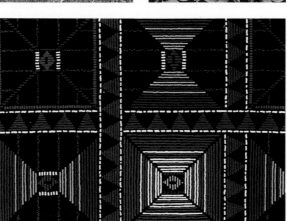

In other words, a motif with bilateral symmetry can be divided into identical halves by a line passing through the center. That's why it is ideal for the patches that meet in the middle of a kaleidoscope block (4). The intricately entwined motifs soften the straight lines of the long side seams and create the illusion of graceful continuity around the important center. In this pivotal position synchronous matching between as many as sixteen reflections is critical.

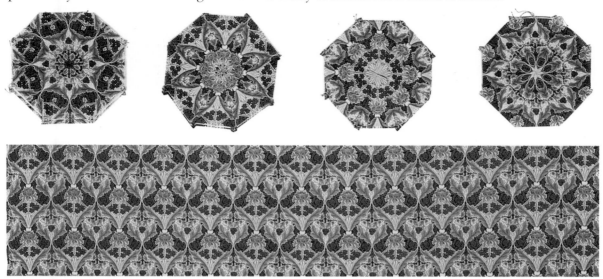

▲ 4 Four kaleidoscopes cut from the same piece of fabric

Intricate patterns arranged in an ordered and formal layout are the treasures of my collection. The interplay of forms caused by the repeat is magical (5). The classic Liberty™ of London designs, which have lasted since the Art Nouveau period, are examples of this kind of pattern. Medallions are another useful device. These circular figures are inspired by star shapes, flowers, Persian tiles. My subjective approach to fabric selection is free of restraints. I like to mix incongruous fabrics. Whether fabrics belonging to different styles and tastes are visually compatible is not an issue. I practice pieceful co-existence.

5 ▶
The prima donna fabric
after patches were cut
from it

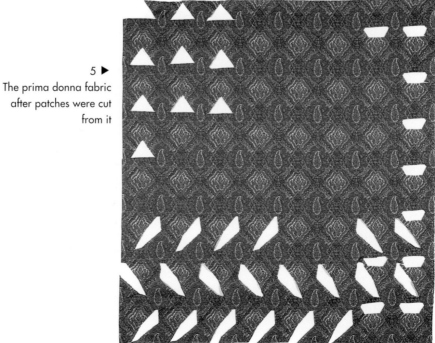

Symmetrically patterned textiles are printed both on and off the straight grain of the fabric. To promote stability, the motif for the first patch in a wedge must be cut on the straight grain. Use enticing motifs printed along the bias for any other position in the piece-of-pie (6).

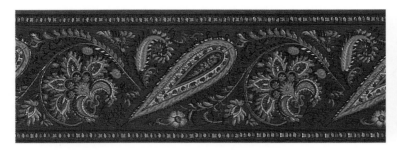 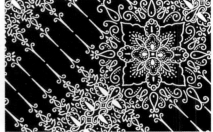

▲ 6 Symmetrical patterns printed on the bias

The textile industry doesn't have a satisfying term for the type of pattern I'm referring to. "Border print" is my personal label because it functions like the border designs printed in long linear runs from selvage to selvage, intended to decorate hems and edgings. Textile mavens would probably call the pattern under discussion a stripe. In this case the term "stripe" does not refer to the straight bands of color called stripes, but to a type of layout where the motifs line up to form stripes.

THE ILLUSION OF SYMMETRY

Sometimes fabrics that seem to be symmetrical at first glance turn out to be pseudo-symmetrical (7). A closer inspection reveals differences between the two sides. Don't use this type of asymmetrical motif for the first patch that ends up in the design's important center. Use it where the patch isn't destined to meet itself. In a position where confrontation is impossible, the discrepancies will not be noticed and it will imitate a symmetrical patch. When motifs inside the body of the triangle are askew, they will still read as identical when the viewer's eye travels around the scope.

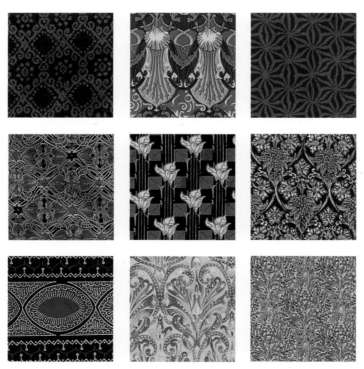

◀ 7
Some fabrics that seem to be symmetrical turn out to be pseudo-symmetrical.

MIRROR IMAGED MOTIFS

A fabric printed with motifs that can be flipped into a mirror image is a useful but rare find (8). Often, figures that appear to be oriented identically to the left and to the right turn out to be the same motif rendered right-side-up and upside-down.

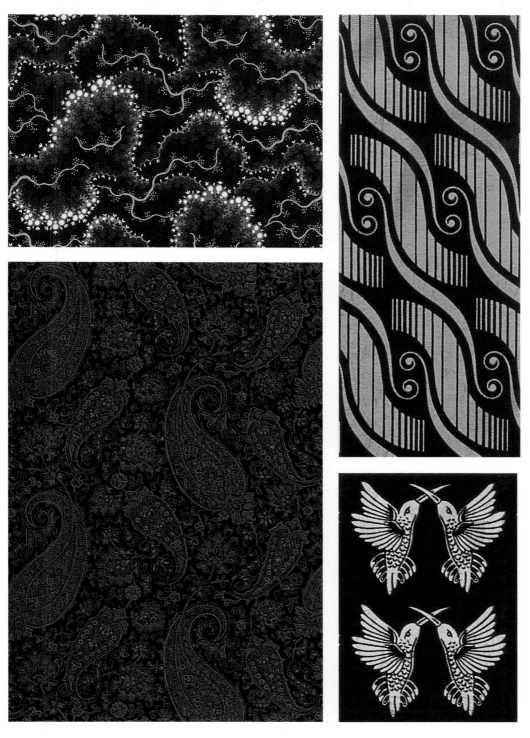

◄ 8
Fabrics printed with motifs that are mirror-images of each other

This category includes the paisley motif, with its characteristic teardrop shape. In its original incarnation, the paisley form was found in set and spaced layouts along the borders of Indian cashmere shawls. The Western preference for all-over layouts in which the forms flow around each other in elaborate profusion eventually replaced orderly patterns.

All-overs

An all-over, nondirectional design looks exactly the same from any angle (9, 10). It has no implicit top, bottom, left, or right. Its layout contains more figure than ground. Sometimes the motif is packed so closely together the background almost completely disappears.

Its forgiving temperament makes it the choice for strip-piecing. You don't have to worry about matching. You can place templates on it quickly without wasting. It is an easy fabric to blend with adjacent prints. This makes it perfect for interjecting slivers of contrast or visual exclamation points. I buy one-half or one-yard cuts.

I covet all-over fabrics that render a sense of luminosity and translucence. They help evoke the glassy, crystalline quality of a kaleidoscope. The current abundance of dyed, painted, and marbled fabrics is a gold mine of sources for shading and transparency.

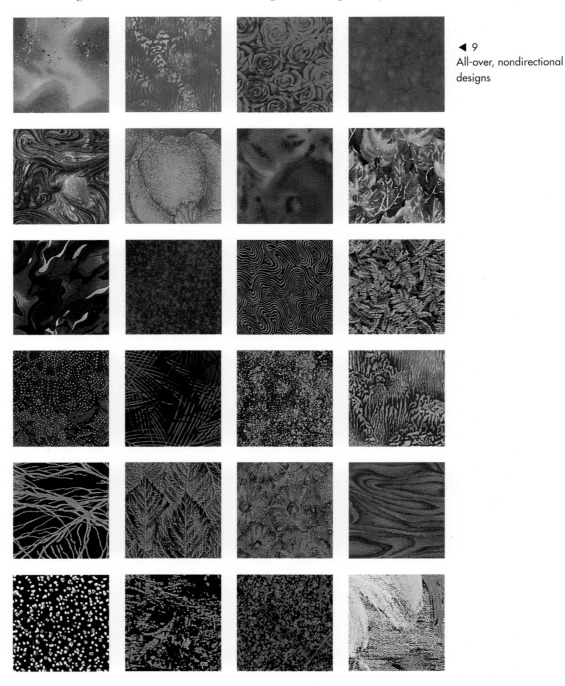

◀ 9
All-over, nondirectional designs

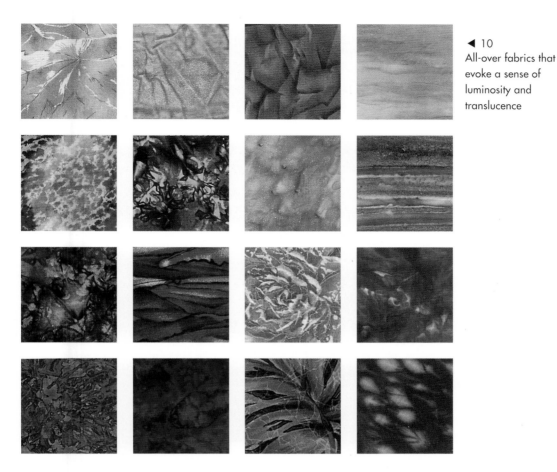

◀ 10
All-over fabrics that evoke a sense of luminosity and translucence

Directionals

One-directional designs have a distinct top and bottom. The patches cut from these fabrics must be oriented in the same direction. This limits your ability to maneuver, and leaves more wasted fabric. Two-directional prints could be turned upside down and no one would notice (11). With a little extra care for identical template placement, directionals become candidates for strip-piecing. It's worth the effort, because they automatically create visual pathways that instill an element of motion. Radiating designs need friends like these.

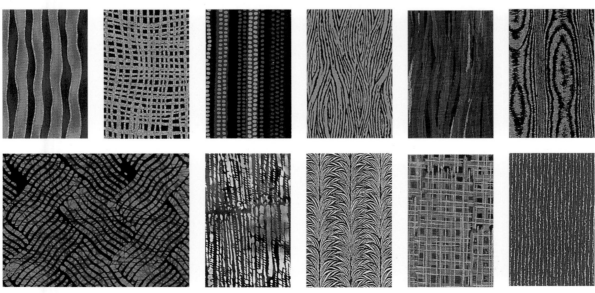

▲11 Two-directional designs

103

Directionals can be neatly arranged in rows, in grids, or on the diagonal (12). Zigzags and serpentine stripes infuse a more lively quality than layouts like chevrons and herringbones, but their erratic behavior makes them difficult to use symmetrically and in relatively small shapes. (That doesn't mean I don't try again and again.) I consider myself lucky when I find a directional rendered as a three-dimensional design. A shadow added to a stripe makes it seem to spring out of the flatness of the fabric.

Patterns distinguished by a gradual shading and blending of dark to light, or one color into another, are worth exploring (13). They are not only great organizers, they also carry the viewer's eye smoothly from one form to the next.

Another kind of directional is fabrics that have a nap, like silks and velvet. I used to practice consistency when piecing fabrics with obvious directional sheen. Now I figure a random approach evokes the subtle sense of shading that I'm after.

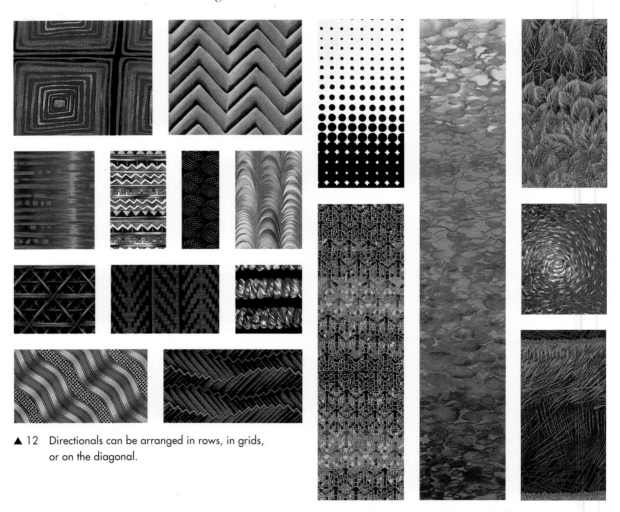

▲ 12 Directionals can be arranged in rows, in grids, or on the diagonal.

▲ 13 Directional patterns distinguished by gradual shading and blending

Novelty Prints: Seek the Unexpected

When you cross over into this way of looking at fabric, your vision alters. The idea is to concentrate attention on the details in a fabric's interior and ignore its total effect. It is analogous to focusing on the twigs instead of the trees or the forest. Paradoxically, this narrow perspective widens the selection. The internal, secondary components of a motif take on an active life of their own (14, 15).

Because novelty prints often depict some real creature or object, they are usually fabric-printed versions of paintings (16). Realistic motifs such as juicy fruits, blooming flowers, and sparkling jewels are rendered with painterly qualities. Patches cut from printed cloth that looks three-dimensional convey the illusion of substance. Borrow shadings and highlights from these resources to suggest the shifting of light in your kaleidoscope.

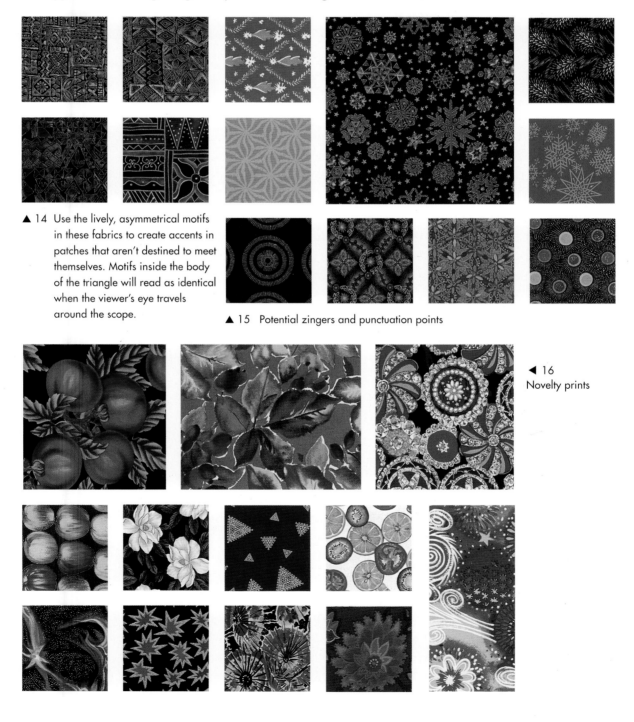

▲ 14 Use the lively, asymmetrical motifs in these fabrics to create accents in patches that aren't destined to meet themselves. Motifs inside the body of the triangle will read as identical when the viewer's eye travels around the scope.

▲ 15 Potential zingers and punctuation points

◀ 16 Novelty prints

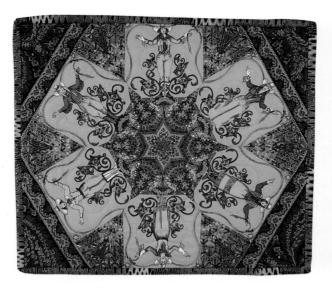

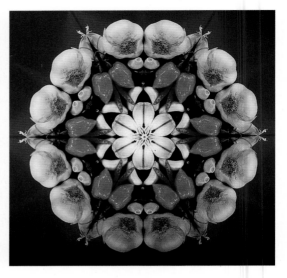

▲ *Even Cowgirls Get Yellow*
This six-sided kaleidoscope was inspired by a cowgirl print.

▲ Is it a scope or is it dinner? Kaleidoscopic image by Mark Reynolds

Check out celestial prints for frenetic zigzags and erupting gases. Falling stars are often depicted with cartoon-like broken lines implying rapid movement. But the sky is not the limit. Take advantage of the faceted sparkle of printed jewels or the twinkling highlights of perfectly round fruits like cherries and grapes. Renderings of feathers bring out the best fine line work and unusual color combinations. Animated, effervescent bubbles suggest transience. The centers of blossoming flowers translate into flickers of glowing light. The tips of the sunbeams in *KALEIDO-SCOPIC VIII: The Sun, the Moon. . .and the Stars* (pages 20-21) were once tropical blossoms. In their new context they burst into scorching flames (17).

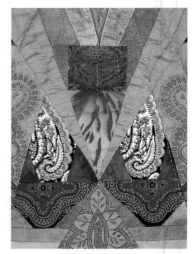

▲ 17 Detail of *KALEIDOSCOPIC VIII: The Sun, the Moon,. . . and the Stars*

DESIGNING: MUSINGS

According to his official biographer, Dr. Seuss thought that writers who knew how a story would end produced an inferior product. A good book has to figure its way out of a predicament. "He wanted his stories to take on a life of their own," she said, adding, "When serendipity pushed itself in Dr. Seuss' face, he recognized it."

This little bit of Seuss lore tickles me. When I first made quilts, I thought the "right" way demanded a design-in-stone before the first scissor snip. Now I know that letting the design suggest other possibilities is an equally valid approach.

The best way to design a kaleidoscope-like image is to think kaleidoscopically. Come to the table with a palette, a concept, and a willingness to revise both. Share control rather than demand obedience from your subject. When the fabric wants to go *that* way instead of *this,* let it. You are supervising a metamorphosis-in-progress. Rearrange fabrics, colors, shapes, and lines into new patterns constantly.

ANGLING FOR A DIFFERENCE

Let's go back to the very beginning. Deciding how many triangles the scope will be divided into determines the angle to be drafted. Our quiltmaking legacy includes many evenly divided six-sided hexagons and eight-pointed stars. A design with eight pieces-of-the-pie becomes a square when a triangle is added to each corner. A six-sided design forms a rectangle. Sometimes one of these shapes works better in the envisioned quilt than another. Other times a "must-use" fabric necessitates choosing one division over the other. Maybe there are only six or seven repeats in the amount of fabric available. Or maybe stuffing a generous design into the wedge defined by a 45° angle causes it to lose its appeal.

Distinguishing each angle's peculiar charms isn't easy, because the differences are subtle. Both can be dressed up or down, becoming formal and grand or spunky and chic. The classic form of an octagon reads slightly more regularly, while a six-sided shape with its wider wedge seems somewhat less sophisticated (18). (See "Conversations with Kaleidoscope Friends" on page 140.)

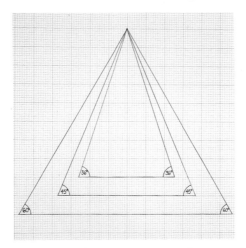

▲ 18   Comparison between 36°, 45°, and 60° triangles

Because visual rhythm is based partly on repetition, a block divided into lots of pieces-of-the-pie automatically inherits a dynamic quality. Rapid, rhythmic visual movements from one repeated element to the next make it throb with activity. The fewer the wedges, the less it vibrates. (Of course, it isn't hard to start a fat wedge whirling with a few well-placed zingers.).

KALEIDOSCOPIC IV: Crystal Canopy (page 16), *KALEIDOSCOPIC XI: Snowfall* (pages 24-25), and *KALEIDOSCOPIC XII: Up Close and Far Away* (page 26) are examples of quilts with hexagonal images. *KALEIDOSCOPIC III: Stained Glass Anthology* (page 13), *KALEIDOSCOPIC VII: The Natural Order of Chaos* (pages 18-19), and *KALEIDOSCOPIC XV: Eccentric Circles* (page 29) are based on eight-sided designs.

I tackled a ten-sided design for the first time in *KALEIDOSCOPIC IX: Public Radio Daze* (page 30), inspired by the dazzling colors and complexity of imagery in a Charles Karadimos scope. The geometric division of 360° into ten created a surprisingly slim 36° triangle, demanding a very different mindset. I had to narrow my mind's eye considerably when I wandered through my fabrics. Big, puffy elements faced being trimmed into slivers of their former selves to fit the slender boundaries. I next explored ten-sided images in *KALEIDOSCOPIC XIII: Random Acts of Color* (page 27), aiming for an informal, spontaneous mood.

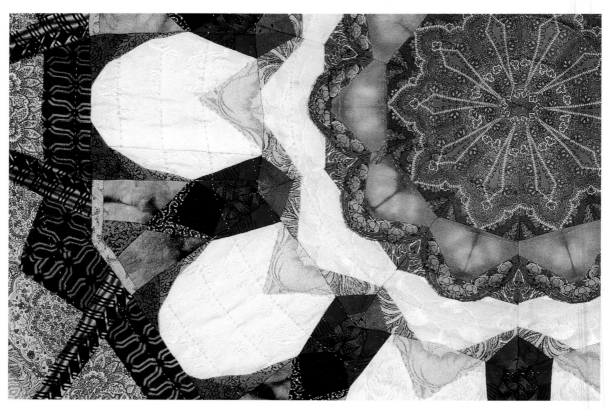

▲ Detail of *KALEIDOSCOPIC IX: Public Radio Daze*

I find I am drawn to state-of-the-art kaleidoscopes that have odd-sided designs. Although an uneven number of wedges radiating repetitively from a common center emerges as a balanced image, its vague irregularity captures my attention.

In 1992 I bartered a fabric kaleidoscope for a dramatic five-sided scope entitled "Twilight" by Randy and Shelley Knapp of Ontario, Oregon. I fell in love the first time I gazed into this scope's opulent interior. But while the colors offered inspiration for a future quilt palette, I didn't think a five-sided design was in my future, because I only sew straight seams. A design divided into an even number of divisions can be constructed much more easily than one with an odd number. In an evenly numbered design, half of the triangles pieced together will form a straight edge (see "Joining Together" on page 77).

For weeks after its arrival, I listened to the evening news, telephone conversations, the sounds of my daily life, with this scope's tumbling images pressed to my eye. Then, in what felt like a second, when I didn't even realize I was focusing on it, I took a creative leap. What if, instead of making ten identical triangular segments, I made five left-sided and five right-sided? Would the resulting image act as a five-sided, odd-numbered design, even though the underlying structure would be an even-numbered division of ten?

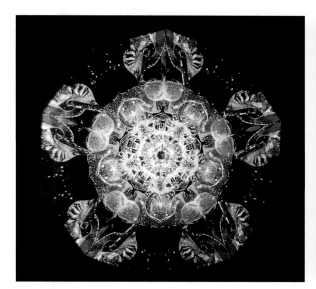 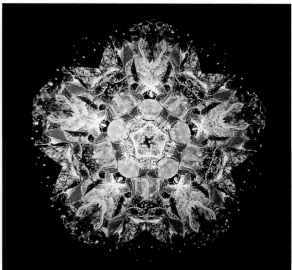

Interiors of *Twilight* by Randy and Shelley Knapp

I played with this idea in *KALEIDOSCOPIC X: Water from the Moon* (pages 22-23). Again I had to revise my thinking. Out went the now familiar central axis with identical elements repeated in the same position on either side. This time I mentally labeled the 36° triangle on ⅛" graph paper with a top, bottom, left ,and right side and forced myself to think of the left side and the right side as separate units. My plan was to create some motifs focused along the left side, and completely different ones directed toward the right, conscious that elements along each of the triangle's sides would connect to their mirror images and blossom into something brand-new. Although for all intents and purposes this design strategy divided a single piece-of-pie in two, the final result is a unified wedge. Smooth connections between the two sides were created by adjusting existing lines (19A, 19B).

Since the left side and the right side did not share a relationship, this scheme forced me, more than ever before, to rely on serendipity to work its magic. I had no idea what the final image would be, or whether I would like it. The good news is, I liked it a lot and now I want to try other odd-sided divisions.

In *KALEIDOSCOPIC XIV: Myst* (page 28) the nine diverse images include one ten-sided, five eight-sided, two six-sided, and one five-sided design, making it a useful quilt for analyzing the effect of different angles.

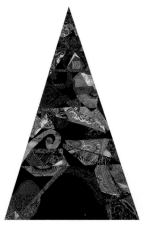 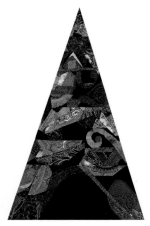

▲ 19A Left-sided piece-of-pie   ▲ 19B Right-sided piece-of-pie

THE NITTY-GRITTY OF THE VERY FIRST PATCH

Begin a tentative palette by choosing likely candidates based on the descriptions in "Our Fabrics, Our Palettes" on page 95. An open mind during this open-ended search can be a real eye-opener. If something tickles your fancy, grab it; don't stop to rationalize your material instincts.

Pick a fabric with unabashed bilateral symmetry for the patch destined to land in the design's important center. Remember, the fabric chosen for this turning point assumes a major role, creating a focal point that sets the mood for the scope-to-come.

Review "How to Make a Template" on page 39. Place the window-like template on the front of the fabric, aligning the center line of the template with the implied center of a motif. Move it up, move it down, turn it upside down. Varying the template's placement ever so slightly alters the final kaleidoscopic effect.

At first the potential for seemingly endless possibilities may be overwhelming. I know it was for me. But I have come to believe in the notion that there isn't a correct or best selection—that fabric choices made today will be different from ones made tomorrow. Embracing the possibilities offered by choice rather than feeling challenged by it can be liberating.

If looking at fabric this way is a brand-new idea, here is a design tip: don't cut the template out right away. Instead, place the entire sheet of template plastic, with the marked 45° angle, on a whole piece of fabric (20). This gives you a chance to adapt the template to the printed fabric, altering it if necessary, before it is cut out, instead of fitting the fabric into the template. Consider this scenario: you plan on a 3" triangle for the first patch, but fiddling with the goods reveals that a 3 ¼" triangle creates a more imaginative image. If you realize the need for this change after the 3" template is cut out, chances are you'll have to scrap the first one and make a brand-new template. Review the discussion on how to shape templates to fit fabric in on page 43.

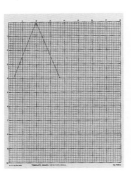 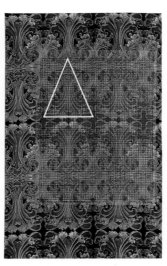

20 ▶
Place the entire sheet of template plastic, with the marked 45° angle, on a whole piece of fabric.

If you don't know where to start, look at the fabric as a whole. What catches your eye? A graceful line, a powerful contrast, a twinkle of brightness? Start there.

Put the template on the eye-catching section and scan its possibilities. It's natural to focus first on the patch of fabric that falls in the middle of the template, along the center axis. Just don't forget that it is as important to analyze what is going to occur along the seamlines. Try to visualize the mirror-imaged consequence. Moving it just a smidgen may transform the result. Identify which of the fabric's motifs center along the axis and which ones land on the seamline, consequently reflecting into mirror images.

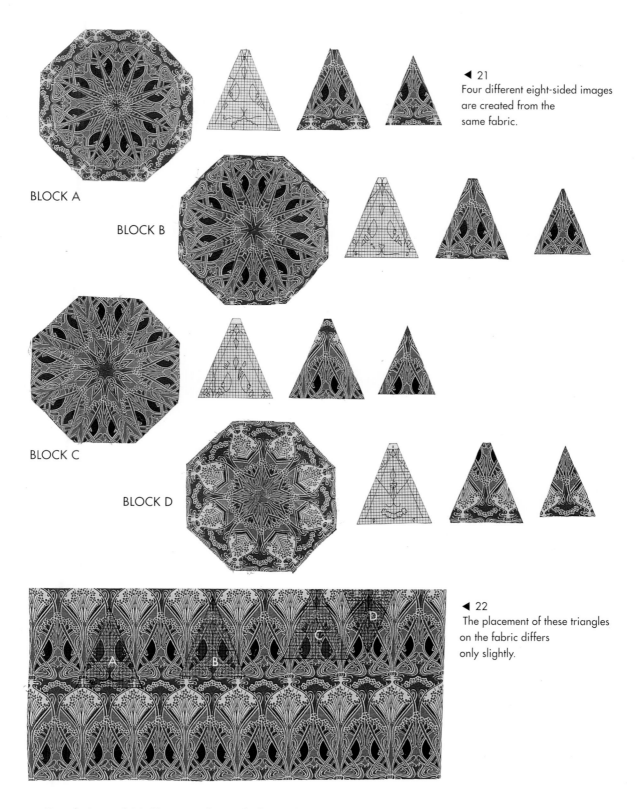

BLOCK A

BLOCK B

BLOCK C

BLOCK D

◀ 21
Four different eight-sided images
are created from the
same fabric.

◀ 22
The placement of these triangles
on the fabric differs
only slightly.

Panels 21 and 22 illustrate how shifting the template slightly transforms the final effect. Four different eight-sided images are created from the same fabric. To the right of each kaleidoscope block is a three-inch 45° triangular template with ¼" seam allowance, a fabric patch created from that template, and the same patch without seam allowance. The exact placement of the four templates on the fabric is shown in Panel 22. Block A's Template sits three-eighths of an inch lower than Template B and one inch lower than Template C. The top/bottom direction of the fabric is reversed for Block D's template. Actually, it is created from the leftovers.

Often my first placement of the template on the fabric renders the least sophisticated result. It seems to be a natural tendency to aim for what appears to be a complete motif. This transparent template technique makes it easy to position an intact motif in a patchwork shape, taking care not to chop off its vital parts. But it turns out that when a design undergoes mirror-imaging, wonderful effects emerge when the motif is cropped. A complete entity ends up looking like the same old thing. It seems expected, a trifle boring, while a little bit reflects itself into something brand-new: a piece of unique, imaginative intricacy that didn't exist before.

Locate the dark blue, circular motifs in the piece of fabric shown in Panel 22. In Block E (23) this shape sits intact in a single triangle, centered along its axis. Because its edges don't touch the sewing lines or extend into the seam allowance, what you see is what you get in the finished product.

Placing the template lower on the fabric alters the outcome. In Block F the circular motif is positioned directly on the sewing line so that part of it spills into the seam allowance. When the triangles are pieced together, the roundness disappears. The dark blue motifs meld into a new, unique shape that is perceived as background from which other colors and lines dance forward.

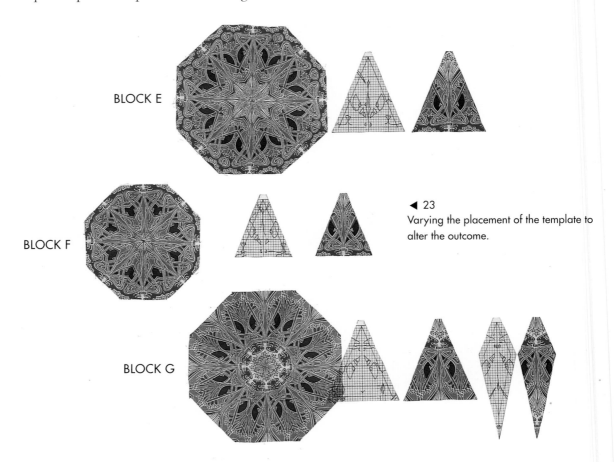

BLOCK E

BLOCK F

◀ 23
Varying the placement of the template to alter the outcome.

BLOCK G

Note the eye-catching, light-catching motif peppering the perimeters of Blocks E and F. As things stand now this lively detail will slip into oblivion, lost in the seam allowance. Revising a piece-in-progress to accommodate serendipity is always an option.

Don't be too invested in your choices. Let the fabric make its magic. Try lots of different things, even the stuff you think might be bizarre. Try out every "what if" idea that pops into your head. Sometimes getting from here to that inspired instance of creativity takes lots of stops in between.

Of course, the first patch doesn't have to be a classic triangle. A predetermined number of degrees forms the angle at the top, but its other borders should be designed to accommodate the fabric. Diagram 21 on page 43 illustrates lots of possibilities for shaping Patch 1.

Block G is composed of eight triangles identical to the one shown to its right. Find the turquoise lines just below the purple doo-dad that sits about 1¼" from the top. In the final version I'm particularly fond of two elements created by these turquoise lines. First, the lines flow over the seamline and merge into an intricate arrangement that continues gracefully from patch to patch. Second, the very slight upward curve at the seams winds up in a neat little circle.

To the far right, the template for Block G is reshaped, maintaining the two elements described above. In this second version the dark blue circular motif is cropped by the sewing line. Compare the bottom shape of the template with the corresponding fabric patch. Because the seam allowance is included, the template extends way beyond the end of the sewing lines. This excess will be trimmed when the template is matched to its neighboring template. (See "How to Match Templates" on page 54.)

At this point I don't know what the final kaleidoscopic image with the revised template will be. For what it's worth, here is my guess. After being drawn into the eye-catching circular center, the viewer's attention will pass gently to the turquoise curvilinear shapes, following these lines away from the center until they gradually dissipate in a tapered point of light color. Of course, this all depends on what comes next.

THE ART OF COUPLING

If possible, don't decide on the final shape and size of the first patch without thinking about where to go from there. The first patch inspires the second. The goal is to create a link between two (or more) fabrics that smoothes the transition, drawing the eye away from its initial fling with the kaleidoscope's center. Find a relationship that binds the two fabrics into a brand-new visual treat. Think in terms of camouflaging seams to encourage an uninterrupted flow of shape or color from one patch to the next.

This search involves physically manipulating the fabrics. Put the fabric intended for the first patch on the work surface. Place a sheet of template plastic with the angle marked on it where you want to begin. Next, look for tempting portions of other fabrics that suggest a possible relationship with the first, perhaps because of similar shapes or colors or something intangible. Investigate the link by folding the second fabric along the motif where you think it might connect to Patch 1. Place the fold along the approximate seamline of the first patch. Fine-tune the connection by adjusting the fold and rearranging the fabrics until one artful combination makes you gasp "aaaahhh!" with appreciation. If this aspired-to revelation seems a long time coming, go on to a different second fabric and repeat this problem-solving routine.

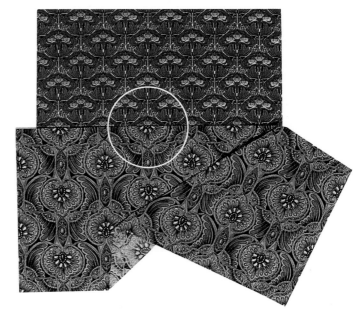

► The art of coupling

Panels 24, 25, and 26 illustrate six different examples of this important juncture. In each case one fabric is used in two different ways. The common fabric connects to two dissimilar ones, unleashing the magic of interlacing patterns every time. The graph paper diagram for each of the two outcomes is displayed, along with its corresponding templates marked with seam allowance, the patches cut from these templates, and the resulting unit of pieced-together patches. These samples offer a chance to try on this new way of looking at fabric. A useful tool to have on hand during the following discussion is a set of mirrors that can be positioned together at a 45° angle on top of a single piece-of-pie.

For homework, find the patches' corresponding places in the whole cloth. Identify where patches are centered along the axis and where they land on the seamline. Visualize the patches without their seam allowances. Imagine the mirror-imaged consequences. Measure how big the first patches are by counting the graph-paper grid.

The twice-used fabric in Examples A and B is from an elegant French Provincial cotton scarf, framed with a four-inch wide block-printed border. A portion of the border can be seen on the left of the swatch. In both examples the scarf is used in Patch 2. In Example A the first patch measures 1⅜" high and is cut from a repetitive stripe with bilateral symmetry. The connection it makes with a motif from the scarf's border obscures the seam and leads attention toward the continuous white lines that scallop around the kaleidoscope. Note the two sets of three black dots in each patch. Visualize the effect when this motif meets itself, without the seam allowance, in a slightly triangular formation at every seam.

In Example B the first patch is cut from an all-over with a spaced layout, meaning that there is less motif than ground. The eccentric circles float apart from each other on an empty field. Extra care must be taken to position the center axis of Template 1 on an on-grain motif. This ensures stability when all the triangles meet in the middle. The template does not have to be cut from the exact same circle each of the eight times, as long as it echoes the curvy line marked on the template. In fact, the effect will be more interesting if there are subtle differences in the shadings and lines that collect in the middle.

There are two reasons why I chose to divide Example B into two separate patches rather than an inclusive single triangle of scarf fabric. The first is practical. I want to use this one-and-only scarf and save it too. By creating a template with a flat end rather than a tapered angle, I conserve fabric. Specifically, the equally appealing, neighboring motif is left intact to use in another scope.

The second reason is motivated by design. When Patch 2 is extended into a taller, single template, the top of the template lands on a murky motif. This would not be an auspicious beginning. Moving the template down to avoid this gloomy center means losing the white leaves at the top of Patch 2. These will bend into graceful arches at the seams. Piecing a new lively fabric to Patch 2 is clearly the answer. Although the first patch measures only three-quarters of an inch, it represents an area eight times as large. Imagine the visual vibrations when eight templates filled with dynamic white strokes pop out of the center. Now that's a charismatic beginning!

At first glance it may seem as though Patch 2 contains an unabridged version of this motif. Actually, the uppermost red and mustard leaves spill into the seam allowances and combine into gracefully curving points. The bottom part of the triangular patch of fabric suggests lots of possible directions for the next piecing sequence. The final shape of the template will depend on these decisions. (See the continuing discussion of this example on page 116.)

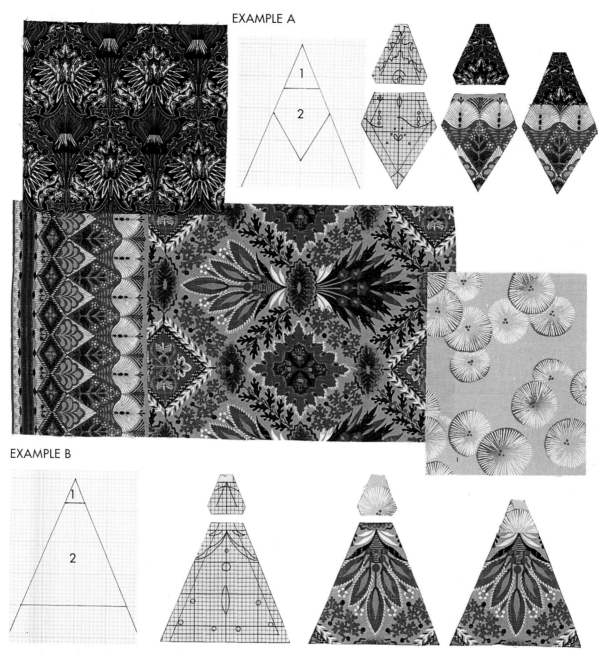

EXAMPLE A

EXAMPLE B

▲ 24 The art of coupling: transitions from the first patch to the second

In Panel 25 the common fabric is used for Patch 2 in Example C and Patch 1 in Example D. In Example C similar (but different) hues of pink unite the patches in a seamless relationship. Visualize the finished result minus the seam allowance. The blue sparks igniting the center end up crowned with golden darts, while each of the olive-colored leaves spills across the seamlines and curls up with its own reflection.

An openwork lace of gold lines starts off the wedge in Example D before disappearing into Patch 2 in an ambiguous shift of color. Patch 2 is cut from an elaborate Japanese-inspired fabric printed on the diagonal. This fabric isn't appropriate for the first patch because it is not printed on-grain, but it is a fine candidate to fill an ensuing position. Also, although the motifs read as bilaterally symmetrical, it ain't necessarily so. A close examination reveals lots of discrepancies from one side to the other. Only the top inch of the motif lines up with the template's grid before losing its correlation with the center axis. When drafting the template for Patch 2, I took care to ensure that this not-quite-symmetrical motif bumps into itself briefly at the seamlines in what will appear to be a flawless connection. The state of being slightly askew works in this design, lending the whole shebang a jaunty, relaxed feel. By positioning the segment that goes awry toward the middle, it doesn't have to conform to the exacting rules demanded by the uptight seams.

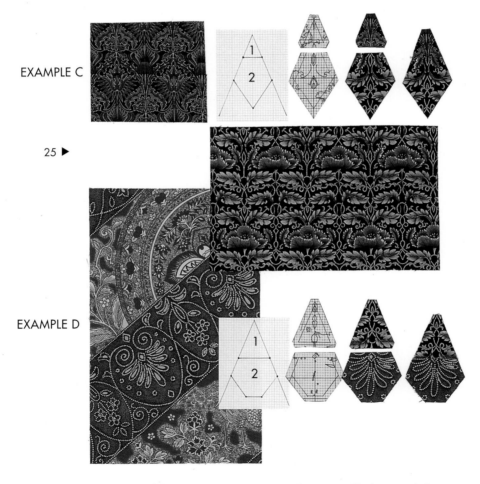

EXAMPLE C

25 ▶

EXAMPLE D

In Panel 26, the common fabric in Examples E and F is a rollicking celebration of color. Goods this good deserve to show themselves off in substantial shapes like the long Patch 2 in Example E. It combines easily with the primary-colored, Gothic-style fabric used for the first patch. The colors and shapes in Patch 1 team up with the hot reds and oranges that encircle the center. The high contrast of green in the next row zaps this junction with a strong, abrupt contrast that starts the focus spinning away from the center.

In this case the template for Patch 2 does not have to be placed at the exact same repeat each time. Utilizing this fabric's exuberant yet somewhat random coloring evokes the radiant yet transient relationships between colors in a scope's interior. To line up the template on the whole cloth, I focused on the zigzagging line separating the color green from the adjacent orange and the arrows marked along the center axis, and let the rest fall where it may.

And now for something completely different. The fabric used for Patch 2 in Example F is a Dutch Java print. The thin yellow lines interspersed with black and purple ones intrigued me. I tried lots of ways to connect these two fabrics before I settled on this one. Visualize the mirror-imaged results. The yellow lines reflect into wings that vanish into blackness. The motif of tiny white lines caught between the stripes may seem lonely and insignificant now, but in the kaleidoscopic version this fringe will become an active component, causing the eye to leap around the circle.

Thanks to a tiny detail toward the bottom of Patch 1, the seam between the two patches becomes unclear. The purple arrow surrounded by the burst of yellow detaches visually from the first patch, looses its shaft in the seam, and connects to the dark vague colors in Patch 2. Meanwhile, the seam is responsible for a wonderful illusion, carving the yellow into a curvaceous edging.

Did I know this was going to be the case when I started the search? No. I can only take credit for the fact that I recognize the gifts of serendipity when they open up in front of me.

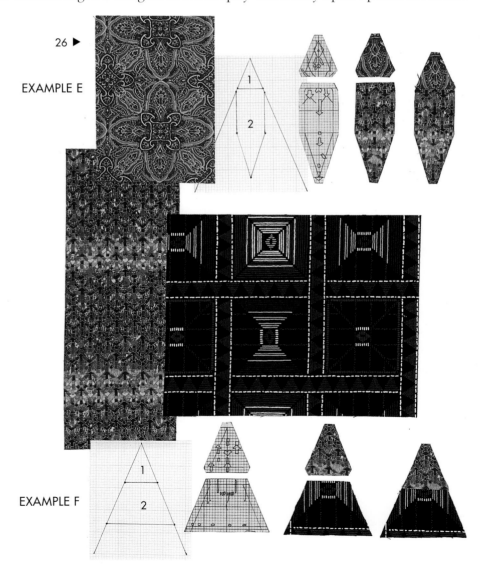

26 ▶

EXAMPLE E

EXAMPLE F

INTERLACING FABRICS AND PATTERNS

Although the kaleidoscopic design is formed against the background of a grid, there is no reason to follow its network of lines. The purpose of this framework is to help organize and discipline the symmetry, perhaps even to influence the proportion of the patches. Best of all, it frees you from a conventional sense of patchwork order by providing the confidence that the finished block will fit together. Here's the chance to create odd angles, the opportunity to randomly facet any shape.

Examples G, H, I, J, K, L, and M, (27, 28, 29, 30, 31) illustrate variations on the theme begun in Example B (24, page 115). Please note, all the following patches and pieced-together samples include the seam allowance unless otherwise indicated.

EXAMPLE G

Sorting through piles (and piles) of fabrics led to a versatile print twinkling with gold outlined patterns on a rich black ground. A session of hands-on experimenting suggested this simple plan: fill the next 1⅜" of the piece-of-pie with a big fat patch of this glittery prima donna. The relation between the ochre-colored doodad at the top center of Patch 3 and the background color of Patch 2 inspired the final choice. The two colors blend into a new motif, visually interrupting the straight line between point c and point d. Seeing the pleasing effect of this relationship gave me the idea to look for other ways to disguise the horizontal sewing line.

Find the red arch in Patch 3 and note its background. I decided to extend this ground, figuratively, across the seam and into Patch 2. This plan involves three steps. Here's the abridged version in a nutshell:

1. Use a template to trim each corner of Patch 2.

2. Strip a piece of fabric similar to the glittery black background to each of the sixteen trimmed corners.

3. Re-mark these pieced-together fabrics with the original template.

Here's the more-than-you-probably-want-to-know version. By placing Template 3 on Patch 3, I found and marked the gridpoint where the red arch ends and the black background begins (*point g*). Counting grid lines identified the coordinates of *point g*, making it easy to mark this point on both the diagram and Template 2. By placing Template 2 on Patch 2, I decided how much of the little red branches to trim off at the corner and ruled a line from *point g* to *point h*. I counted grid lines and transferred this line to the diagram and to the other corner of Template 2.

Check out Template 2. See how the left side of the template is different from the right side? The left side is revised according to the new scheme and correlates with *points g* and *h* (including seam allowance). The right side, marked with seamline *g-h,* sits intact on a strip of all-over fabric with metallic highlights. This versatile template is now two templates in one.

First, use the revised corner of Template 2 to trim both corners of Patch 2. Align Template 2 to Patch 2, mark and cut the left corner, flip the template over, and trim the other corner. Repeat with all eight patches.

Next, cut two strips of Fabric 4. Use the right side of Template 2 to figure out how wide the strip has to be. Stitch the eight patches along seamline *g-h* to the strip. Press. Again, place Template 2 on Patch 2, positioning template line *g-h* directly on seamline *g-h*. Make sure the center axis of the template lines up with the implied center axis of the fabric. It's OK to fuss with the fabric to ensure the template is correctly aligned. Mark and cut each of the eight patches. Repeat this sequence on the other side of Patch 2.

In the pieced-together version of Example G, the left side is the original idea and the right side is the revised version. Lively interlaced patterns are already starting to emerge. The black prints link together and seem to recede behind the red arch, establishing a dimensional quality to the design. The eye will loop rhythmically around the scope as it follows the recurrent motifs.

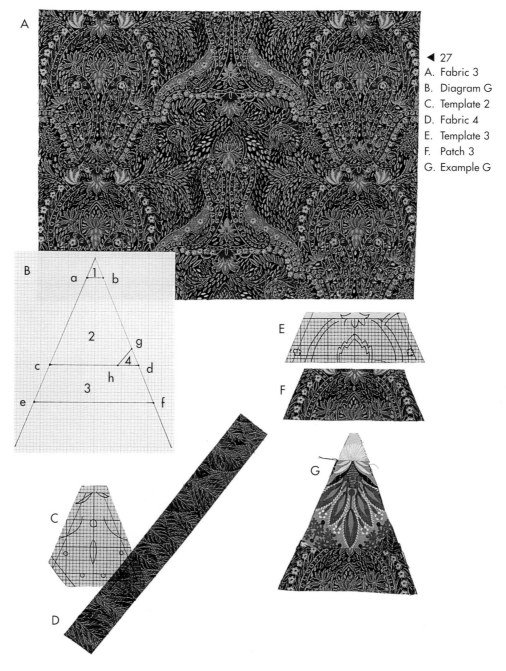

◀ 27
A. Fabric 3
B. Diagram G
C. Template 2
D. Fabric 4
E. Template 3
F. Patch 3
G. Example G

EXAMPLE H

Example H illustrates a second seamless connection with the little red coral-like patterns in Patch 2's corners. The new motif draws the patterns down into a slightly curving V. Imagine the arc of visual movement as the eye veers along these gently bowing contours.

Here's the sequence for this design process. To map out the shape of Patch 3, align a sheet of template plastic to Fabric 3. It is important the motif in Patch 3 is centered symmetrically along the axis, so make sure to match a bold inch line on the template material with the implied center of the motif. Looking through the transparent stuff, focus on what portion of the fabric you want in the patch. With a ruler, outline the motif using grid lines to guide the placement of the lines. These lines define the template. Trace bits of the motif onto the template, add seam allowance, and cut. Counting grid lines, transfer the shape of the patch to the diagram.

The lines defining Patch 3 on the diagram suggested a simpler way to piece the patches together. Find line *g-h.* In the revised version, shown on the right side of the diagram, this line is extended. It becomes line *h-i,* trimming off a bit of Patch 2 in the process. Reshape Patch 2 to the new dimensions by aligning Template 2 with the revised diagram. Trace the lines that alter its shape and add seam allowance. Match the edges of Template 2 to Template 3 for accurate piecing alignment.

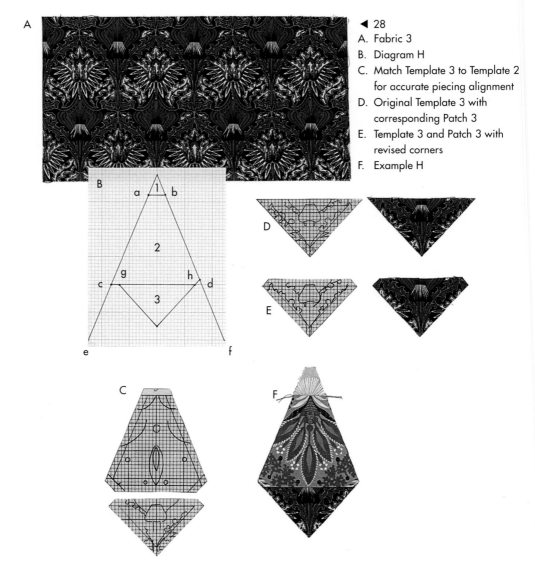

◀ 28
A. Fabric 3
B. Diagram H
C. Match Template 3 to Template 2 for accurate piecing alignment
D. Original Template 3 with corresponding Patch 3
E. Template 3 and Patch 3 with revised corners
F. Example H

EXAMPLE I

In Examples G and H the design spotlight aims toward the center axis. In Example I, resolving the how-to-continue-the-design-dilemma returns to the same impulse that motivated the previous two examples: to visually play off the red patterned motifs in Patch 2's corners. But this time, instead of pursuing the piecing sequence in the center, the design focus is pointed at the seams.

In this experiment, two very different fabrics fill the same shape. The temperamental personality of the prima donna on the left requires its own template, adorned with clues for accuracy. Note the elegant result as this motif joins its mirror image in a pointy formation along the seam. The delicate nuances contribute to a well-mannered, organized visual pattern. The second fabric, a sparkling all-over print, achieves a similar result in both shape and color but in a less compulsive way.

The significant difference between the two fabrics is that each requires a different piecing technique. In terms of the design sequence both fabrics can be considered Patch 3. But, regarding the piecing sequence, the two deviate completely. The left patch's fastidious personality demands its own template. The right fabric gets cut into long two-inch strips and strip-pieced to the shape labeled Patch 4, regardless of whether this space is filled with a single fabric or faceted into many. Instead of making Template 3 and Template 4, make one Template (3+4)(plus seam allowance). Use the fabric randomly to capture the momentary and transient nature of a kaleidoscope.

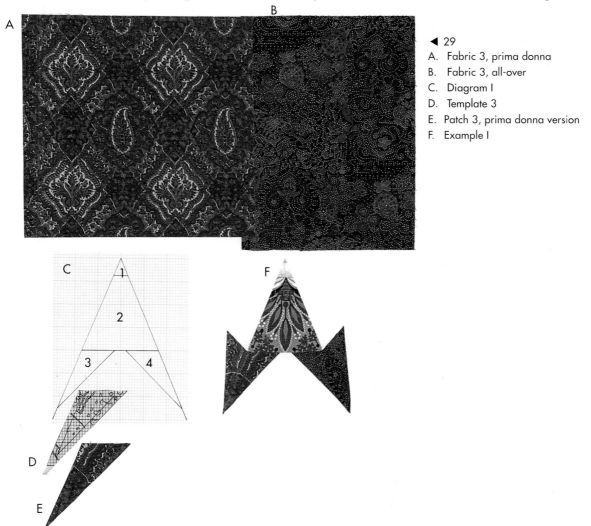

◄ 29
A. Fabric 3, prima donna
B. Fabric 3, all-over
C. Diagram I
D. Template 3
E. Patch 3, prima donna version
F. Example I

121

EXAMPLES J AND K

In Example J the complicated fabric, with undulating motifs and a strong sense of movement, is one of those rare finds with perfectly mirror-imaged patterns. Any of its off-grain motifs reflect into exciting kaleidoscopic effects brimming with animated details. The elegant wiggles of gold seem to dance before our eyes. An accommodating fabric like this deserves to show off its goodies in a big patch. My problem is, I get so tempted by this kind of potential that sometimes I create a patch so generous in its dimensions—it seems to cross the line from enticing into boring.

Here's the thought process behind the search for the perfect piece of print. During this exploration I viewed the fabric through a sheet of template plastic marked with the center axis and shape *e-c-d-f,* pivoting it on the fabric. My goal was to position a strand of wine-colored seaweed along line *c-d* to visually merge with Patch 2's little red branches. The template revealed I could let the seaweed attach to itself at the seams or keep a twinge of black background exposed that would form slight but dramatic rays. I went for both: a small stab of dark drama toward the top of the template and continuity from a merging maroon motif near the bottom. A bunch of white bubbles convening at the center axis slip into the visual rhythm set up by the white details in Patch 2.

Anticipating the movement of the viewer's eye around the composition-in-progress suggested further design possibilities. At this point the lines of seaweed connect in a continuous coil around the scope. The effect is definitely pleasing. But maybe it would be even more interesting if this much sameness was interrupted. I decided to pierce the winding flow of pattern with a stab of color, choosing an all-over luminous fabric because it works well with the background color of Patch 2.

These new considerations required modifying the diagram. I added line *j-k* to Example K. To trim Patch 3 identically, make a new Template 3, tracing the shape from the diagram. Don't cut down the original template. Keep it intact, place it on the diagram, and trace line *j-k* onto it. Use the new template to trim the eight left-sided and eight right-sided Patch 3s. Strip-piece the new fabric to Patch 3 along seamline *j-k.* Press. Now use the original template to reshape the patch by aligning line *j-k* with seam *j-k.*

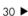

30 ▶

A. Fabric 3
B. Diagram J
C. Template 3
D. Left and right Patches 3
E. Patches 3 sewn together
F. Example J
G. Fabric 4
H. Diagram K
I. Revised Template 3
J. Revised left and right Patches 3
K. Template (3+4)
L. Patches (3+4)
M. Patches (3+4) sewn together

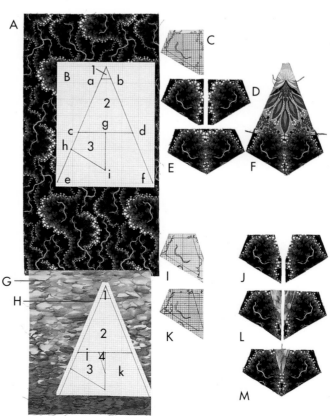

EXAMPLE L AND M

A Patch 2 missing a corner inspired the last two samples. Template 2 fits the available fabric, allowing for the seams. The leftover shape created by transferring the lines to the diagram becomes Patch 3. Choosing a prima donna for this position establishes the need for a separate Template 3. After marking this irregular triangle with directional clues for instant orientation, match its edges with Template 2 for accurate piecing alignment. In the case of an all-over, the drill is to strip-piece Fabric 3 to Patch 2 and outline shape with Template (2+3). A separate Template 3 is not needed.

In Example L Fabric 3 zaps the junction between Patches 2 and 3 with a sharp contrast. This reinforces the effect of the straight line and generates another area of interest along the seam. In the finished block the combined result of Patches 1 and 2 will be an eight-pointed star surrounded by scallops of Patch 3.

In Example M a similar sense of color between the fabrics in Patch 3 and Patch 2 softens the straight seam without camouflaging it. (The background in Patch 2 takes credit for this impression, but I think it's really due to the tan oblong-shaped projections surrounded in red.) The chevron pattern printed with three-dimensional qualities aims its V, and the viewer's eye, toward the seam. Please note that the piece-of-pie in Example L is shown without the seam allowance.

In both examples Fabrics 3 are energetic patterns that infuse a quality of motion into the design with a minimum of effort. The diagonal lines imply movement, evoking the impression that, just like in an actual kaleidoscope, change is imminent.

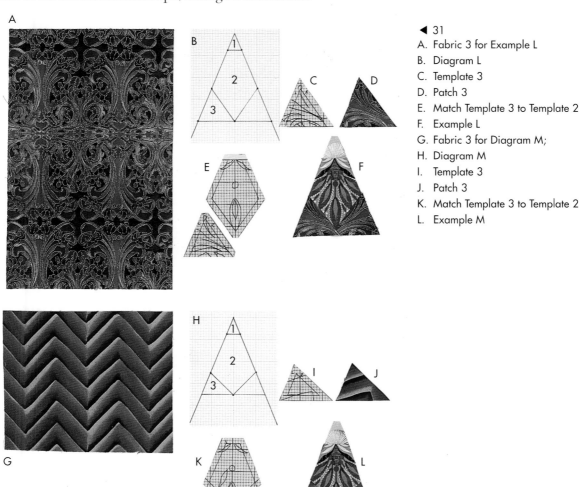

◀ 31
A. Fabric 3 for Example L
B. Diagram L
C. Template 3
D. Patch 3
E. Match Template 3 to Template 2
F. Example L
G. Fabric 3 for Diagram M;
H. Diagram M
I. Template 3
J. Patch 3
K. Match Template 3 to Template 2
L. Example M

UNLOCKING QUILTER'S BLOCK

Everyone involved in creative work has experienced that uncomfortable period when she stares, clueless, at an empty canvas, a blank page, an unruly pile of fabric. Sudden solutions are instances to appreciate, but since we can't explain how an idea "appears out of the blue," we can't rely on spontaneous insights or serendipity to rescue us in the nick of time.

The best way to overcome quilter's block is to do something. Doing something, even if you have no clear direction in mind, stimulates the thought processes. The idea is to visually brainstorm. Let your mind wander freely, unrestrained, uncensored, and alert to what might develop. Play with the idea, letting it guide you to a unique solution. Brainstorming, by nature, may lead to some strange pathways. However, as complex as creativity seems, in the final analysis a successful design can begin with one simple idea.

Ask people you consider artistic what they consciously do to stimulate the creative process. Some will mention making quick "roughs" or sketches. Turning neatly stacked fabrics into textile mud pies seems to be my way of doodling. My viewpoint ping-pongs between eye-catching, chance combinations. A cloth peeks out, igniting a relationship with the stuff over there, which prods my memory of something I know is in here somewhere, but wait, maybe this. . .or this. . .hey, maybe *both* will work instead.

(If, at birth, I'd been given a choice between being naturally neat or having naturally curly hair, I'm sure I would have picked the first. As it turned out, I am a curly-haired messy person. Things may look pretty neat on the surface, but my closets are a mess. I used to think it was a worthy effort to hide my disorganized tendencies. But in the past couple of years, as my art has empowered me, I've given up the facade. To my family's dismay, the clutter that used to stay tastefully tucked out of sight is following me out of the closet. After all, so many quilts. . .so little time).

Gazing into kaleidoscopes is my research. When my attention is caught by a particularly effective image, I stop to figure out how this was achieved. My intention isn't to reproduce it exactly. Instead, my goal is to develop a personal vocabulary that describes the radiant yet transient relationships between colors in a scope's interior. This will help me translate these serendipitous displays into fabric for all my future quilts, whether kaleidoscopic in design or not. Leaf through the color photos in this book, in any quilt book, in any book of art. When something catches your eye, explore the element that hooks you.

CONSCIOUS ACTS OF DESIGN INTERVENTION

When you're trying to decide "where to go from here" you are looking for a creative solution to a visual problem. Although there is no strict list of "do's and don'ts," there are lots of basic design standbys to consider that will jump-start the brainstorming juices.

Start with the graph paper diagram. Let your mind wander around the network of lines, unhampered by color. It can suggest ways to elaborate on already existing themes or visually connect patches that aren't necessarily next to each other. Sometimes interrupt, other times continue, the prevailing pattern. For example, when most of the shapes are horizontal, throw in a couple of vertical ones. Designing the kaleidoscope is a developmental process. It evolves gradually, becoming larger, fuller, richer.

The relative values of the patches in the design will arrange themselves into areas of sharp and mild contrast. This will happen in spite of you so don't agonize too much. It's a useful device when you're trying to decide "where to go from here." Check out the background color of adjacent patches. When the color that functions as the ground connects to similar hues, seamlines will be disguised, while the printed elements appear to advance and float on the fabric. Try on the option of a comparable value or temperate deviation in the next patch for a gentle transition.

Or, zap this junction with a strong, abrupt contrast, disconnecting the tranquil flow and introducing a new element. Remember: the eye is drawn to sharp contrasts. A valuable use of dark and light contrast is to create an accent or visual emphasis. High dark and light contrast instantly grab our attention. So by planning high contrast in one area and subdued contrast in adjacent patches, you can predict that an accent is in the making.

An alternate way to achieve dramatic impact is by introducing black (see page 12—peacock pillow). Black makes adjacent colors seem rich and clear. Slip in a single striking element, or intersperse several black patches. In *KALEIDOSCOPIC X: Water from the Moon* (pages 22-23) it seems as if a whole cloth of black sits behind the lacy network of patches, peeking through here and there. Actually, the openwork effect is due to the many instances of strip-pieced shapes of black, using the basic technique described on page 50.

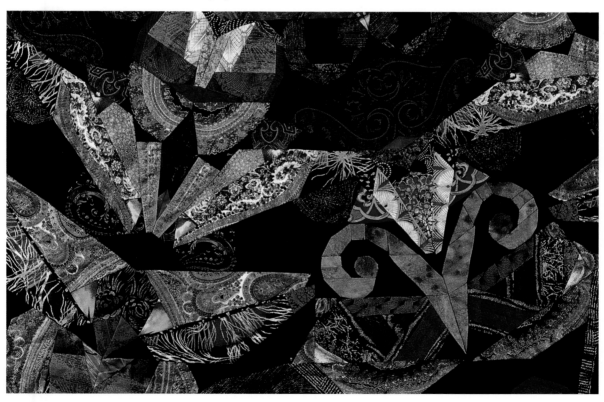

▲ Detail of *KALEIDOSCOPIC X: Water from the Moon*

Ask yourself, is this a good time to throw in a zinger? Remember, a pinch of something unexpected becomes a symmetrical sprinkle when it is peppered identically throughout the design. A motif that seems unrelated in a single pie-slice sector is often responsible for achieving visual rhythm.

Take another look at the samples in this book. This time, observe how fabrics that look like they landed from different planets often unite in flawless connections, usually because an incidental doodad from one makes an unexpected link with the middle of a motif in the other. Instead of looking at the whole pattern of your fabrics, notice the individual elements. You will probably discover more relationships than you can use.

PHILOSOPHICAL KALEIDOSCOPING

As the designer, your job is to capture attention with a unified image that offers visual satisfaction. The good news in a kaleidoscopic design is that there are often happy coincidences that make it even better. The even better news is that the viewer is on your side. She doesn't want to see unrelated chaos. She works with you, looking for organization, searching for coherence, uniting the different elements.

Aim for the creation of a harmonious pattern with related elements by applying a unity-with-variety principle. Shapes may repeat but in different sizes, colors may echo in analogous hues that vary in value. Irregularity and variations all serve to maintain the viewer's interest. Resist the temptation to line up elements neatly, such as perfectly parallel lines that wind up looking like stripes. Vary lines from thick to thin instead of aiming for evenness and consistency.

Match seams, not colors. Don't even think about matching colors; matching is boring. Comparable colors that bear a resemblance to each other make more sophisticated visual connections. Gradations and shadings convey the impression that some patches are closer than others or that the light source is unevenly distributed. Color helps establish a relationship between parts. Even if each and every shape is colored without regard to the others, the final version will be seen as shapes and areas which overlap and interweave.

The time involved in developing an idea differs from problem to problem. Two of the kaleidoscopes in *KALEIDOSCOPIC XV: Eccentric Circles* (page 29) are opposite examples. In spite of its extremely complex image, the top right scope is really a streamlined design. Seven different fabrics make up the twenty patches that comprise the nine-inch piece-of-pie (32). (To get the desired effect in its neighbor to the left, a single wedge is composed of forty-one pieces, multiplied by eight. . . .) (33). At the other extreme, the left, bottom scope was unruly. It took almost a week, and three major ripping sessions, to create a satisfying design (34).

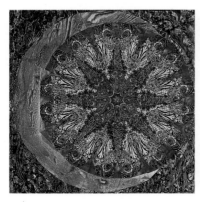
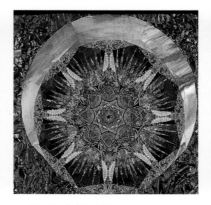
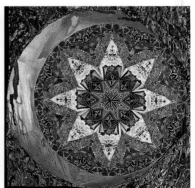

▲ 32   Top right kaleidoscope   ▲ 33   Top left kaleidoscope   ▲ 34   Bottom left kaleidoscope
The details of *KALEIDOSCOPIC XV: Eccentric Circles* form a harmonious pattern with related elements.

When your designing instincts point you in another direction and a revision is called for, don't think of the original idea as a mistake. This puts a negative slant on a natural event in the design process. Relish the kinds of ideas that propel you further along a path of creativity. Be grateful that your critical thinking skills kicked in. Personally, I'm a fast talker but a slow thinker. More often than not it takes me lots of mulling before I sense where I'm going and feel in control. The Sample (page 128) is a case in point.

MIRROR, MIRROR

To use a mirror or not to use a mirror, that is the question. My answer is: you're the boss. Do what makes you happy.

The idea here is that two mirrors, hinged together at a 45° angle or a 60° angle and placed on top of a fabric, serve as a crystal ball, unfolding the final mirrored-image reflection before your very eyes. Veritable abracadabra. You see the result before you go through the tedious steps of cutting and sewing.

It's a seductive way to design. My fear is that it can seduce us into thinking that we can't create spectacular effects on our own. Personally, I like the promise of surprise. I want to believe I am teaching my mind's eye to instinctively see the same thing from lots of perspectives. To me the image seen through a mirror seems more predictable, less fluid than the real thing.

However, I use my bias to form guidelines, not rules. Mirrors find their way onto my work surface every so often, because I recognize their potential as a design tool. I reach for them when I'm dissatisfied with the outcome of a close-to-being-finished scope or when I suspect that an alien element has invaded and taken over a design. It helps me investigate whether this component overpowers the rest of the design or looks totally out of place in the final version. In this case I'm inclined to take something out (as long as it is along an accessible seam) and add something else. On a single piece-of-the-pie, I put a scrap of new fabric on top of the offending one, and let the mirrors reveal the scrap's potential to rehabilitate the design. Sometimes, after obsessively enacting this ritual with a wide range of fabric snippets, I decide to leave it as is. Other times, I change what I didn't like by appliquéing something new on top of it.

Which brings me to another interesting discussion. . . .

THE CONCEPT OF CHEATING

Tell the truth. Just now, when I said that sometimes I solve a problem by appliquéing, did you think: "Ooh, that's cheating"? Excuse me while I take a brief stand on my personal soap box. Who am I cheating? The audience? The quilt? Where did this sense that real quilters always take the hardest route come from?

OK, I admit I used to think this behavior unbefitting a quiltmaker. But this judgment doesn't seem valid anymore. I want to encourage people to create in their own styles. Please, let's not allow external pressure to dictate that we conform to an imaginary standard based on the mythological perfection of the quiltmaking legacy.

KALEIDOSCOPE

THE SAMPLE

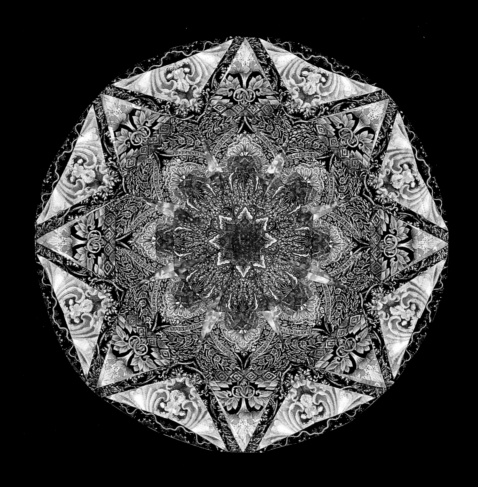

THE SAMPLE

The Fabric Made Me Do It

Over ten years ago I named my first one-woman quilt show "Serendipity." This word succinctly defines my love affair with quiltmaking: the merging of control and spontaneity to spark something unexpected. The eight-sided sample block is a case in point. No matter how sincere my intent to toe the line and create a representative cross section of the preceding guidelines, the design danced off in its own direction. I envisioned completely different fabrics and more strip-pieced contributions than the mix that wound up in the grand finale. Few remnants of the original pastel palette survived the metamorphosis (35).

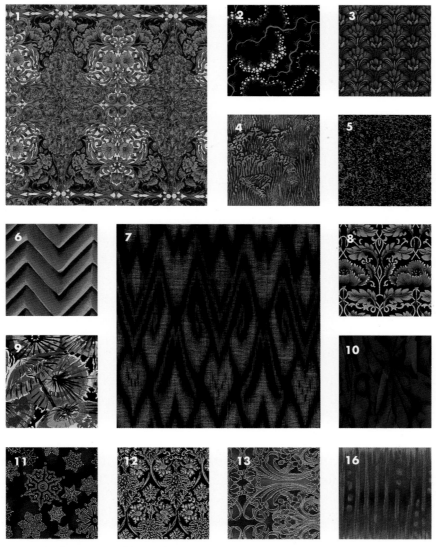

▲ 35　The final palette of fabrics for The Sample

The following play-by-play directions offer a dry run, a chance to rehearse the process of a kaleidoscope block from start to finish before setting off on your own. They assume the reader is now familiar with the tools, techniques, terminology, and design guidelines described in the preceding pages of this book. Please note that seam allowance is immediately added to every template.

1 The search for Patch 1 began with a 45° outline of the piece-of-pie marked symmetrically on a sheet of template plastic, and ended with a long thin spoke of charming trellis. The prima donna fabric purchased expressly for this purpose did not even end up in the block. Trimming the 45° triangular shape to conform to the on-grain motif created Template 1 (36A).

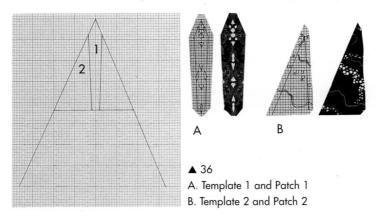

▲ 36
A. Template 1 and Patch 1
B. Template 2 and Patch 2

2 Extending the horizontal, bottom border of Patch 1 on the graph paper diagram defined Patch 2. This patch is not positioned along the center axis. Therefore when making Template 2, it is not important to match a bold line of the template grid to the grid of the graph paper. For instant orientation I marked L and R on this asymmetrical template. Since it is nonreversible, I planned to cut eight left-sided patches, flip the template over and cut eight right-sided patches. To ensure accurate alignment come piecing time, I invented a new angle at the right-bottom corner of Template 2, preserving approximately one-quarter inch seam allowance, and transferred the new angle to the corresponding corner of Template 1. After aligning the templates right sides together, sewing line to sewing line, I used the edge of the just-cut angle to copy the identical shape onto Template 1. Trimming off the excess plastic created identical corners.

3 I explored lots of potential Fabric 2s by rotating window-like Template 2 on a variety of candidates. Placing an actual Patch 1 on the fabrics was also effective. When Patch 1 made an eye-catching connection with a motif, I positioned Template 2 as though it were sewn to Patch 1 and checked out the portion of fabric that landed within the template. I played with the possibilities, wriggling the template a little bit this way, turning the fabric a little bit that way. Hints from the winning version were traced onto the template (37B).

■ TECHNIQUE TIP   At this early point in the design process I usually cut out only one patch per template. Things change; ensuing decisions lead to future patches, hindsight, and revisions. Also, now my design instincts are in full gear. I can do the mundane stuff when I'm slowing down.

4 I had second thoughts about Patch 1. It might be a lovely single entity, but I was afraid it would be too much of the same sweet thing when multiplied by eight. A lively motif printed on a vivid royal blue bonded smoothly to an altered Patch 1 and perked up the effect. After marking the modification on the diagram, I used it to trim Template 1 and make a template for Patch 3. And, of course, I matched the revised version of Template 1 to Template 3 (37A).

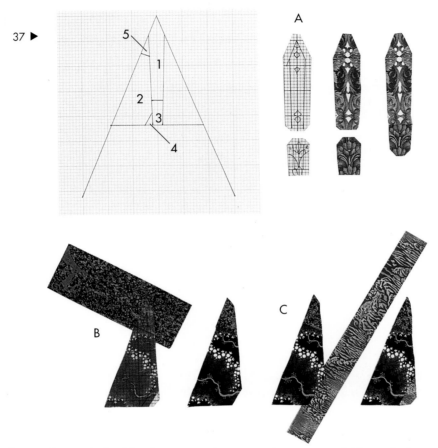

37 ▶

5 The design focus shifted back to Template 2. Perhaps it would benefit from a similar review. I wanted to reinforce the ambiguity between Patches 1 and 2. The relationship between Patch 2's white bubbles and the lattice of white along the central axis worked well. The wonderful royal blue in Patch 3 gave me the idea to spill similar color across the seam from patch to patch. I used see-through Template 2 to find the best site for this new element. Counting grid lines, I transferred the seamline to the diagram and to Template 2. Fabric 4 is stripped on Patch (2+5) (37C).

6 A similar operation at the top of Patch 2 offered an easy opportunity to punctuate the design with a pinch of something different. This time, rather than introduce an unexpected element with an eye-popping disposition, I chose a sparkly all-over on a dark ground for a gentle transition (37B).

■ TECHNIQUE TIP   Instead of pruning Template 2 to its pared-down dimensions, I made a new Template 2. I kept the original "as-is" and traced the seamlines for Patches 4 and 5 onto it. Now this two-in-one template can be used to mark patches after strip-piecing all-over Fabrics 4 and 5 to Patch 2.

7 From this point on I will cut and sew eight of these units whenever it is convenient. For future reference let's call this collection of patches Unit A.

8 The motifs in Patches 2 and 3 set off the next chain of design events. The idea to continue the design in a color family similar to the brown "seaweed" at the left bottom corner of Patch 2 resulted in a chevron pattern with three-dimensional qualities. Following the contour of the chevron generated a form that worked well along the seamline. I planned to let half a V meet itself at the seam and unite into a complete chevron.

To map out the shape of Template 6, I traced the potential space revealed by the diagram onto template plastic. Then I aligned the template plastic to Fabric 6 so that the left border of the piece-of-pie met the middle of a chevron. Tracing the right diagonal outline of the motif's V produced the shape of the patch (38). I transferred the line to the diagram by counting grid lines.

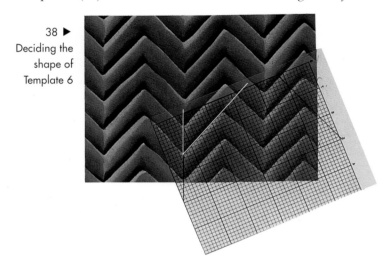

38 ▶
Deciding the
shape of
Template 6

9 Peeking out of my pile of fabric was an elegant Indonesian ikat on a rich indigo ground. Combining the non-native textile with domestic prints piqued my eclectic tendencies. In spite of the disparities, the ikat's woven pattern continued the theme of strong directional V-shapes, and its deep background color blended effortlessly with the ground of Patch 2. I created a template by following the pattern's triangular contour and transferred this shape to the diagram. Because this patch falls on the center axis, I made a template with a bold inch line down the center to ensure that the motif was centered symmetrically. The compatible backgrounds of Patches 2 and 7 gave me the idea to extend the margin of Patch 7 so that its color flowed across the seam into Patch 2. Now Patch 6 bumped into Patch 7. I transferred these lines to the diagram, trimmed off the excess seam allowance at the template's bottom to one-quarter inch, and matched the top corners of Template 7 to the top-right corner of Template 6 (39).

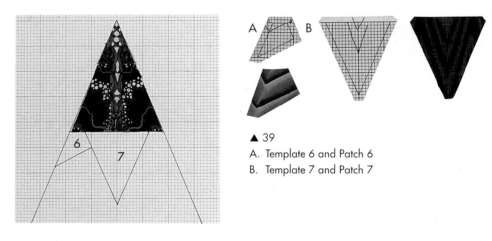

▲ 39
A. Template 6 and Patch 6
B. Template 7 and Patch 7

10 Having introduced strong angular features, I now sought to soften all that straightness with something elaborate and flowing. After trying lots of stuff, I was surprised to find a comparable feel in color between the leaves in Fabric 8 and the discreet greyish hue in the ikat. I made the most of this resemblance, using my very best matchmaking skills to maneuver the two fabrics into sync (40A).

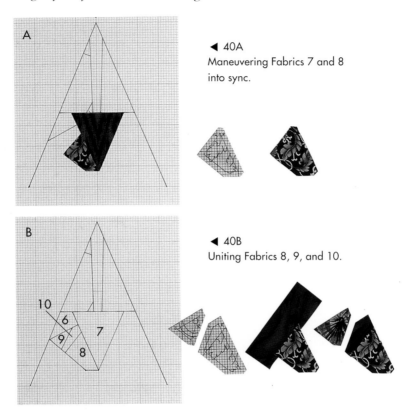

◄ 40A
Maneuvering Fabrics 7 and 8 into sync.

◄ 40B
Uniting Fabrics 8, 9, and 10.

11 The result was Patch 8, connected to Patch 7 on one side, surrounded by empty graph paper on the other three. Using a ruler, I extended the left boundary of the patch up toward Patch 6. After meeting the demands of a pack of prima donnas, I wanted the relief of a forgiving fabric. I found an obliging all-over printed with shadows and highlights, opting to continue the ground color. By now it was apparent that the dark common ground played a major role in this design, visually uniting the piece-in-progress, carrying the viewer's eye smoothly from one form to the next.

12 How much of this moody blue to use was the next question. Fill up the rest of the section? Fracture it into a couple of patches? Extend the lines of the diagram in alternate ways? I postponed this decision until I knew where the design was headed.

I can't explain why, but a certain fabric kept slipping into my peripheral view. A sea of brightly colored overlapping umbrellas, the bamboo kind that perch on top of drinks with names that evoke the South Pacific, wanted my attention. Why not exploit its spokes? After selecting an appealing motif, I held my breath and counted the number of identical repeats in my piece of fabric. There were only fifteen. I borrowed a couple more from the Phabric Phantom, a.k.a. Diane Rode Schneck, a master fabric shopper and accomplished collector. Fitting a wedge of umbrella next to Patch 6 created the leftover shape that became a strip-pieced patch of blue (40B).

■ TECHNIQUE TIP   This is a good time to take a break and tidy up the templates. First, match Template (8+10) to Template 9. Next, according to the diagram, the top of shape (8+9+10) must match the bottom of Template 6. However, there isn't a Template (8+9+10). You can either make one, or match (a) the top-left corner of Template 9 to the bottom-left corner of Template 6 and (b) the top-right corner of Template 10 to the bottom-right corner of Template 6. If you make another template, it will probably come in handy during the succeeding design process. It's also useful to check if Patches 8, 9, and 10 are sewn together accurately.

There are a couple more matches to make. For clarity's sake, let's label the section comprised of Patches (6+8+9+10) Unit B. The right corners of Unit B have to match the left corners of Template 7. And, if this was not already done, trim the bottom-left corner of Template 2 to fit the top-right corner of Template 6.

13 Now I switched from studying the patches individually to reviewing the piece-in-progress as a unified image. The result: I decided the design was too somber. The ikat seemed too big, too formal, too defined.

The V shape lent itself to modifications at the corners. I searched through the piles for glitter, glamour, contrast, surprise—and came up with snowflakes. I cut out a few, tried each in the left corner bordering the golden chevron, and placed a bit of snowflake at the ikat's pointy bottom. Suddenly patterns emerged, entwined, and interlaced where there wasn't a link just a second before.

I returned to my piles to continue searching for relief from boring corners. I looked for an all-over remedy, but returned with a prima donna flashing gold, curvy lines. Patch 7 became a trio of fabrics. I made a new trim Template 7 and matched it to Templates 11 and 12. After cutting eight Patch 11s, eight left-sided Patch 12s, and eight right-sided Patch 12s, I pieced eight of these units together (41).

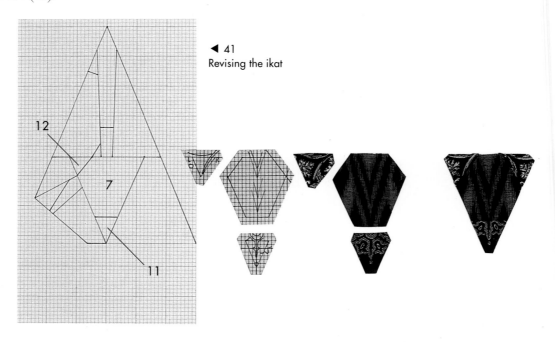

◀ 41
Revising the ikat

14 The next section to sew together was eight left-sided Units B to the left side of Patch (7+11+12). Repeating this step on the right side produced the segment we'll call Unit C. I sewed eight Units A to eight Units C.

15 It dawned on me that I had used completely different fabrics from the ones I had originally planned on. I pulled these out from the bottom of the pile and gave them a chance to audition. A sheaf of gently bowing lines won the role, circling the block like a garland.

After matching Template 13 to Unit B, I cut eight left-sided and eight right-sided Patch 13s (42). I sewed the sixteen patches to the piece-in-progress. Although I intended the block to be bigger, it occurred to me that Patch 13 made a graceful ending. The problem was, it was not on grain.

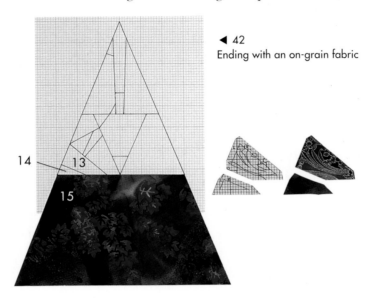

◀ 42
Ending with an on-grain fabric

16 The solution was to ensure that the remaining shape, Patch 14, was cut on-grain. This required making an individual template for Patch 14 and treating it like a prima donna. However, the plot thickens. To maintain the circular effect created by Patch 13, the fabric in Patch 14 had to make an almost flawless match with the fabric it abuts in Patch 15. This camouflage caused the seam between the two to disappear, figuratively. The result was a kaleidoscopic image sitting wreathlike, encircled by a muted background.

This ruse was achieved by using the same fabric selected to square off the block in Patch 14. A typical all-over print would render this effect automatically, but in the case of this randomly dyed batik I had to hunt for sixteen different relationships. This required cutting out the four Patch 15s before Patch 14. I found where the two patches encountered each other by positioning the two templates as if they were pieced-together patches. After matching the edges of Template 14 to Template 13, I used Template 14 to cut out sixteen on-grain patches that correspond colorwise to their southern neighbor. Once all sixteen Patch 14s were pieced to sixteen Patch 13s, I sewed four Patch 15s to four pieces-of-the-pie (42,43). Voilà.

17 No, wait. The kaleidoscope seemed a tad. . .quiet. It lacked heat. What if I stripped in a burst of light at the left-bottom corner of Patch 2? Let's call this addition Patch 16 (44). Here's how to finagle this altered state.

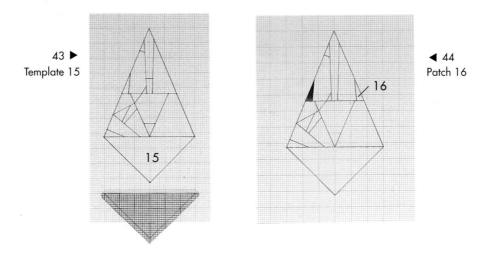

43 ▶
Template 15

◀ 44
Patch 16

Luckily, I still had both versions of Template 2 from Step 5. By positioning Template 2 on its corresponding Patch in the piece-of-pie, I figured out a pleasing place to insert the new fabric. Although it darts into the darkness of Patch 2, its color clings to Patch 6 and creates a unified presence. I drew the seamline on the template, transferred it to the diagram, and traced it onto the already revised version of Template 2. I trimmed this template to fit the new dimensions. Using a seam-ripper I unraveled about one and a half inches of both ends of the seam connecting Unit A to Unit B. I used the modified Template 2 to crop Patch 2 accurately and, once the new fabric was strip-pieced on, the original Template 2 to reshape the patch. After sewing the seams between Units A and B together again, I carried out the final piecing sequence for an eight-sided design. And the block was finished (45, 46).

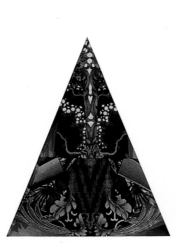

▲ 45   A single piece-of-the-pie

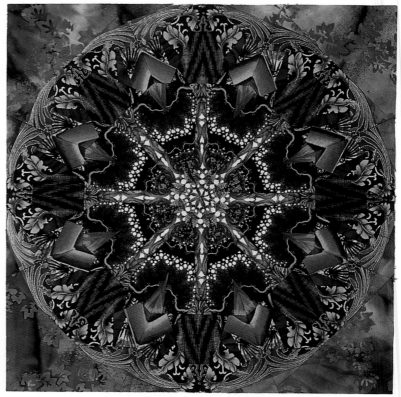

▲ 46   The finished block

KALEIDOSCOPE

THE KALEIDOSCOPE RENAISSANCE

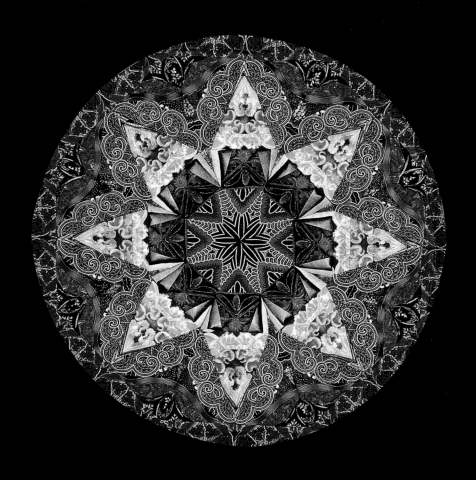

THE KALEIDOSCOPE RENAISSANCE

THE HISTORY OF THE KALEIDOSCOPE

The past decade has witnessed a renaissance of interest in the kaleidoscope as a dynamic art form. Invented in 1816 by Sir David Brewster, a Scottish scientist and philosopher, it was originally labeled an instrument of philosophy and intended as a design tool for artists and others who worked with patterns. However, it was soon widely recognized as a form of adult parlor entertainment, and later as a children's toy.

On this side of the Atlantic, the first kaleidoscope made in America appeared as early as 1818. By 1857 they were produced and marketed in quantity, with prices ranging from twelve cents to as much as twenty-five dollars for an elaborate model attached to a lantern. The earliest existing American scopes are attributed to Charles Bush, a resident of Boston, who secured several patents for his work in the 1870s. Selling for two dollars and mounted on a wooden stand, this handsome instrument had a barrel of black cardboard. Its object case contained about thirty-five glass pieces and was rotated by a spoked brass wheel. Because some of the pieces were liquid filled, air bubbles inside the liquid continued to move even after the object case was at rest.

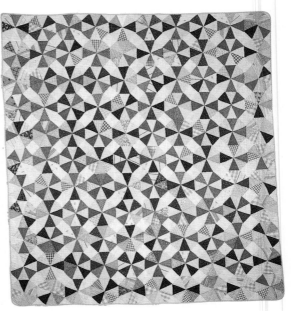

▲ *Kaleidoscope*, 72¹/₂" x 67", circa 1910.
From the collection of Jonathon Holstein.

It is likely the kaleidoscope was the inspiration for the versatile traditional quilt pattern called "Kaleidoscope" (circa 1869). Eight equal triangles radiate from the center of the block to form the overall pattern. Because it seems to create curves where there are only straight seams, this simple pattern using only two templates encourages design exploration through the deliberate placement of dark and light fabrics.

KALEIDOSCOPES 101

Like quilts, kaleidoscopes retain a relationship to the tradition from which they descend. Contemporary scope makers have created a new state of the art by combining their tradition with modern technology. A basic kaleidoscope consists of an eye-piece, an object case containing items to be viewed, a tube, and either two or three mirrors along the length angled toward each other in a V-shaped triangular configuration.

The mirror system organizes the light rays into images. A two-mirror system provides a reflection of the objects in the form of one central image (1) while a three-mirror design produces reflections of reflections. By duplicating the pattern to infinity, innumerable images are created throughout the entire field of view. This is the version we fondly remember as childhood toys (2). In both formats changing the angle of the "V" determines the number and complexity of the patterns.

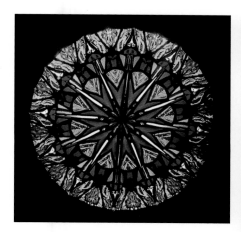

▲ 1   The interior of a two-mirror kaleidoscope by Allen Crandell

▲ 2   The interior of a three-mirror kaleidoscope by Carolyn Bennett

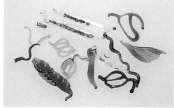

◀ 3
Pieces of glass used in a Charles Karadimos kaleidoscope

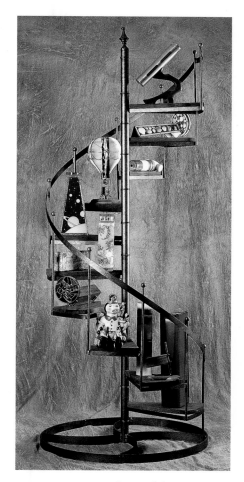

▲ 4   An assortment of state-of-the-art kaleidoscopes from the collection of Cozy Baker

Although all kaleidoscopes are composed of the basic elements, there are many styles and variations (4). The pattern changes when either the scope or object case is rotated. The end pieces fall into four main categories. "Wheels" are made of glass or acrylic and can be embedded with stained glass, gemstones, and all types of found objects. "Cells," or object cases, are filled with free-falling items or liquid filled with floating items. The stuff inside the object cases is limited only by imagination. Along with beads and gemstones, twisted threads and shards of lampworked glass, there can be dried flowers, feathers, or shells. "Marbles" or "crystals" are often hand-blown especially for the scope. Lastly, the array of color can be derived totally from polarized white light. Often confused with a kaleidoscope, a "taleidoscope" uses only a clear lens at the end and fractures whatever it is pointed toward into a kaleidoscopic image.

THE BREWSTER SOCIETY

In 1986 Cozy Baker, of Bethesda, Maryland, founded the Brewster Society, an international organization of designers, collectors, and lovers of kaleidoscopes that has served to revitalize this important art form. The organization publishes a quarterly newsletter to keep enthusiasts up to date on kaleidoscope events and holds an annual convention. Along with writing four definitive books on the subject, Cozy has acquired the world's premier collection of over one thousand contemporary and antique kaleidoscopes (5).

In her book *Kaleidoscope Renaissance* Cozy writes, "As the demand for customized scopes increases, the innovations keep pace. Kaleidoscopes are being installed in ceilings and skylights of homes, built around fish tanks and water fountains, constructed into silos and formed from balloons." And, as this book attests, these magical devices have become the design inspiration for quilt artists as well.

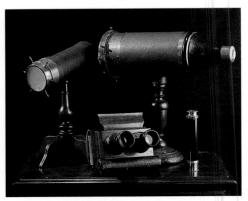

▲ 5   Antique kaleidoscopes from the collection of Cozy Baker

CONVERSATIONS WITH KALEIDOSCOPE FRIENDS

An unexpected consequence of my interest in making kaleidoscope quilts is my friendships with kaleidoscope makers. Our mutual admiration society yields opportunities to barter kaleidoscope-inspired quilt blocks for the real things and conversations that often turn to our shared inspirations (6, 7, 8, 9). At first I was so bewitched by their handiwork I assumed they were either geniuses or wizards. Gradually I began to decode the technical stuff behind the magic, and I found the artistry.

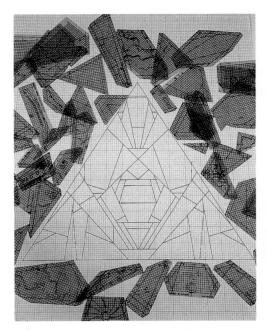

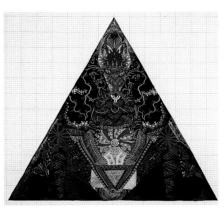

▲ 6   The graph diagram for Peggy's Piece surrounded by the templates for this block

▲ 7   Peggy's Piece: A single piece-of-the-pie

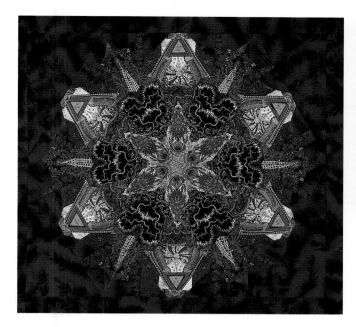

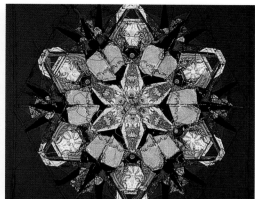

▲ 9   Back of Peggy's Piece

◀ 8
Peggy's Piece: pieced kaleidoscope exchanged in barter for kaleidoscope by Woodland Glass

Our media are so different, yet the design strategies focus on similar considerations. The two major ingredients in a kaleidoscope are the mirror system, which determines the number of reflections, and the pieces in the object case. I liken these components to the number of triangular-shaped wedges that radiate from the center of the quilt block and the fabric.

Some scopemakers approach their found objects in a manner similar to my own attitude toward fabric. For example, Charles Karadimos' description of the effect he aims for as "controlling the randomness" mirrors my fabric manipulating tendencies. Coordinating the interior colors to harmonize with the exterior casings reminds me of choosing the "just-right" backing. Working out successful design solutions by trial and error turns out to be a learning style common to both of our creative processes.

Realizing that over time I had formed an opinion about the differences between six, eight, or ten divisions made me curious about whether scopemakers had a preference for different angles of symmetry. Of course they do! Charles Karadimos and Kay Winkler like a thinner wedge. Charles considers this effect more apt to maintain an adult's attention longer because it is subtle and sophisticated. "The more intricate the patterns, the longer you want to sit and look at it," say Charles. "It gives you the feeling that something even better is going to happen next."

In his opinion, it is easier for scopemakers to achieve color balance and randomness than intricacy and refinement. His scopes range between eight- and fourteen-fold symmetry. He considers the magic lost if the viewer can recognize the pieces in an endcase (10, 11). Kay specializes in 15° two-mirror kaleidoscopes made of stained glass. This mirror configuration gives a multifaceted twelve-point image that resembles a rose window (12, 13).

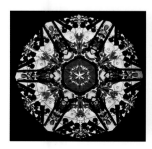

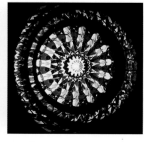

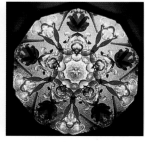

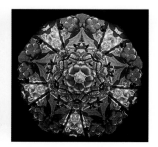

▲ 10   Interior of Charles Karadimos kaleidoscope

▲ 11   Interior of Charles Karadimos kaleidoscope

▲ 12   Interior of Kay Winkler kaleidoscope

▲ 13   Interior of Kay Winkler kaleidoscope

And then there are those, like Peggy Burnside of Woodland Glass and Shelley Knapp of Knapp Wood, who prefer a larger section. Both scopemakers are known for object cases filled with refined pieces of flame-worked glass that have lots of texture. A vast palette of colors and dichroic glass gives the scopes Peggy makes with her partner, Steve Kittelson, their characteristic range of tones and jewel-like images (Figure 15). She favors six points because it allows stronger interplay between the colors and enables the viewer to see the definition of the pattern. In addition, she prefers an even, rather than an odd, number of points.

Shelley, known for her instinctive use of color, dedicates extra time to creating a diverse array of deeply defined pieces in the object case. This is the part of scopemaking she likes best. Her favorite division is five or six, because the generous size shapes a view that accommodates glass sculpted pieces. For her, the magic derives from how the pieces react together.

You see, my instincts were right in the first place. Kaleidoscope makers may use the rituals of science rather than spells and charms to produce their extraordinary effects, but the results are pure magic.

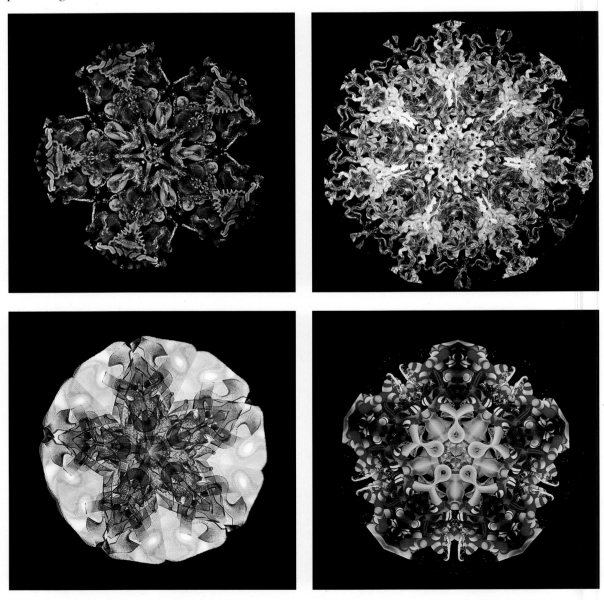

▲ 14 Interior of *Evolution,* by Randy and Shelley Knapp

▲ 16 Interior of *Falling Star,* by Randy and Shelley Knapp

▲ 15 Interior of *Mystic Rapture* by Burnside/Kittleson

▲ 17 Interior of *She Dances With Fire* by Randy & Shelley Knapp

INDEX

Titles of quilts and kaleidoscope images are listed in italics. Photos are referenced in bold face type. Lower case "d" indicates a detail.

SOURCES

▲ KALEIDOSCOPES

The Brewster Society
Studio B
9020 McDonald Drive
Bethesda, MD 20817
(301) 365-1855

▲ PRODUCTS

The Cotton Club
P.O. Box 2263
Boise, ID 83701
(208) 345-5567
e-mail:
Cotton@micron.net
Mail order source for textile designs with repetitive/
symmetrical motifs by
Paula Nadelstern for
Benartex, large protractors
with easy to read numbers,
see-thru template material,
rulers and graph paper
pads with eight-to-the-
inch-grid, books, notecards,
and gift wrap by C&T
Publishing.

▲ BOOKS

Snow Crystals
by W.A. Bentley and W.J.
Humphreys
Write for a free catalog.
Dover Publications, Inc.
Dept. 23, 31 East 2nd Street,
Mineola, NY 11501

▲ FABRIC

Benartex
1460 Broadway
New York, NY 10036
http://www.benartex.com
Inquire about textile prints
designed by Paula
Nadelstern for Benartex.

**International Fabric
Collection**
3445 West Lake Road
Eric, PA 16505-3661
(800) 462-3891
Write for free catalog,
including Liberty of
London tana lawn and
fusible interfacing.

Pieces of Eight (Dianne
Smith)
P.O. Box 4306
South Colby, WA 98384
(360) 871-7756
e-mail: silk@silverlink.net
Hand-dyed machine
washable silk.

Skydyes
Mickey Lawler
83 Richmond Lane
West Hartford, CT 06117
Write for price list of
hand-painted fabric.

B&J Fabrics
263 W. 40th Street
New York, NY 10018
(212) 354-8150
(212) 764-3355
This is my favorite store
in the garment district.

**Batiks Etcetera & Sew
What Fabrics**
200-B West Main Street
Wytheville, VA 24382
(800) 228-4573
FAX (540) 228-9297
www.batiks.com
e-mail: info@batiks.com
Write for swatches of
unique batiks including
repetitive symmetrical
motifs.